Next to You

Gloria Hunniford was born in Northern Ireland and was the first woman to have her own daily radio show on BBC Radio 2, which she presented for thirteen years until 1994. She had her own television chat programme, *Sunday Sunday*, on London Weekend Television. She has appeared on and presented numerous other shows, including *Gloria Live*, *This Morning*, *Holiday*, *Songs of Praise* and *Open House with Gloria*, which gave Channel Five some of its highest ever ratings. She has won several prestigious awards, including TV Personality of the Year, Radio Personality of the Year and a Lifetime Achievement Award, and has an Honorary Doctorate from Queen's University Belfast. Alongside Caron she has two sons – Paul and Michael – is married to Stephen and between them they have eight grandchildren.

D0230381

Next to You

Caron's Courage

Remembered by Her Mother

GLORIA HUNNIFORD

PENGUIN BOOKS

PENGUIN BOOKS

Published by the Penguin Group
Penguin Books Ltd, 80 Strand, London WC2R ORL, England
Penguin Group (USA) Inc., 375 Hudson Street, New York, New York 10014, USA
Penguin Group (Canada), 90 Eglinton Avenue East, Suite 700, Toronto, Ontario, Canada M4P 2Y3
(a division of Pearson Penguin Canada Inc.)
Penguin Ireland, 25 St Stephen's Green, Dublin 2, Ireland (a division of Penguin Books Ltd)
Penguin Group (Australia), 250 Camberwell Road,
Camberwell, Victoria 3124, Australia (a division of Pearson Australia Group Pty Ltd)
Penguin Books India Pvt Ltd, 11 Community Centre,
Panchsheel Park, New Delhi – 110 017, India
Penguin Group (NZ), cnr Airborne and Rosedale Roads, Albany,
Auckland 1310, New Zealand (a division of Pearson New Zealand Ltd)
Penguin Books (South Africa) (Pty) Ltd, 24 Sturdee Avenue,
Rosebank, Johannesburg 2196, South Africa

Penguin Books Ltd, Registered Offices: 80 Strand, London WC2R ORL, England

www.penguin.com

First published 2005
Published in Penguin Books 2006
1

Typeset by Rowland Phototypesetting Ltd, Bury St Edmunds, Suffolk
Printed in England by Clays Ltd, St Ives plc

ISBN-13: 978-0-141-02377-9
ISBN-10: 0-141-02377-5

For Charlie and Gabriel,
our pride and joy.

Caron's wonderful spirit
lives on through them.

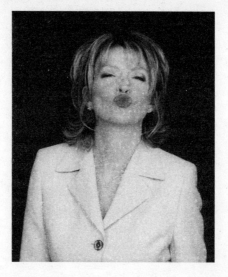

Next to you

You cannot see or touch me
    But I'm standing next to you.
Your tears can only hurt me,
    Your sadness makes me blue.
Be brave and show a smiling face
    Let not your grief show through
I love you from a different place,
    Yet I'm standing next to you.

April 2004

Contents

Biography

Caron Keating was born in Fulham, London, on 5 October 1962, but she was brought up in Northern Ireland. She was educated at Methodist College in Belfast and graduated from Bristol University in 1982. She worked on *Blue Peter* from 1986 to 1990 and went on to work on other high-profile television programmes including *After 5* and *This Morning*, where she stood in for Judy Finnegan. She was married to Russ Lindsay in 1991 and they had a son, Charlie, in 1994. Caron was diagnosed with breast cancer in September 1997, shortly after the birth of her second son, Gabriel. She spent the next three years at her home in Barnes, London, juggling the private battle with her illness and her public television career. Following a mastectomy, she moved with her family in May 2000 to Fowey, Cornwall, during which time she had an aggressive course of chemotherapy. In December 2001 Caron flew to Byron Bay, Australia, where she lived for the next two and a half years. She returned to Switzerland for treatment in March 2004 and died at her mum's home in Kent on 13 April.

After Caron's death, when we read through her notebooks and observations about dealing with cancer, it became very clear that she really wanted to write a book and indeed had started to do so. Sadly she never got the opportunity to finish it.

This is her story.

Prologue: Next to Me

Caron and I never talked about death – only about life. All during Caron's courageous seven-year battle with breast cancer, the child became the teacher as I watched in admiration, and sometimes desperation, the way she fought for life, to live in the 'now', having whatever treatment her oncology team recommended but, parallel to that, continuing her worldwide search for a cure or miracle to rid her body for ever of cancer. She just wanted to get on with 'living' instead of 'living her cancer'. She wanted to return to normal family life, the joy of looking after her gorgeous boys, Charlie and Gabriel, alongside her ever-supportive and loving husband Russ. The closest Caron came to discussing the possibility of death was to reiterate, time and time again, that she didn't want her boys to grow up without their mum.

Yes, of course she was angry and frustrated at times, racked with pain later and, no doubt, besieged by fear, particularly in the dark hours in the middle of the night when the mind races beyond all reason. However, all through that period of fighting her cancer she could always smile and her impish strident sense of humour constantly found its way to the surface. Despite the turmoil raging inside her, she made it easy for the family to be around her, and when we visited in Cornwall or, subsequently, in Byron Bay in Australia, she always had a busy itinerary of things lined up for us and places to go. So much so that we could hardly keep pace with her. She was always busy in mind and body, passionate about everything around her – constantly searching for a new challenge in life. Boy, did she face it!

As a mother who had loved and treasured my beautiful daughter from the moment of her birth, I was faced with the most heartbreaking helplessness at not being able to 'fix it'. The sticking plaster and the 'There, there, Mummy will kiss it better' routine suddenly wore as thin as a wafer. Yes, I could envelop Caron in my love as I'd always done, I could shop and cook for her, be supportive, help with the children, look for doctors and treatments and talk endlessly, but for the first time I couldn't take away the illness and soothe, as I had done hundreds of times in the past.

Nothing can prepare you for the second someone confirms, 'Your child has got cancer.' I remember thinking, No matter how well this story turns out, life will never be the same for Caron or the family ever again. Cancer patients tell me that although they have in essence beaten the condition and been declared 'clean', with every pain and ache the question comes: 'Is this it again – has it moved somewhere else to attack me once more?'

This is how Caron described that fateful day of diagnosis:

It was John Lennon who said, 'Life is what happens when you're busy making other plans.' At all devastating moments in life, I find I am usually doing something really mundane. In my case, I was lying in bed at my mum's in Sevenoaks reading about Debbie Daniels in the *Daily Mail*, when Russ walked in with a really strained smile on his face. It's a look I've seen a couple of times before, actually – complete nerves outrunning what to say. A sort of look a five-year-old boy has when his mother has caught him out in a fib.

Anyway, what he'd just found out was that a lump I'd had removed from my breast had cancerous cells in it.

I think it's safe to say I went into complete shock. It's like one of those situations you never ever think will happen to you.

I'd been convinced that the lump they'd taken out was completely harmless and in fact I only had it out to placate Russ and my mother. It had been examined by several specialists, all of whom said, 'Well, it's soft and evenly shaped and seems OK.' Even needle biopsies were inconclusive and so that lump had been there for about five months without me doing anything. Had I known then what I know now, I'd have started really looking at my lifestyle and getting my body cleansed immediately – I would have seen a herbalist, holistic dietician, etc., but the only advice I'd been offered was to cut down on caffeine and chocolate – it could affect your hormone levels, they said. Having just had a baby, it might have been a good place to start – with something a little more effective than a chocolate ban.

So my pleasant lie-in suddenly took a severe turn for the worse and I was immediately plunged into appointments with breast surgeons and the introduction to my oncologist.

Oncology is not a word I think I'd ever come across before and now is one with which I am all too familiar – still don't really know what it means, other than someone who has a variety of invasive treatments at his disposal. A sort of Attila the Hun of the medical world. Other doctors offer pink medicine or innocuous-looking capsules; an oncologist has at his fingertips all manner of disturbing treatments, red liquids which have to be kept under cover until the very last moment before they enter your veins, destroying all in their pathway and wreaking havoc with your hair on the way. Huge machines which you lie under in splendid isolation, whilst disembodied voices tell you to breathe in and a ray of invisible energy invades your body. The comforting thing is, the treatments are often accompanied by cheery, lush nurses, who exude confidence and warmth and have done this kind of thing so many times before and tell you of all the patients who are still around twenty-five years later – so much so, you relax, believe them and start having a laugh with them.

The thing I love about the human spirit is that, no matter how dire the circumstances, there always comes a point when you can have a laugh and forget about what's happening for a minute – realize you are still alive and all things are possible. But I am galloping ahead of myself . . .

There wasn't a huge amount of laughter as I recall – not even a snigger – as the doctors talked about another operation following my revealing lumpectomy, so back in I went to have the area cleaned up – like a garden, I suppose, and lymph nodes taken out, just to make sure it hadn't wandered off anywhere else.

In the year since then, I have spent many, many hours trying to figure out why and how it happened. It's often one of those things we ask ourselves, 'Why this? Why me?' I found myself thinking of other people who had had stuff to cope with and thinking, Well, I didn't cope any less well than them. Why should this happen to me? The simple truth is, often we don't know. We can have a few ideas why but there are some things that are plain and simple mysteries, and it's a waste of energy trying to figure it out.

Also, often it's a combination of reasons – stress – life situations – diet – environment – genetics – spiritual – emotional trauma – who knows? Our soul's learning.

One thing I do know is that it comes with an onslaught of fear. Unfortunately all fear is ultimately a fear of death – some of us have been forced to face it sooner than we'd anticipated.

ILLNESS ISN'T THE ISSUE – HOW IT MAKES YOU FEEL IS . . .

I was in the garden that day. Caron was resting after her first lumpectomy and at the back of my mind I had a niggle: 'I trust and pray everything is clear.' Nevertheless, I still thought, as Caron and the doctors had predicted, that it would turn out to be a milk lump. I was to relive that split second of confirmation from Russ many, many times. And what it does in one swift swoop, is to take away the carefree aspect of your life, because in your soul you just know there will be dark days ahead of doubt, fear and struggle.

I just couldn't absorb the reality. My beautiful, intelligent, feisty, loving daughter had been stricken with cancer. In my head I kept thinking, This doesn't happen to a thirty-three-year-old wife and mother, a young woman balancing a hugely successful career. My mother had died of breast cancer some eight years earlier at the age of seventy-two, and even though it was deeply sad to lose her and I was bereft, it was in the right order of life. If I could, I would have changed places with Caron to keep the natural order of the generations – after all, I had had a good innings. However, when Caron was first diagnosed the doctors were going for a complete cure, and even when the cancer had moved through her body to her bones, some six years later, we were still going for 'management'. Somehow, through her courage, Caron had clung to that hope of life and we clung with her. It's amazing how one can condition the mind to say, 'There's always hope, whatever the doctors predict.' Miracles do happen and new treatments are being developed all the time. Whatever the outcome, it's all you have: to live for the second and live every second of every day. Now that she is dead, I am still doing it. It is the only way I can seem to survive this. You have to have faith. Caron believed in angels. She believed that when they had visited they left a white feather. She said it was their calling card. I don't think I can ever accept that my daughter is no longer with me, I carry her in my heart. Like Caron's total conviction in angels I hold on to the belief that she is here, somewhere, next to me.

1. The Sun Never Sets

It was Easter Sunday, 2004. Caron had wanted to go up to a café in the mountains. It was a stunning spot that had become her favourite place during the month she'd been in Switzerland, receiving pioneering cancer treatment. But her strength eluded her. Instead, she settled into a chair back at the hotel to paint Easter eggs with her family. But halfway through the painting, something in her changed. She seemed to run out of steam again, so Russ took her back to her room. We tried to massage some comfort back into her legs, but they were cold and completely unresponsive to our touch. We had a family conference in the corridor and decided it was time, after a two-and-a-half-year absence, to get Caron home. Michael, my son, flew the boys, Charlie and Gabriel, back and took them to Russ's parents. My husband Stephen and I returned to Sevenoaks to get the house ready. Because of Caron's deterioration, we decided that it was best she avoided the airports and Russ would drive her home the following day. That night, Caron was in a huge amount of pain. Russ listened to her agitated torment as she tossed and turned and mumbled in her sleep. At times she was almost delirious. There was nothing unusual about the pain – by now, Caron had tumours up and down her spine – but despite experiencing some harrowing times during the previous few months, it seemed to Russ that this was worse.

The following morning Caron couldn't get out of bed but looked brighter. Still seeking help, she persuaded Andrea, a reflexologist from the Paracelsus Clinic to come to the hotel and give her a massage in her room. There was no way she could make the journey to the hospital. Andrea confirmed that

Caron had started to 'shut down'. Nothing was responding. It was as if all her vital organs were beginning to pack up. The nurse told Russ to get her home as soon as possible. It was eleven thirty a.m. on Easter Monday.

Russ packed the bags and carried them down to Stephen's car. He, Caron and the boys were supposed to be in England for four months and Caron had brought a lot of stuff. It took until four o'clock that afternoon to get Caron dressed and packed and all the bags out. It was a very tough time: she was still in great pain, virtually immobile, and had to keep getting back into bed for some relief, then couldn't get out when the worst had passed. She didn't want to eat; she couldn't sleep. She was struggling with everything. The decision was right. It was time to get her home.

When it came to leaving the room, Caron couldn't walk, even with the aid of her cane. Russ suggested she get on to one of the porter's trolleys so that he could push her to the lift, but she couldn't even raise her leg to step on to it. They had no option but to walk. Which they did. Step by agonizing step, until they reached the lobby. It took almost an hour. In the car, Russ had laid out loads of blankets, then reclined her seat. Caron was so relieved to get in that she told Russ, 'I'm not getting out of this car until I get to Mum's house.' They set off for England.

For the first four hours Caron slept. She mumbled a bit, and sometimes rolled her head to and fro, but apart from that she was peaceful. At no point was Russ certain that Caron was dying, but he knew he had a monster journey ahead of him. To cope he set himself little hurdles: get out of Switzerland; cross France. He was praying to get back to England. He admits now that his goal was to get his wife through the Channel Tunnel alive. He thought about what he would do if the worst happened and she died in the car on the way back. Should he just go through, pretending she was asleep? He decided that was exactly what he would do. He couldn't bear the idea of having to leave her body in a French morgue. The temptation to put his foot to the floor was overwhelming, but he didn't want to be stopped so he stuck to the speed limit and just kept on driving.

It was horrendous. Caron lay either too still at his side, or moaned with pain, yet an amazing sunset guided him westward and home. He followed the burning sun all the way through Switzerland and France. Every hill they crested, there it was again, the sun that never set.

Halfway across France, Caron suddenly came to: she rose from the brink, looked at Russ and smiled. There had been numerous times over the last six months when Russ had thought, This is it, then watched in amazement as Caron got up the following day, smiling again, better. On that car journey, something somewhere had given her a boost. Russ doesn't know what it was, but suddenly she was back with him and, miraculously, seemed fine. Outside the car, the flat, wide-open expanse of the battlefields of France spread out to either side of them. Hovering above the ground a gossamer thread of mist reflected the indigo-orange light of the setting sun. There was no one on the road but them. It was an extraordinary cocoon, a Tardis, taking them home. A quiet moment to share after all the panic that had come before. Time stretched out, then concertinaed, then stretched out once more as Caron slept again, then came to. Russ knew that as a unit they were unlikely to be alone again. When they reached Sevenoaks they would be surrounded by the rest of the family and, more intrusively, doctors with strong medication and nurses with damning prognoses that signalled the end of their journey together.

They started to talk about the very fabric of their life together. As Russ says, there was never a time that they didn't chat, and this was no different. Except that Caron was dipping in and out of consciousness in what was an honest, heartfelt, albeit dislocated conversation. He would be talking to her, then notice she'd gone back to sleep, fall silent and concentrate on the hurdle ahead. Forty minutes later, she'd stir, or reach for a drink, answer the question or continue where she'd left off.

Although he can't remember the specifics of what was said, he knows it still never reached a dramatic 'I am dying' moment. It was softer than that. Kinder. What they did was reminisce. They laughed about some of the strange and funny things they had done together. Their time in Cornwall. Their adventures in Australia. In this magic capsule, suspended in time, they discussed all they had achieved. They had enough time to say things to each other that they wouldn't have said at any other time in their relationship. Caron was incredibly loving and more than that, appreciative of everything Russ had done for her – and, as this book will show, he did more than was ever expected of any man. She said some wonderful things to him that will stay with him for ever. Was she finishing things off, tidying up life's loose ends? We will never know for certain, but Russ feels that somewhere in her system Caron knew she didn't have a lot of time left. There was pride in what they had done together, the love and support they had given each other and everything they had achieved. In fact, what took place between them was communication on such a deep level that nothing had to be spelled out. They didn't have time for that: Caron would drift off to sleep again.

Once they had crossed the channel it was almost as if Caron knew she was home. Her body relaxed. It was a surreal experience for Russ: it wasn't as if their 'lives had flashed before them', but somehow they had said goodbye, without ever voicing the word. Mainly, of course, they talked about their two wonderful sons, about the joy, light and pride Charlie and Gabriel had, individually and together, brought to their lives. They talked about what special souls their two sons seemed to have, what they might contribute to the world, and their wonderful personalities. Throughout Caron's illness, she had been searching for a miracle to extend her life. During that car journey they finally recognized that the miracle had been there all along. Charlie and Gabriel, their phenomenal children, would take Caron's spirit into the future and beyond. They were the miracle. They were Caron. Against the backdrop of seven years' soul-searching, trauma, questioning and pain, Russ and Caron had striven to remain a happy family unit. They had succeeded in doing that. Caron had only ever asked for one miracle: to live. But she was granted a second: a happy life.

The hardest part for Caron throughout the relentless march of her disease was the threat that she wouldn't see the boys grow up. She couldn't even think about it – the prospect of her boys growing up without their mother terrified her too much. It also gave her the extraordinary strength to go on defying the MRIs and the X-rays, and keep going. She hung on as long as she did for her sons; the strength of character and courage, the wilfulness and tenacity, the bottomless pit of maternal love is the legacy she leaves her children. They may never understand what she went through to be with them because their memories of her won't be of a woman dying of cancer – she made sure of that. But we who were on the sidelines know that Caron dug as deep as a human can to stay alive for her children.

It was just gone midnight when Russ and Caron reached our house in Sevenoaks. After nine hours in the same position, Caron had seized up and we couldn't get her out of the car. In the end Stephen and Russ lifted her on to a chair and carried her through to the kitchen. It was not an easy task: even a fractional movement caused her incredible pain. Physically her body betrayed her, but even then her mind was so alert. She looked around the house she knew so well and had been absent from for so long. She noticed that I had put up the painting she'd done for me at Christmas and said, 'That looks lovely there.' She sat at the kitchen table, as she had so many times before, had a cup of green tea in her favourite pink spotted cup and ate a little of Stephen's home-made vegetable soup. I was overjoyed to have her home, but terrified by what I saw. It was only later, as I wrote this book, that I realized I had experienced a similar midnight tea-party once before: on the night that Caron was born.

The next hurdle was to get her upstairs. Russ and Stephen put her in a sturdier chair to carry her to the room in which she had recuperated so many times before. It was some time around three a.m. when we finally got her into bed. Then Russ, Stephen and I returned to the kitchen and, for a short while, just stared at each other. No one slept that night. I paced the corridor. Russ lay alongside his delirious wife. It was a terrifying, dark night.

As soon as it was light, I was back in organization mode. I rang our lovely family GP, who promised to be there as soon as surgery ended. I had slept for ten minutes but Caron was finally home with me, although the nightmare had not passed. I was so excited that she was back in her room, but terrified of what lay behind the door. Caron woke at about ten thirty and I heard the soft voice I had been waiting for since dawn.

Finally Russ came out and told me I could go in. Caron was sitting up in bed, and it was a wonderful sight. But looks can deceive – the top of the bed lifted at the touch of a button. After a little chat I went downstairs and made Caron breakfast. When my children were sick I used to make them tea in the 'magic teapot'. It was tiny with a tiny cup, and I made tiny squares of toast to go with it. After her father Don died Caron took the original magic teapot home with her, so I bought another for my grandchildren. It was that teapot that I took up to her on a tray that morning. Sliced melon and tiny squares of rice bread. It was wonderful to be able to do something. It was wonderful to have her home. I sat beside her and held her hand, afraid that if I let go, I would wake and discover that this was yet another wishful dream, and she was still twelve thousand miles away in Australia. But it was real. Her hand was warm in mine, but her breathing wasn't so good.

When Dr Richard Husband arrived he gave us little to hold on to. 'I'm so sorry,' he said to me. 'I had no idea how ill she was.' He said he was going to send over his surgery nurse, Cathy, who could administer a drip to help ease Caron's breathing. He told us then that, as the experienced nurse she was, with a great inbuilt instinct, Cathy could probably give us an idea of just how serious a condition Caron was in. We were in turmoil. What did he mean? How bad did he think Caron was? She'd been here before. She'd rally again. Wouldn't she? *Wouldn't she?* The doctor couldn't answer our desperate questions. Nurse Cathy arrived. She gave Caron a bed-bath and made her comfortable, then came out to tell us her prognosis. 'She doesn't look good,' she said, and promised she would return with the equipment for the drip. We probed and questioned, got an answer, then dismissed it. We had heard those words before from almost every practitioner we'd met on this journey: every time she had got better. I said what I had said many times before: 'You don't know my daughter. You don't know Caron. She is a fighter and she will win.'

Russ called my eldest son Paul, who was skiing with his family in France. Paul had decided not to go on to the slopes that morning, almost as if he was waiting for the call. As soon as Russ suggested he should come home, Paul set things in motion. Michael had gone to work in London, but when Russ called and told him Caron was asleep, something made Michael walk out of his office and go straight to Charing Cross station. An intuitive decision he will remember and be grateful for as long as he lives. Both of my sons had started their journey home to their sister, although sadly only Michael made it in time to see her alive. Caron continued to rise and fall out of a sleepy haze throughout that day.

★

During the day Russ and Michael, Stephen and I sat on the end of the bed and chatted to Caron, or to one another, then left her to sleep. At other times I just stood and watched her. At one point Michael spent a little time on his own with her, held her hand and talked to her. Then he went downstairs to get a cup of tea. When he came back he put his head round the door and Caron was absolutely still. For a split second he thought the worst had happened. He stared at her, willing it not to be so, then heard a gasp, and her chest rose again. He didn't tell us – he thought maybe he was being paranoid. But he did come and get me and Russ. We didn't leave that room again until her last breath had left her body. The nurse came back: Caron's breathing had become even more erratic and heavy. Again we probed. 'She hasn't got long at all,' said the nurse. Well, we knew that, but we were all thinking three, maybe six months. The summer in Cornwall, at least? Russ was terrified and decided to send for the boys. His parents had taken them to a fairground and they didn't have a mobile. Eventually he got hold of the owner, persuaded him to track them down among the throng of other happy families, and told his parents to bring the boys to Kent straight away. It is a strange irony that a day that became so monumentally important was taken up with so much organization and decision-making.

At about six, two extraordinary things happened. Caron's breathing changed again, and Charlie and Gabriel arrived at the door. The nurse told us that Caron was starting to slip away. We all looked at each other in terror. I saw my own boundless fear reflected in Russ's eyes. Inside my head I was shrieking, 'This can't be happening! Stop it! Stop it!' Caron had just got home. It wasn't fair. This wasn't how it was supposed to be. Russ raced downstairs to the boys. He told them on the way up that Mummy was going to find it really hard to pull through this, then brought them into her room. As incredible as it seems to me now, although she was dying, an extraordinary smile had spread across Caron's lips. The little boys hugged and kissed her, talked to her for a little while, said goodbye, then went downstairs. It was unbearable to behold. Russ, Michael and I stayed with Caron, clinging to her until her last breath had left her body, and still this amazing, enigmatic smile held fast.

It was peaceful. It was diabolical. There is not a word in the world to describe how it feels to watch your child die. It wasn't that my heart was breaking, rather that my soul was shattering. I was dying with her but, unlike Caron, my body wouldn't let me go. Despite the terrible carnage in my heart, Caron radiated a still, quiet peace. Finally the nurse said, 'She's gone . . .' But she hadn't. Not quite. Her body was warm. She lay there, smiling reassuringly as if to say, 'It's okay, everything is going to be okay . . .' No, she hadn't gone. Not then. Not ever.

Michael went downstairs to calm the boys and cuddle them. Charlie said, 'Is Mummy going to wake up?' and he replied, 'I don't think so, darling . . .'

Russ and I stayed upstairs, still clinging to Caron. He looked at me, lost. It had all happened so quickly. 'How are we going to tell the children?'

The doctor was there – I had not been aware of his arrival. He took us aside and said, 'You watch, the children will lead you . . .' They were incredibly strong and prophetic words. Because they did.

Together we went downstairs, and I watched Russ say the hardest, most awful words any father might ever have to say to their child. Mummy was not coming back. Hearing him speak so gently to his beautiful boys, hearing him try to explain the inexplicable, was almost equal to watching my daughter die. I know that for Russ it was the hardest thing he has ever had to do in his life. All the fear, confusion and pain we had felt upstairs was transferred to them in that second. It was too shattering to watch.

Outside it was an incongruously beautiful day and the house

was filled with shafts of amber sunlight. I remember Michael taking Charlie and Gabriel to the window. He said, 'Every time you feel the warmth of the sun on your face, Mummy is with you.'

I didn't think any of us would survive that day. But the doctor was right: the children do lead us. They are the future. They carry Caron deep within them. Every time I look at the boys I know that her spirit is alive. I can see and feel her, I can sense her presence. I watch them do what adults find so hard. They live fully in every second. In one breath they will say, 'I miss Mummy,' and in the next they are on the trampoline, bouncing their way back to happiness. They were the reason for us to get up the very next morning. They are still the reason to get up in the morning. Even though we couldn't stomach food, they needed feeding, same as always. Somehow we provided food. I can't remember the details. I was in shock. We were all in shock.

I wouldn't let them take Caron out of the house. I couldn't bear the idea of her in some impersonal funeral parlour, with people she didn't know looking at her. So she stayed at home, in her room, and all of us would go and sit with her. We filled the room with flowers, photographs of Charlie and Gabriel and lit candles everywhere. Last thing at night I went in, sat beside her on the bed, and said goodnight to her as I'd always done. She looked so beautiful and pain-free.

Paul arrived in Sevenoaks an hour after Caron had died. He knew something was wrong from the moment he set foot in the house, and after his chaotic dash from France could not accept that he had missed her. Like the rest of us, he spent a lot of time sitting with her. Other friends came too: she was rarely on her own. Sometimes we'd all sit in her room with her, drinking tea, reminiscing – her favourite pastime. At others we'd walk around like zombies, shocked and stunned that Caron could die like that, suddenly, or so it seemed to us. Nothing had prepared us. Not the seven years that had passed since she was diagnosed with breast cancer, not the prognosis two years later that she had eighteen months to live, not the mastectomy, the chemotherapy, the radiotherapy, not even when the cancer went to her bones and she had to walk on a cane. Not even the laboured breathing and crippling pain she suffered in those last few days. She'd always come through before. The songs and good times came back. The cloud passed. The positive stand she had taken had infiltrated us all, so when her death came, as it tragically did, we were as shocked as if she'd been run over by a bus.

If I could I would have kept her at home for ever. The crippling pain that seared me on the day of her funeral was because I knew I would not see my beautiful daughter again. Words are futile. The pain is boundless.

2. An Irish Girl

Now that I look back it's as if Caron was in a rush from the very beginning. I should have known from the rude interruption halfway through *Oliver!*, the musical, that nothing was going to be predictable about this birth, this child, or her subsequent life. My husband Don and I had decided to go to London for a final fling before the baby came. Not quite eight months pregnant, I had nearly reached the point when I couldn't fly. I had been singing and performing since I was eight and loved anything to do with the theatre and performance, so naturally my treat was to take in a show in London's West End.

I didn't even make it to the interval. In the middle of the first half, I had an overwhelming desire to go to the loo – I simply couldn't wait. I had to get out. So, I squeezed myself along the row of seats and just as I got to the ladies' my waters broke. It took me completely by surprise, even shock. Here I was in a strange city, knowing no one and nothing about what was to come.

I found my way back to my seat in the dark and told Don what had happened. He did a triple-take, then said, 'What now?'

For a moment we sat there, frozen, while the musical played on. Then Don panicked. He fell off his chair in his hurry to get us out of there. It was the classic thing – going out to the foyer and saying, 'Help, my wife's having a baby,' then a short pause, as I stood there, seemingly with nothing wrong, 'We think –' The theatre staff called an ambulance.

In its own way it was scary: I was only twenty-two, and while London was an exciting place to visit, it wasn't where I wanted to have my first baby. I wanted to be with my mother and family, at home. So, it was frightening to be bundled into an ambulance that screamed across London, lights flashing, weaving through the traffic. And then the most awful thing happened: having reached Charing Cross Hospital, we were turned away. There was literally no room at the inn. I remember thinking, This would never happen in Northern Ireland! Nobody would ever turn you away, ever. So here we were, in this big, wide, impersonal city, being sent off on another mad dash to another hospital. Not only did I not know where I was being turned away from, I had no idea where I was being taken to next. Now, if it had been a department store we were trying to locate, I might have had more of a chance, but beyond occasional retail therapy, London was completely unknown to me. We ended up in the maternity hospital in Fulham. The birth was quirky. So was my girl.

In those days husbands were definitely not encouraged to stay for any of the labour or the birth, so at about twelve thirty a.m. the nurse told Don to go home: nothing would happen before morning, she predicted, since this was my first baby. As Caron continued to do until her death, she defied the doctors and their predictions and was born just two hours later. Don barely made it back in time. I don't remember a great deal about those two hours, except that I was given some pethidine, a pretty strong drug, which isn't used quite so liberally today. It was as close as I ever got to being high. Zipping along on cloud nine, I rabbited on about how marvellous *Oliver!* had been, how I was only visiting and was due home the following day. I thought it was lovely to be having a tea-party in the wee hours of the morning. I was really quite oblivious to what was going on.

Having had the joy of seeing Caron's sons Charlie and Gabriel born, I know how different birth is these days. Parents are consulted, birth plans are adhered to, men even attend antenatal classes. I can't imagine Don practising his breathing exercises with me. Back then, you did as you were told and you did it on your own. Only when it was all over did the proud father come in and get passed a clean little baby, neatly swaddled in white cotton. He was not told of the extraordinary toil that had come before.

Once Caron had arrived, I went from the shock and surprise of being in a strange city to the most amazing feeling that nothing else mattered. She was safe and sound, and although she went into an incubator for a while, she was in good shape. In fact, considering she was five weeks early, she was amazing. As I said, she was in a rush from the beginning, which makes sense to me now as she had a lot to do and only forty-one years in which to do it.

From day one, premature and tiny, she looked incredible. Although her body was small, she had this wide, knowing face, more advanced than you'd expect a newborn to have. Of course, I believed she was the most beautiful girl ever to be born and, of course, I still do. I remember when my father saw her for the first time, he just said, 'She has the most perfect rosebud mouth I've ever seen in my life.' And that summed it up. That's what she had: rosebud lips. Wonderfully full, right from birth.

I stayed in hospital, on the ordinary ward with all the other mothers around, and the talk was of what we were going to call our babies. I loved the name Karen, it was the 'new name' then but when I wrote it down it looked too hard next to the K of Keating. So I thought of spelling it another way. I was really keen on all Leslie Caron's films, my favourite being *Gigi* and, like many women of my generation, I wanted to be that girl. So I rewrote the name, using Leslie's spelling, and for evermore Caron had to spell it for other people. But I didn't think about that: I just thought how lovely it looked on the page. As for the inspiration behind her second name, Louisa, I have no idea. I have a funny feeling that all the girls around me were talking about it and I just liked it.

I have no recollection of those other women, except that

there was a great deal of camaraderie on the ward, which was an instant support for me. I was high on the birth being over successfully, Caron was all right, thank God, so beautiful and a girl, but I missed my mother and the rest of my family. The Irish are very family-oriented. Nowadays, of course, you would hop on a cheap flight without much of a thought, but it wasn't so easy back then and certainly not as cheap. Travelling anywhere in those days was always more of an excursion, so for a little while it was just Caron, Don and me until Don had to go back to work. Then it was just the two of us.

Suddenly the two friends of Don, Fen and Harry, who'd been expecting to put us up for a couple of days, had to convert their sitting room into a nursery. I didn't want to fly with Caron too quickly and felt I should stay on and gain a bit of strength. I'd been sick throughout my pregnancy and, as unbelievable as it is to me now, I'd actually lost weight: the day after the birth I weighed only six stone ten. When I look at Caron's baby pictures I seem to be all eyes, staring out of an emaciated frame. Believe me, it was the last time I ever weighed so little. As I said, a flight to Belfast then was a big deal, a real event, and I didn't feel up to it. It was a different era, and attitudes to childbirth were different. You had a lot more bed rest afterwards than you do today: now women are up and home within hours of delivery. So I stayed on in London alone with my baby. My life shrank. I had two points of reference: the house I was staying in and the clinic six blocks down on the left. I was the small-town girl lost in the big city. I followed the route I knew, visited the clinic, then turned round and followed it back.

I breastfed Caron: I had lots of milk and she was a little gulper, which was great – although she ate so much, so fast, that she often had projectile vomiting. Baby sick isn't fun at the best of times, but in someone else's house it was a source of real worry. I remember being mortified that Caron had been sick over Fen and Harry's furniture and was terrified of staining something. In the end I put towels across the settee and bed and covered the carpets: if they took a hit I would wash them myself, so my kind hosts wouldn't know.

Towards the end of Caron's life I found myself doing it again. Caron refused to stay in hospital so when we visited the clinic in Switzerland we stayed in a nearby hotel. Without the assistance of nursing staff, I found myself washing towels and sheets once again in secret. I see so many patterns to Caron's life now, so many themes that have repeated themselves, some as thought-provoking as premature birth and premature death, others more mundane, like washing those towels. But there is another.

Those first few weeks after I had Caron were tough – relentless, actually. The feeding, changing, being sick, feeding again because she'd been sick and was hungry meant there was no break. It was endless. And there was no back-up. We got on with it, though. We had to. I wonder where that strength came from. I still wonder where Caron's strength came from when she was fighting a far harder battle. Looking back, it was odd having experienced something so momentous, then having no one to share it with. Cancer is like that; Caron's illness was like that. Just after she'd been born, there were times full of fear, determination and loneliness, but they provided something else too. Something profound. A magical cocoon for Caron and me, and despite the tears, we bonded hard and fast. There were times like that later, in hospital or when she was recovering at Sevenoaks. Many times in Australia too.

Just after she was born and we were locked in to each other, I got to know her baby nuances, those little expressions and noises that meant she was thirsty, hot or bored. Like the changes in her breathing at the end. In fact, throughout Caron's life I observed her, and I could always tell if something was out of kilter just from a change in her routine or voice. Perhaps it started then, during those strange days in London when it was just the two of us against the world.

Because I was breastfeeding I didn't leave her with someone else to give her a bottle – anyway, there was no one to leave her with. The two people we were staying with worked during the day so it was just us. She had my complete attention, with no one else to divert it – nobody whatsoever. When I was in Australia with her she and I talked about that time. We talked about when she was born and when we were together. Although I was frightened and tired as any new mother is, it was, with hindsight, a very special period of my life that was completely suspended in time. I relive it time and time again, and look back on it now with tremendous gratitude, particularly since she's gone.

There was no such thing as paternity leave, but as soon as Don had checked in with work and got things tied up, he came back for us. It was probably only a couple of weeks, but at the time it felt like a year. We decided to go to Manchester to see his family before we made the journey home to Ireland. So, off we went. I remember the pride of going north to Don's parents – I hadn't spent much time with them but they had welcomed me warmly into their family. They were fantastic. Don's sister-in-law, Mary, had given birth to Janette only three months previously, so we had a lot in common, and there was great excitement about the two little girls being together.

Someone suggested we should have a joint christening service while we were there and Caron was duly baptized into the Catholic Church with her cousin. But it wasn't her only christening. When we returned to Northern Ireland she was christened again, this time into the Church of Ireland, in St Mark's, Portadown, with my parents, sister Lena, brother Charles and all the family in attendance and my mum and sister as godmothers. This may seem strange, but you must understand the time in which we lived. Don was not a practising Catholic but came from a family that was. I came from a Protestant Ulster family and my father took his role within the Orange Order very seriously, so our marriage had initially caused upset to my family. In fact, my father, a highly principled man, had refused to attend our wedding and my mother had to follow suit, though in later years she confessed it was the greatest regret of her life. Strangely enough, I was able to accept my father's views at the time because he had always stood by his principles and had never held a grudge.

By the time I came home with Caron, though, all that was forgotten in the dim and distant past. We were an even stronger family. My parents idolized her from the moment I brought her into their house and throughout her childhood they would do anything to get their arms round her and have her to stay. They lived about twenty-five miles away from us in Portadown. In those days there was no motorway: like flying, any car journey had to be a well-planned expedition. It took about two hours to travel through all the little towns by the country roads. You didn't really go for a day, you went for the weekend or over-night. So, because Don was a cameraman and worked odd hours, I went quite often. My mum and dad got to know Caron extremely well. At that point they had only one other grandchild, Lawrence, and Caron was the first girl. She was a much-loved baby – she was an easy child to love: she was always adorable to look at, cute and bright, and could twist you easily round her little finger. She always had a strong connection with her grandparents, as I feel I have with my grandchildren.

I realize now that it was only when I had experienced what birth was and had a child of my own that I understood the true value of my own parents. The moment Caron was born I could see why my parents had been protective. I knew why they hadn't wanted me to do certain things. I knew why they had lavished so much love on me, and I knew how it felt to have the treasure of a child.

Don and I were living in a rented house in Marmont Park in Belfast, near Hollywood in County Down. There were some people living opposite whom I hadn't really had a chance to get to know. We had really bad snow in the winter of 1962 – it fell to waist deep – and I remember going across to the woman opposite. 'I'm wading my way down to the shops: is there anything I can get for you?' I asked. Roberta McConville was her name and she became a great confidante. She and her husband Ernest are friends to this day, and Roberta was one of very few people I talked to about Caron when she got sick.

So began this wonderfully happy period. We were young, I wasn't working and enjoyed being at home all day with Caron. She was a good baby, slept well and, although she still threw up, always seemed well satisfied. They were special times, which never happened again: by the time Paul was born, I was working more and had Caron to care for too. We were saving to buy a house of our own and Don would get irritable if I spent money on things he didn't think reasonable, so I had resolved to start making my own and got a job as an Avon lady. It was brand new in Ireland at that point. I would settle Caron into her pram, then load up the cosmetics and go calling, 'ding-dong', from house to house. Needless to say, the profits were negligible, but the doorstep chats more than compensated for that.

If that seems odd for the time, allow me to put my desire to earn money into context. I had been earning since I was nine, performing with my father, a part-time magician, singing at Ham Suppers and Daffodil Teas held all over Northern Ireland in various halls and schools. The tables were laden with home-made local produce, 'ham so thin you could see the pattern of the plate through it', and a whole variety of cakes and sand-wiches. They were simple times. The entertainment came after everyone had eaten, Dad doing his magic tricks, me singing. So, I was used to my ten shillings a night. In fact, when my parents said I couldn't go to grammar school because the uniforms were too expensive, I told them precociously I'd pay for them myself – not very gracious, perhaps, but going to grammar school was what I really wanted to do and I was prepared to fight for the right to further education.

Stubbornness runs in our family and Caron had more than her fair share. As Michael has said on many occasions, she tended to get her own way. And when she wanted to do something, the rest of us seemed to toe the line. Most of the time she did it with charm and got away with it, but that didn't mean she wasn't prone to the odd tantrum. Stubborn and wilful: traits in Caron's personality from the very beginning. And thank God, because they kept her going right up to the very end. In fact, the last oncologist we ever saw in Switzerland couldn't understand how she was still walking, let alone living.

Until I got married I had been working at Ulster TV but I couldn't go back to my old job because in those days they had a strict policy about husbands and wives not working in the same department, which we had done before we were married, me as a production assistant, Don as a cameraman. The reason for the rule was that Don would have been on the camera with headphones and I would have been calling the shots and working out the timing, but if things didn't run smoothly the director was likely to mutter, 'Stupid b***h got the time wrong', which, of course, Don would have heard. Once again, different times, so off I went and played house. The books I read, on how to have a child and stay happily married, recommended old-fashioned things, like 'Even though you're now a housewife, make sure you dress up and put on your makeup before your husband comes home. Make enough time for your husband and try, if you've got well-meaning parents, to have a weekend on your own to make sure your relationship stays kindled.' My mother couldn't wait for our rekindling weekends. They must have worked, too, because when Caron was only nine months old, I was pregnant again.

Now it was definitely time to move, and we did, into a bungalow in Marnabrae Park, near Lisburn. It was the first house we owned and it was where Paul, my gorgeous eldest son, was born in 1964. It was an American-style open-plan bungalow, which we thought was stunning, and cost us the princely sum of £2800 with an additional £300 for central heating. You can't buy a kitchen for that money now, let alone a house. Professor Billy Thompson and his wife, Anne, were the first people we met when we moved in. They became instant friends and Anne and I saw each other every day. Because we were at home, she'd ring up and say, 'Your place or mine?' So we'd frantically do all our housework in the morning, then go round to one house or the other, throw the kids into the garden and let them play while we sat drinking coffee and chatting. We have fourteen grandchildren between us now, and we often dissolve into giggles when we watch young parents constantly finding ways to entertain their children. Our mantra was 'Go out and play, we're talking . . .'

Part of our routine was visiting the baby clinic. We'd walk there to buy baby milk, with the current infant in the old-fashioned Silver Cross perambulator and an older child sitting on the end. The shopping would be under the pram cover. It was a four-mile round trip and we'd be starving by the time we headed back, so we often bought fish and chips, hid them under the cover too, and ate them as discreetly as we could on the way home. In those days it was not done to eat in the street. They were innocent times, I suppose. We often talk now about how sorry we are that we didn't know then how fantastic and carefree things were. Instead, we spent all our time talking about when we could afford a car so that we wouldn't have to walk the roads with those big prams. You spend a lot of your life wishing it away. Then we were living for the future. My daughter spent a long time living in the past, searching for reasons that would explain why she had got ill. In time she and I learnt to live in the present, make the most of the moment, live for *the now*. It is a hard thing to do. But it is still the only way that I can survive this. I have no option but to live hour by hour, day by day. I can't seem to get through it any other way.

The trips to my parents' house continued. Caron and my dad would make the bus journey together, leaving me time to give Paul some undivided attention. Those bus journeys became legendary, and Caron wrote about them in later life:

Music has always been a constant in my life. I grew up to the sounds of everything from Hollywood musicals and Irish rebel songs to Tom Jones and my mum's cabaret numbers. Having begun her singing career at the age of nine, Mum was still working as a nightclub singer when we were small and used to rehearse around the house all day. As a result, by the age of three, I was word perfect and had a repertoire Debbie Reynolds would have been proud of.

Who knows what is simply an outpouring of genes or gently cultivated and moulded by interested parties around? All I do know is it's not every small girl who's encouraged by her doting grandfather to stand on her seat at the front of an Ulster bus belting out 'Bye Bye Blackbird', 'Won't you Come Home, Bill Bailey?' and 'Queen Of The Road' for the benefit of the entire bus.

We're not talking about a few stops along the road here – at that point there wasn't a motorway between Lisburn where we lived and Portadown where my grandparents were – the journey took at least an hour and a half, and I went to stay with them regularly. I have absolutely no recollection of these impromptu performances. No recollection of the other passengers' faces. Did they really love it and applaud, as family legend would have it, or were they inwardly cursing the fates for incarcerating them with the Shirley Temple of the no. 11 bus route? No recollection of how I felt – of the joy or horror it engendered in me. It's just when I recall moments of extreme shyness just a few years later that I find it hard to believe we're talking about the same child. Still, there are a lot of things that seem a good idea at the age of three, that somehow lose charm later on . . .

Caron would be sent off with food parcels to make my mother's life easier, including tinned spaghetti, one of her favourites and a good standby for lunch. When I went to collect her, my mother, who was a wonderful cook and always made everything from scratch, would tell me she'd used up all the food but couldn't bring herself to open that tin of spaghetti. Once Caron must have been at my parents' for a while because when I went to pick her up she called my mother 'Mummy'. I remember gulping and thinking, I'd better not leave her here too often. It was an embarrassing moment and my mother felt terrible. But, you know, seeing one's parents' pride in one's children is intoxicating. I understand why Caron felt so bereft when her beloved father died just days before her second son was born. She had enjoyed such a close relationship with her grandfather, while he and my mother took such joy from her, as she did from them, that she was sad Charlie and Gabriel wouldn't know their grandfather as she had known hers. So, if I was a little jealous in that moment when Caron called my mother Mummy, it was short-lived, because I was delighted they were so close.

Caron was wonderful with Paul when he was a baby. She'd help carry the nappies and want to pour out the Napisan and shake the talcum powder. But, as with everything, she soon worked out how to use her brother to her advantage. Neither of them was a great eater and used to say, 'What can I leave?' when I put down a plate of food. Not a great endorsement of my culinary skills. But before Paul could 'talk', I would have them sitting up at the table with boiled eggs and I would say, 'You can't get down until you've finished your eggs and toast.' A few minutes later I would see Paul running around and ask, 'Have you finished?' and he'd nod and run off to play. In the meantime Caron would have switched her uneaten egg for Paul's quickly devoured one and I would chase after Paul saying, 'You haven't eaten your egg and Caron has finished hers. Get back up to the table,' so the poor boy would end up eating two eggs and Caron, as was her wont, got away with murder. I only found this out in later years. At the time poor Paul couldn't tell me about his elder sister's devious trick, which, of course, was what Caron was relying on. She was naughty, yes, and most of the time was up to something. But always with charm and a broad grin, which remained with her until her last moments.

Perhaps she got away with more than most because, from the start, she applied herself. She was naturally bright and intelligent. She was always drawing and painting, just as Charlie and Gabriel do now, and she loved reading. She would never have had a bag without a book in it – no matter where she was, she was knee-deep in a novel. School came easy. I never had to pressurize Caron. Maybe girls are easier than boys to manage, but Caron had this knack of making you think she was doing everything *you* wanted when half the time she was really doing exactly what *she* wanted. She always had a delicious sense of humour, and I have a photo of her chasing her cousin around at a wedding, which epitomizes her impish streak.

Although she was an outgoing child, as the story of the bus shows, Caron developed a certain shyness in later life. Although she wasn't shy about the job she did, she was shy when she had to walk into a room where she didn't know anyone. She didn't like going in alone, always wanted someone with her. When someone is naturally beautiful, as she was – and, forgive me, she was – and naturally bright, and things appear to come easily to them, perhaps they don't feel worthy of praise, or feel that they don't deserve their achievements. I found it hard when she questioned her worth. I didn't understand her lack of confidence, which became more apparent as she got older. Maybe when you are struggling with potential death you put everything under a microscope. She asked a lot of questions about her childhood and I'd say, 'I don't know why you're even querying any of this. You were adored, idolized, loved, treasured, every

adjective you can think of, from the moment you were born.'
Maybe that in itself caused the problem. As I said, there was
never any pressure on her – I never had to say 'You get in there
and do your homework', none of that, because she just did it
and wanted to do it. But as a consequence she set herself very
high standards – maybe too high. She was a great child and had
a great childhood. But the holistic approach to healing is to
scrutinize everything, so she did – her father and me, her childhood, her husband, her relationships, her self, her self-worth.
At times it was exhausting for all of us, because sometimes there
just isn't an answer to 'Why?'

3. Belfast Brogue

Every day was an adventure

That was how Caron described her childhood. In her own words. As well as all her notebooks, Russ found pages of writing on the computer after she died. 'Every day was an adventure' was her opening line of a book she called *All of Me*. I love it because I know my little girl was on that adventure until the end. She didn't get bored, nor was she boring. She was always doing something, off on a challenge. I know that one of the things Russ missed most is that Caron kept him so busy. At their home in Byron Bay she was forever putting him to work – trimming trees, making a beautiful English rose garden, painting tables, building a new deck round the pool. Even when she could hardly move, she was up to something, living every minute. Her great friend in Australia, Melinda, says she couldn't keep up with her. Ironic, really, because by then there were times when she couldn't walk without a cane. But that was Caron. Always doing. Always busy. Always on an adventure. And it started young.

One of her favourite activities was setting traps for the 'Marnabrae Boys', and wrote about it:

The Marnabrae boys were the children who lived in the road that ran parallel to ours in Lisburn in Northern Ireland, which of course automatically relegated them to the enemy. There was a piece of wasteland in between our roads, a patch of scabby grass that became the battleground for the local kids. We spent hours planning how to get them – digging holes and painstakingly covering them with sticks and twigs, and grass on the top.

Then we'd lie in wait, hoping that the boys from the next road would fall in. I don't think we were after mass injuries, but a twisted ankle would have been very satisfying.

The funny thing is, I can't remember who they were and whether they ever retaliated – they were probably blissfully unaware of our intentions. None of them ever did succumb to the traps, though we had much fun planning them. I often look at my own boys spying on the grown-ups – spending hours stealthily tracking us round the house, peering round corners – it's like a parallel universe from the one we inhabit. It's been one of the aspects I've most loved about bringing them up in Cornwall and Australia. I can't give them the freedom I had as a child – but we're lucky enough to have the space to let them run fairly wild around home. For most of the year they're outside building cubbies, making fires and roasting marshmallows, discovering possums under the house and coming in at night ruddy-faced from their adventures, covered with mud and very happy . . .

Not so different from my memories of Caron, Paul and Michael's childhood, except there were no possums in Northern Ireland. In the beginning, as I said, I was a stay-at-home mum, but soon I was working again at Ulster Television, this time singing in front of the camera. Viewers would call up with requests and I would burst into song. On top of that I was doing more and more cabaret, and singing on a number of radio shows. I was branching out and, though I didn't know it then, singing would eventually lead me to the doors of Dan Gilbert, a forward-looking producer at BBC Northern Ireland.

Music was a mainstay in our house at Marnabrae Park and our subsequent home in Hillsborough. Even Paul was in on the act, first serenading the cows with his trumpet, then progressing to the drums, as Caron remembered:

The trumpet was consigned to the second-hand shop and instead he was fuelled by a passion that few parents would willingly choose – drumming.

It is safe to say he was obsessed and spent every Sunday washing the neighbourhood cars for 50p to add to his drum fund. Bit by bit, a kit that Ray Cooper would have been proud of grew in the 'roof space', the part of upstairs that my dad always planned on turning into a proper room and somehow never did. Now it echoed with the endless thudding of the bass and the clatter of snare drums. A drummer by himself is lonely and soon he decided a band was what was needed. I don't know where they came from, but it grew organically, up there in the rafters. Guys with the obligatory long, permed hair, tight jeans and electric guitars started clumping up and down the stairs, laden with gear and trailing leads, dreaming of world fame.

This turned out to be not so far-fetched for one of them. Vivian Campbell, who lived down the road and played bass guitar, went on to play for Thin Lizzy, Dio and eventually Whitesnake. And one glorious Wednesday morning he did the great rock-star thing of roaring up to our house in a Ferrari. Red, naturally. It was a magical moment for all of us and proved that dreams can come true. It was possible to get from our roof space to Wembley!

Unfortunately for the rest of the band Vivian was alone in his pilgrimage to musical fame and fortune – although they did end up supporting Dexy's Midnight Runners at Queen's University in Belfast and went through the great support-band ritual of being booed off the stage. It didn't matter: they'd made it that far.

All of this lay in the unknown future when they were starting out and didn't help with the immediate problem of who was to be the lead singer. I had high hopes of applying for the position but had no chance. The thought of having his sister in his band was complete anathema to Paul. Desperate to be near them, I had to settle for making the coffee for the endless Sunday morning try-outs. A trickle of rock chicks would make their way up to the roof space and sing the standard audition piece Fleetwood Mac's 'Dreams', and week after week Mum and I would stand in the kitchen while the song was murdered above us . . .

Paul remembers this slightly differently. He said the person murdering the Fleetwood Mac number was Caron, and it was 'Rumours', not 'Dreams'; she auditioned every Sunday, and every Sunday she was ruthlessly dismissed by her younger brother, who was now rather enjoying his new-found power. If those dismissals proved too harsh, Caron retaliated: she would sneak downstairs and switch off the mains electricity so none of the equipment worked.

Like the panel from *Pop Idol*, we would give our appraisal, me erring on the more Simon Cowell view of their talent, complete with my view of how much better I would have been. Mum, harbouring no secret desire to perform in the band herself – well, none that she confessed to, anyway – was rather kinder. Though for her, as an ex-professional singer, it was just as painful.

For now my own singing career was confined to the bathroom mirror and those glorious moments when everyone was out and I had the upstairs to myself. I would switch on all the microphones and amplifiers, light up the place with Paul's carefully constructed light-to-sound unit made from bolted-together biscuit tins lined with tinfoil and covered with coloured gel, and would sing my heart out to all my favourite tracks. It was fantastic, my own private karaoke bar, and I sounded incredible – to me . . .

Caron's passion for singing never left her. What she loved best of all was singing round the kitchen table with her mates and she did it at every kitchen table she ever owned and many more besides. Whether she was in Ireland, at Bristol University, in London, Cornwall or Australia, there was always a song to be sung. She found music lifted her spirits, soothed her soul and made her heart soar. No wonder, then, that the further the cancer progressed, the more music Caron made.

Much later, near the end when they were living in Australia, Caron and Russ had a really good friend called Khaleed. If he called up and Russ had to confess that Caron was not having such a good day, had been resting in bed and that the pain was taking its toll, Khaleed would reply, 'I think it's time for "The Horse" . . .' Minutes later he would arrive with his guitar and start strumming Caron's favourite song. That Christy Moore piece and all the other Irish songs that Khaleed had perfected would give her the strength to get out of bed, despite the pain, and together they would all sing 'The Horse' until they were hoarse and Caron's smile had returned.

When Buddhist monks came to stay at Russ and Caron's last home in Byron Bay, they were made to sit through family renditions of 'The Boys From County Armagh'. You have never seen a more confused-looking line of faces as we belted out the chorus. Caron loved singing in a group, regardless of natural talent. She believed that, just as organized religion had lost its appeal, the ritual of community singing had been forgotten and, with it, the feeling of connection and togetherness that goes with it. She wanted it back.

One of the perks of my singing career on the cabaret circuit was the costumes and my aunt Myrtle could copy any designer dress I cut out of *Vogue*. With the ever-present cigarette in one hand and a cup of tea in the other, I would explain my latest fancy, and she would whip it up out of nowhere. I kept scraps of material left over for dressing the other important women in our house: Caron's dolls. Hundreds of them.

Mum, who was then quite handy with the sewing-machine herself, would make outfits for my dolls. I had the best-dressed mother and dolls around. Often when I woke up in the morning, Susan (a long-haired raven beauty) or Diane (cute with blonde curls) would be perched on my bedside table, decked out in some fabulous new sequinned number. They had tweed coats with matching hats and capes, trouser suits, ponchos, any number of evening dresses, all bang up to date fashion-wise.

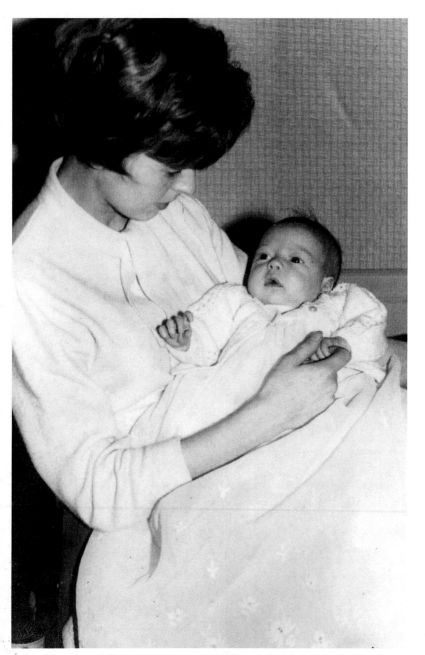

Gloria aged twenty-two at Caron's first christening in Manchester.
The second was in St Mark's Church, Portadown, Northern Ireland

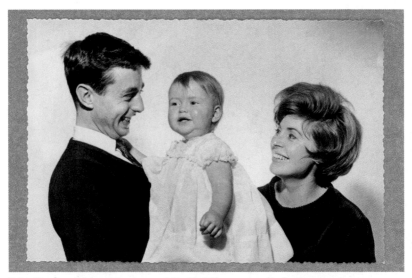

Baby Caron, with her Mummy and Daddy. What an angelic face!

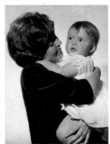

My treasure – a very bonny girl

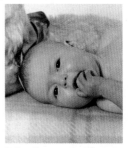

Baby Caron, taken by a cameraman friend of ours, Will Armstrong

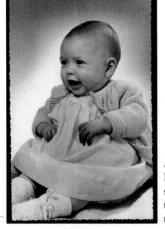

A real-life doll. Look at that smile – it was there right to the end

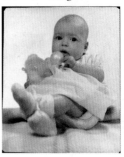

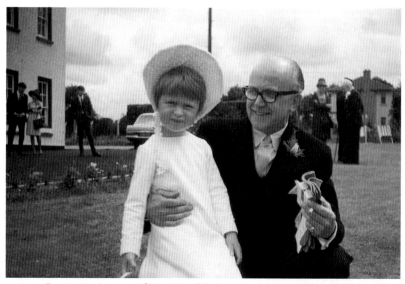

Caron, wearing one of Aunt Myrtle's dresses, at my cousin Rosalind's wedding. Note Grando's adoring look of approval

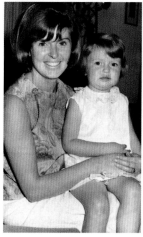

Winners of the 'Mother and Baby' competition at Butlin's. Silver cup and £100 prize. Caron always said I never gave her the prize money

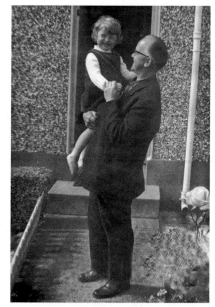

Caron and her lovely Grando – at the front door of the house where I was born in Portadown – during those singing days on the bus

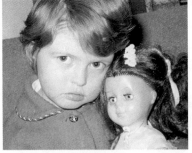

Caron and her favourite dolly, Susan

Our first kitchen in the first house we owned, Marnabrae Park, Lisburn.
Paul and Caron helping with the washing-up. As always, Caron with a dolly in hand

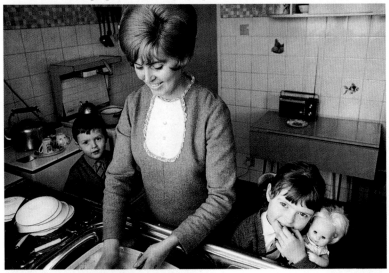

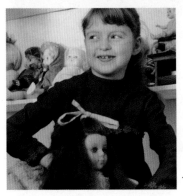

Susan, the long-haired
raven beauty.
Just one of Caron's
dozens of dolls

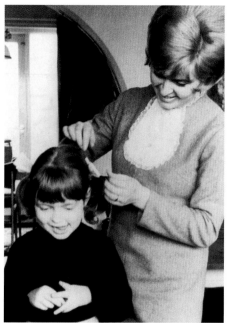

Cheeky pigtails, going off to ballet lessons

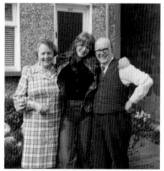

Armagh Road, Portadown. With her much-loved Nanny and Grando, May and Charlie Hunniford

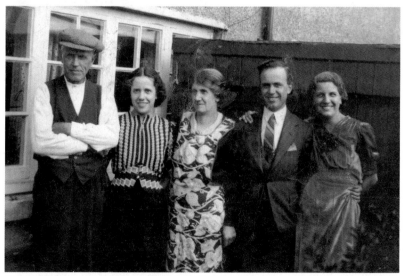

Alexander Gardens, Portadown. The Hunniford clan. *From left to right*: Caron's great-grandfather who lived to ninety-six; Aunt Myrtle, who made all those frocks; Granny Hunniford, a gentle soul and a great homemaker; Charlie (Grando), part-time magician; Aunt May, like a second mum to me

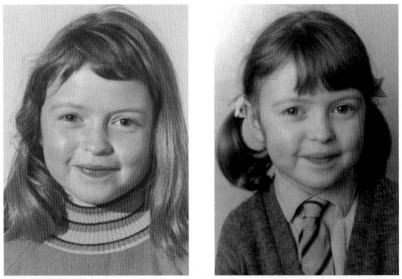

That impish grin – always so appealing and beguiling

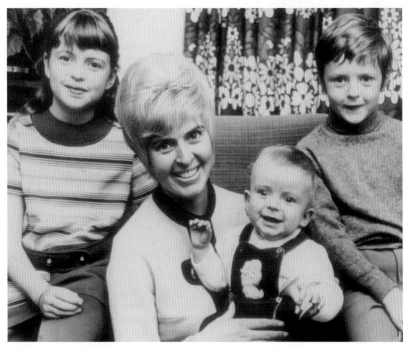

Taken at Marnabrae Park – our first house

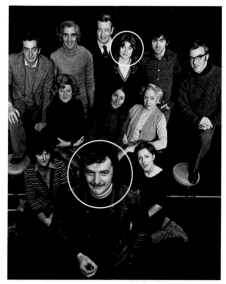

Caron at the Arts Theatre, Belfast with
Roy Heayberd, Artistic Director. Spot a young
James Nesbitt to the right of Caron

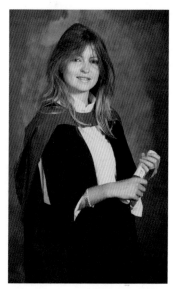

A landmark occasion:
Caron's graduation in English and
Drama, Bristol University, 1983

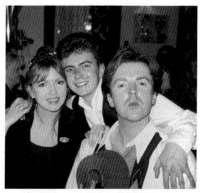

Caron and her brothers, Michael (*centre*) and
Paul (*right*). One of many happy New Year's
Eves in St Paul de Vence, France

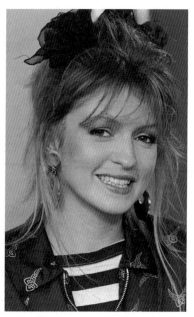

The ultimate pin-up *Blue Peter* girl

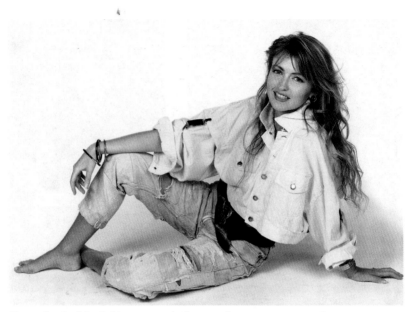

Caron ahead of the fashion game – before torn jeans were even trendy

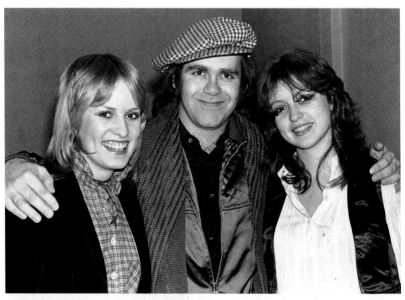

Good Evening Ulster scoop – live appearance from Elton John. Caron was usually around the UTV studios, particularly if pop stars were there

Aunt Myrtle made dresses for me – royal children-style velvet dresses with lace collars. I hated them. They were the clothes of children who had to keep themselves clean and behave. I was much happier in stuff I could grub about in and explore. Mum had other ideas and so began 'Clothes at Dawn with Glo'.

It happened once a month. She would come into my room and go through the wardrobe, hauling out things I'd shoved to one side, then shaking them on the hanger proclaiming, 'And why do you never wear this? If you didn't like it when I bought it why didn't you tell me?' There was the famous pink broderie-anglaise gypsy skirt and matching scarf, which came out with alarming regularity for about two years. Truth is, when it came to dress sense we were galaxies apart.

Mum is one of those people who is pretty much always groomed and well dressed – ready to plunge into whatever smart occasion life may throw at her. I used to think it was something that would happen to me one day – a sort of rite of passage, like my periods starting. I would wake up one morning, desperate to don a tailored suit and encourage my hair to behave. I'm still waiting.

My brother and I used to follow Mum round supermarkets at a discreet distance, listening to what people said about her: 'Oh, she's smaller than she looks on the telly'; 'Isn't that Judith Chalmers?' and then, when my own TV career was under way, 'Gloria always looks so lovely, but have you seen that daughter of hers?'

I ended up making two records, the second of which did quite well. The cover featured me clutching a small muddy lamb. I am actually wearing a wig in the picture because I hadn't had time to have my roots done. As my daughter so eloquently put it, 'Given her subsequent addiction to hair salons, this seemed a whopping oversight on Mum's part . . .' There's no doubt about it: only children can get away with saying such things. And Caron, like me, was never one for mincing her words.

A housewife in the top-ten charts was news, and I was subsequently interviewed on *Good Morning Ulster*, the equivalent of the BBC *Today* programme. Dan Gilbert, the producer, was looking for a female interviewer, liked what I had to say and offered me a job. The timing couldn't have been more perfect. Driving around the country at night to sing at gigs had got increasingly dangerous – I was once stranded beside the road late one night and the police circled the car several times to make sure I was a genuine breakdown, not some IRA or UDA decoy. It wasn't unheard-of to travel to a booking, only to arrive and discover that the club had been blown up the night before, or to take a turning on the way home, find yourself in the middle of a riot and have to turn the car round before you got swamped. I had seen cars set on fire, too, so when Dan Gilbert offered me a job, I said yes on the spot. But, like singing, broadcasting had to be fitted round family life. We didn't have nannies or babysitters, and although Don was supportive in those macho times before the New Man had been invented, it was only up to a point. The singing had been fine because it didn't interfere with bringing up the children – he babysat when it suited him – but broadcasting was different: it was a daytime job and I had to work very hard to do it all.

Before my first year was through, I discovered I was pregnant with Michael. I asked my producer if it would cut short my broadcasting career but he smiled and said, 'Not at all. I'll just cut a hole in the desk so you can reach the microphone.' I had juggled work and motherhood before so I could do it again. I worked right up to the wire.

Caron was eight when Michael was born in 1970, and she wasn't very well. It was just before Christmas and she had a terrible cold. Michael was due on Christmas Day but Billy Thompson, the doctor who would deliver him and the husband of my best friend, knew I was heartbroken at the prospect of being away from the children at Christmas. He proposed having the baby induced so I could be back for the holiday. Inducing babies was getting popular at the time and the idea seemed attractive. He assured me it was safe and there would be no problems.

When I finally brought my eagerly awaited and precious second son Michael home, Caron was completely uninterested in him. When we talked about this later in life, she always said, 'It was only because I was ill, Mum.' What she was extremely concerned about at the time was whether or not she would get a bicycle from Santa. So, a week after I'd given birth, just out of hospital and not very steady on my feet, off I went to the shops to buy the pink bicycle she wanted so much. However, if I had had any doubts at that point about her relationship with her new brother, I had only to remember her dolls: as I said, Caron had hundreds, and discovered now that she had the real thing too. Until she died, Caron was like a second mother to Michael. She was his confidante, and although he and I are close I know there was stuff he wouldn't talk to me about but could always tell Caron and vice versa. They could communicate with a look. When Caron was undergoing chemotherapy, it was often Michael she wanted to accompany her. She thought I was too recognizable and that Russ would be too worried, which might irritate her, but Michael could breeze in and put the humour back into the room. They had an understanding. They were always quite similar. A couple of Irish mavericks.

I was still working for the early morning news, which consisted of putting together *ad hoc* interviews. At that time if I managed to have one interview on every day, I was over the moon because it meant I was building my presence on the radio. I kept my Uher tape recorder at home and would wait for the call. Sometimes there would have been an explosion in Lisburn, or nearby, and off I'd go. I was forever saying to my friend Anne across the road or my sister Lena who lived nearby, 'Could you look after the kids for a while? I've got to dash.' It was always a juggling exercise because, as I said, we didn't have a nanny and I was expected to be able to do it all without compromising anything. Often I'd be in the middle of frying eggs and bacon, get a call, switch it all off and go.

Sometimes I had to take the kids with me but I stopped doing that after one particular experience. I had had to take Caron with me because she was off school and we were on our way to an army camp in Londonderry when the Land Rover we were being driven in was caught in heavy crossfire. We huddled on the floor of the vehicle as bullets and bricks flew overhead. It was a terrifying ordeal, and I felt terrible that I'd put Caron in harm's way. It may have seemed to an outsider that just living in Northern Ireland was putting children in harm's way, but it wasn't like that to us. It was home. Yes, I knew more about the front line because of my job, but Don and I never considered leaving. Most of the time we lived an idyllic rural life and, apart from that one incident, the children didn't experience terrorism first hand.

However, it seeped indirectly into their consciousness. We were in Scotland on a holiday, visiting the twelfth-century ruin of Sweetheart Abbey near Dumfries, when Paul, then eight, asked innocently, 'Aah, who blew it up?'

If you lived in hard-line areas like the Falls Road, Shankill Road or the Derry ghettos, you were obviously more affected by the Troubles, but the rest of us simply had to be careful not to drive into the wrong spot, go into the wrong pub or get involved with the wrong people. Having said all that, a lot of what took place was indiscriminate. For example, the Abercorn restaurant was in the centre of Belfast and everyone went there, so when it was blown up one Saturday afternoon the damage was horrendous: children, men and women, Catholic, Protestant and visitors, were injured there that day, two killed. There was absolutely no logic to it.

In a strange way the Troubles worked to a parent's advantage. When we lived in Hillsborough, a village fourteen miles outside Belfast, and the kids were older, they would naturally go into the city for nights out with their friends. With the backdrop of pubs and clubs being blown up, we *had* to know where they were at all times. It wasn't me being heavy-handed, it was just safer if I drove them to where they were going and safer if I picked them up. In fact, we had more control than we might have had ordinarily. Often we would say to them, 'Bring your friends home.' That was why our house was the rehearsal space for the band. Neither the endless dirty coffee cups nor the relentless murdering of Fleetwood Mac's 'Dreams', or whatever it was, by the continual procession of hopeful rock chicks could convince me to change my mind about that. When the children were home, I knew they were safe.

Having said that, when Caron was older she confessed that in her mid-teens she was up the Falls Road on many a night in one of the less-salubrious political drinking dens. That was Caron to a T. With her butter-wouldn't-melt looks, and childlike smile, she could convince us that she was nothing less than perfect. But that look turned coquettish when it suited her. I'm sure with hindsight – and perhaps he would agree – that Paul unfairly received the lion's share of our discipline, though he would probably have known exactly what his sister was up to. It is testament to him that he never told tales. I know that when Caron, aged sixteen, was presenting *Green Rock*, the Irish equivalent of *Top of the Pops*, Paul, who was a bit of a roadie back then and quite a serious musician, often hauled equipment for visiting bands to earn extra cash. Thin Lizzy was his favourite, and they played in Ulster while 'The Boys Are Back In Town' was at number one. But while Paul was outside in the van, it was Caron they asked out, Caron who drank with Paul's hero of heroes, the drummer Brian Danley, and Caron who had the perks while I was sitting in the kitchen doing my nut trying to work out where she was at midnight. Oh, yes, she got a great deal past me.

This is how Caron analysed that side of her personality while in Australia:

How fabulous to be able to live like innocent children but then again at some point in our lives we start to discover that other people will react to our behaviour and we start to ignore how we're truly feeling and what needs to be said in favour of gaining something from the other person. In my case, I can see clearly now that I wanted my parents to love me, not be cross with me, and so I took on the role of being 'a good girl, doing things right'. 'Right' amounted to what I can see now meant not making too much trouble. What I hadn't realized is that I didn't actually have to do anything to gain their love – it was mine automatically. The other problem was I was a child with very strong views as to what I wanted and resorted in the end to my vivid imagination to get there. So, although it seemed to the other persons that I was going along with them, I was actually trying to work out how to get to where I wanted to go, because I wasn't able to say 'no' or 'that's not for me' – 'that doesn't work for me' – and bring things out into the open where they could be sorted out in a way that suited everyone and consequently knowing on some level that determination and a vivid imagination was not a great way to behave, pretending all the time to be this 'good girl'. A dichotomy arose with me when I was 'good' on the outside and feeling horrible on the inside and every so often spikes of frustration would shoot from me. I would be saying one thing and thinking another and fondly imagining that the other party had no idea what was going on.

I was given a daily radio programme of my own on the BBC in 1971. It was called *A Taste of Hunni*. What an original pun! I did that show for years. It was perfect for me: no more mad dashing around, I simply worked within school hours and for a long time that was just how family life continued. The children came everywhere with me: I'd bring Caron and Paul into the BBC offices, where they would happily play cricket in the corridor with a screwed-up ball of paper, or be given the latest pop record or simply hang around the studio. You wouldn't get away with that in London, but it was totally accepted in a small area like Northern Ireland. Most of the time it was simply to drop off a tape, but even so, I was lucky to have that freedom.

Eventually the house in Marnabrae Park got too cramped and we moved to Hillsborough, a proper Ulster village, surrounded by lush green fields and endless possibilities for the kids. It was inhabited by many an eccentric character and there was real community spirit and an open-door policy. The children and our dog took full advantage of it all. Once, the owner of the antiques store took a client up to inspect a four-poster bed and found Che, our family Labrador, peacefully asleep on it.

Caron, Paul and Michael all loved Irish Christmas in the village: ever since Michael had been born we'd go to one neighbour every Christmas Eve, another on Boxing Day, and have them all over to us on Christmas morning. That sums up life in Hillsborough. We knew all the kids in the area and, considering the times, it was incredibly free. Caron loved all that 'traditional Irish stuff', as Michael calls it: despite her forays into alternative therapies, her Byron Bay lifestyle, she was a traditional girl at heart. As a family we loved a good time, having a joke, a sing-song and long chats round the fire.

If community spirit was in her nature, it was nurtured in Hillsborough, where the adventure continued. She was a regular in the pub – behind the bar, of course, earning her Saturday-girl money. People still talk to me about the welcome sight of Caron serving food at the Hillside pub. That was another thing about Caron – and this is not just her infatuated mother talking: she made an impact wherever she went and is remembered with extreme fondness by everyone who spent time with her. At her funeral, flowers arrived from all over the world and some from the stars she'd worked with, but the ones I really appreciated came from places like the local deli Jolly Jacks in Cornwall although she hadn't stepped foot inside it for over two years.

As the children got older and my job became more time-consuming, Caron probably took on, or felt she took on, more responsibility. I was now working full time in Belfast during the day, which meant that Caron, and often her then boyfriend, Shaun McIlrath, escorted Michael home from school. Michael's directness probably got Caron into trouble more than once. On one memorable journey home, he asked a girl on the bus if she shaved. 'Yes,' she replied. Her legs and armpits . . .

'Well,' said Michael, 'you've missed a bit above your lip.' I'm sure Caron and Shaun hid.

Caron's entry into Shaun's life had been typically full of flair, as he recalled: 'I first became aware of Caron at our prep school, Fullerton House, because she'd impaled herself on the railings that went all around the grounds. Then I remember kissing her at a party when I was about ten, and as she trotted off, I thought, Hey, that's the girl who speared herself.'

He had to wait another six years for his next kiss. They were at the Newtownards Flying Club Valentine's Dance. Apparently Caron kissed him, which I now understand was her *modus operandi*. Cheeky little monkey – but, once again, you wouldn't think it to look at her. Shaun remembers her as spectacular, even then – but slightly aloof. It came from the shyness she was developing: some people mistook it for snootiness because I was in the public eye. I suppose I was a reasonably big media name by then in Ireland, but in my mind I was only ever Mum, and never had to deal with other people's misconceptions of us as Caron did. I believe that that was where her mistrust of fame was rooted. No doubt her head was turned later, during the heyday of *Blue Peter* when she was new on the scene and fresh to the possibilities that fame allows you, but not long afterwards she seemed to close herself off from it. She never courted fame. She didn't love the showbiz side of life, which I have always quite enjoyed. She didn't do first nights and premières. She experienced the loss of anonymity very young, and that was my fault, an unintentional by-product of my career, and I believe she spent her latter days hauling it back.

But it wasn't complicated back then. The complications and questioning came later. In the beginning, I know from her friends, she was so proud of what I'd achieved. I was a small-town Portadown girl who'd gone on to bigger things. And don't forget the perks. Caron came with me to meet many famous faces, which was exciting for a teenager. She would come to the studio when some of the star names were there. If Elton John or Rod Stewart was on – particularly Rod Stewart – I couldn't keep her away. In fact, in the car I had to pretend I was Rod Stewart and she would hold an imaginary mike and interview me: 'So, Rod . . .' Caron said that as I had the right hair colour and was partial to the odd bit of fake leopardskin, it didn't demand too big a leap of her imagination. She could always make me laugh. Sometimes she would come to the studio after school, do her homework in my dressing room and just hang out on the set. Often all three of the children were there. She was never fazed by the studio or the famous faces, and I suppose it became second nature to her. I'm certain that's why she could always look a lens in the eye: she'd been around them for most of her life.

Paul remembers the BBC canteen food almost more fondly than the guests he met: chips and fried onions, which he swears he can still taste.

Caron also loved to accompany me to the Arts Theatre in Belfast to interview the actors. She loved the atmosphere and it became a regular haunt. One of the few times that I returned to the stage was when Roy Heayberd, the artistic director, asked me to be in a production of Stephen Sondheim's *Side by Side*. I agreed. Caron remembered it vividly:

Sondheim, wordy and precise – a bugger to learn. Again desperate to be part of it all, I went to rehearsals – eventually knowing the show better than Mum. We spent hours in my bedroom going over the lyrics – which was not quite the same as stepping into the spotlight, feather boa draped around my neck, expectant audience waiting for that first perfect note. Instead I rose to the dizzy heights of piano page-turner, partly fuelled by my love of the show, but mainly by my lust for the male lead. A tall camp Ulster farmer, blessed with the voice of an angel – I had little idea, at that point, of his sexuality. I sat there night after night feverishly hoping for two things – a date with the farmer and that my mother would get a terrible cold and lose her voice so that I could step in and save the day. Mild flirtation and a bit of a kiss on the cheek in his car after a party was as good as it got. Mum stayed resolutely healthy – inwardly I was relieved not to have to launch myself on another unsuspecting audience . . .

Caron adored the whole atmosphere of the theatre. Her room was decorated with the comedy and tragedy masks, but I think she loved the camaraderie of the theatre more than performing: she never really wanted to be an actor. In a way Caron was always a slightly reluctant performer: she loved the idea of it, was brilliant at it and wanted to be asked to do it, but would then decide that she didn't really want to. I remember she was mad at me because I wouldn't let her work on a stage production every night, even though I had been out entertaining with my dad from the age of nine. Looking back, I don't know how I did that three or four times a night, then got up for school. Of course I didn't think it was a sensible thing for Caron to do when her O and A levels were coming up. She accused me of being hypocritical and said, 'You did it, why can't I?' Eventually we reached a compromise and she was allowed to work there at weekends and on one night during the week. Needless to say, I believed my rules were being kept, but not a bit of it. Shaun now tells me that he and Caron, dressed like Kate Bush meets early Boy George, would sneak out of school at any opportunity and hang out at the theatre. As ever, Caron, by hook or by crook, had her own way.

But she wasn't irresponsible: she never swayed in her duty to her youngest brother. When he was at Fullerton House Junior and she was at Methody, the senior school, I was presenting a nightly news programme, *Good Evening Ulster*. Caron would wait for Michael outside the school gates, the same ones she'd impaled herself on, and catch the bus. When they got off they had a five-minute walk home and she was in charge until either Don or I got home. As Michael puts it, 'Caron, being the oldest, made the coffee and peanut-butter sandwiches for *Grange Hill*.' Did I put too much responsibility on her young shoulders? No more than was expected of any sixteen-year-old of a working family at that time. It happened all over the country. And there was always something impish about Michael: he was born ahead of his years. I swear he could hold court at nine. As Shaun remembers it, Michael never came across as needing mothering – in fact, I think at times he terrified Shaun with his imperious interrogations. I remember Michael, aged nine, staying up for one of our parties and asking a six-foot broker what was happening in the stock market. So, maybe asking Caron to make a few peanut-butter sandwiches wasn't too much and the responsibility she felt for him was in her own head.

It wasn't as if they were on their own: as the money situation improved, I could afford help and we had two wonderful afternoon nannies, Gilly and Quinny, who took it in turns and adored the children. But still, like a lot of working mothers, I felt guilty. Maybe it just goes with the job of being a mother. It doesn't matter what you do for your children, it never feels like enough. I went to Australia seven times in two years, a 24,000-mile round trip every time, yet I ask myself, 'Was it enough? Should I have gone more? Stayed longer or even lived there to be more supportive?' Stephen tells me I'm beating myself up unnecessarily, that for Caron and Russ to have us there all the time would have been a burden in itself. We would have tired out an already exhausted woman: Caron needed space and time to heal and meditate. I know, when I'm feeling rational, that he's talking sense. Trouble is, I don't often feel rational.

Because my weeks were busy, weekends at home were sacro-
sanct. Even Shaun remembers them as a big deal in the Keating
household. In the morning, after Don had left to play golf, which
was every weekend, the children and I would go shopping and
end up at the bakery in Hillsborough, where we would buy a
wonderful chocolate and cream roulade, which we'd take home
and eat while we watched old black-and-white movies and
musicals by the fire. Caron remembered this clearly, and towards
the end of her life often talked about those chocolate-coated
afternoons. In those days we were easily pleased, and once the
'off air' sign came on, it was back to village life for me. Yes, I
had a sophisticated job in broadcasting but, more than that, I
am, and always will be, a family person, a mum and now, thank
the Lord, a grandmother – a role I take seriously. Caron had the
same ethos. She was a lovely mum right up to the end. She
was very family-conscious, mad about the kids knowing their
grandparents, uncles, aunts, cousins, and everything else that an
Irish family brings with it. I know if she'd been spared she'd be
getting together the Irish side of her family and the Scottish side
of Russ's. She was keen that the boys should know their heritage
and what Ireland was like because it was so much a part of her.
As Janet Ellis, her co-presenter on *Blue Peter*, said later, 'Her
Irishness was strong. I thought she was lucky to have it – it
looked fun, the spontaneity, her ability to get people together
and always have a good time.'

Before Caron could drive she spent a lot of time knocking
around Hillsborough, but most of the other kids lived in Belfast.
Shaun would come up on the bus and was with us most weekends when life, as always, centred on the kitchen. He remembers
Caron as full of life and massively fascinated by everything. He
says her endless interest in people made life more interesting for
him – it gave him another perspective. He learnt to see the
world through her eyes. For instance, they would go to a party,
and while he would think it was a bit rubbish, he would hear

her describing it to me as I drove them home and think, Were you at a different party from me? It was infectious and part of what made Caron so attractive: that she got so much out of people and situations, whoever and whatever they were. She could always go exploring and find something interesting. And once you pick it up, it makes everything feel like an adventure. Shaun says he does it to this day. Caron inherited many traits from her father, but her interest in people and places, I think, might have come from me.

Not only did Caron locate the interesting, she noted it, observed it and often drew it. Shaun says he always thought she'd have been a good writer. I have many notebooks that she filled when she was ill, and some of the content is in this book, so I know she could express herself beautifully on paper, sometimes heartbreakingly so. Later, Shaun thought that her TV career was a distraction, that she should have nurtured her love of poetry, literature and art. He was wiser, perhaps, than we realized at the time: I know that during her endless search for purity of soul she discovered a lasting regret that she hadn't been a writer and had always wanted to write 'that book', the one she felt was inside her. Was the family propensity for life in broadcasting too tempting to resist? Caron certainly saw the up-side of that lifestyle. It's glamorous. You get to meet really interesting people. And it must have looked easy. I admit I am a consummate performer: I can't remember a time when I wasn't out there, strutting my stuff. And although Caron was best at looking the camera in the eye, perhaps Shaun was right when he said there was never any real difference between me at home and me at work. With Caron there was: as natural as she was on screen, perhaps she kept back a part of herself.

Caron never talked about having a 'so-called' famous mum to Shaun or her friends. All Shaun remembers is a couple of arguments between her and me but he viewed them as part of a typical mother–daughter relationship. Remember, Caron was a teenager, which by definition causes problems. Once she made a joke about me not being there, which I took badly because I worked hard to manage and balance my career and my family. The joke showed me that Caron didn't understand how hard I worked to maintain a strong family core and educate them. But the arguments were rare. Even through the dark ages of teenage rebellion we got on well and were always very close. Probably because I thought she was doing everything that was expected of her and had no idea – still don't – of what she was really up to. I'm not stupid: even now I know her friends are only going to tell me so much . . .

But she couldn't have been up to that much because she got two As and a B at A level and, as Shaun says, she was always conscientious. In fact, he claims that the only reason he passed any exams was because Caron was studying and he had nothing else to do – if he went to see her she stipulated that he had to bring a book. So, although she might have delighted in minor wickedness, I don't believe she was up to anything major. It was simply a case of spreading her wings and finding her individuality – hence those extraordinary clothes.

I have endless memories of her childhood – they would fill a book on their own but my final one is this: apart from when Michael was born and she had flu, and when she had her appendix out, I cannot, and I have racked my brains about this, remember her being ill as a child. She was not a sickly person. In fact, she was a strong, healthy girl. What came later came without warning. Her childhood was indeed an adventure.

4. A Sea Apart

When her father Don died, Caron fell apart: his shockingly premature death came just days before she was due to give birth to her second child. In all the searching that followed her diagnosis and the apportioning of blame to which Caron subjected herself and the rest of us, we as a family are agreed on one thing: if anything might have triggered the cancer, it was that juxtaposition of birth and death, and the subsequent havoc that it and her hormones played on Caron's psyche.

To understand that havoc, you need to understand the background to our divorce. Don and I agreed we would never publicly discuss our separation, and until now I never have. I would still prefer not to – divorce is never in anyone's plan and certainly wasn't in mine. Dissecting it is uncomfortable but I realize it needs to be addressed here. Don did not have to endure Caron's illness, but he was never far from her thoughts and therefore, spiritually, he was with us throughout. Caron made sure of that.

Don was born near Cork in southern Ireland and soon after he arrived his family moved to Manchester. Despite his English upbringing he was Irish at heart. He was a raconteur, an accomplished debater, traditional, self-contained, respected and thoughtful, but with that came a fairly hefty amount of machismo and structure. As I have said, it was fine for me to work as long as it didn't interfere with my ability to bring up the children and run the house. Yes, he did the babysitting while I was out singing, but only when it suited him. And he cooked, which set him apart from most of the men I knew at the time: if he got home before me he would start cooking dinner without a second's thought. But in essence he was the man of the house and he did as he pleased. And that never wavered.

Although I loved him for a long time, liked him to the end and respected him always, he and I were very different. Among his children and friends, Don's frugality was legendary and always the butt of a few jokes. In Ireland the custom is that everyone gets a round in whether it's needed or not and drinks soon stack up on the table. Don was teased for endlessly finding excuses to leave when his round came up. When he did open his wallet, his mates would flap away the imaginary moths. Once we took the children to New York, a big deal: trips to America from Northern Ireland were unheard-of at the time. It was a real budget family holiday, but an adventure, and we drove to New York from Toronto where we'd been visiting family.

We hadn't eaten properly for a few days: we'd been living off cheap fast food and an ever-diminishing kitty. I wanted to go out and eat something substantial and healthy, but when we got to the restaurant, Don kept saying, 'We can't afford this and that,' and 'Don't order the vegetables, they're too expensive.' Well, I got cross and it turned into a stand-off between us, with me refusing to eat at all. What Don didn't know was that I snuck off to the ladies', wrapped my steak in paper napkins, took it back to our hotel and ate it in secret, locked in the bathroom. Stubbornness and hunger don't go hand in hand.

Clearly I did not share Don's attitude to money. Of course you must live within your means, but you have to live too. I spend money, it's true. Caron and I together were frighteningly efficient consumers. I've been earning money since I was eight, that's a hard habit to break. I've always believed if you earn it you can spend it. However it wasn't all frivolity. Don paid the mortgage but all the extras were from me – private education being one of these extras.

Don tended to do his own thing. Every Saturday and Sunday he went to play golf. You wouldn't get away with that now: it simply isn't acceptable to leave your wife and three kids all weekend. Of course you can go for a round, but not all weekend, every weekend. In later life Caron asked me why I let him get away with it. Well, you just did, in those days: it was the way of our world. Men didn't do the bottles or change nappies – it was macho Ireland!

He did an evening news programme too, the BBC Northern Irish version of *Nationwide*, so he'd saunter into work quite late, set up the day's programme, and afterwards go to the BBC club for a drink before he drove home. He wasn't the only one working either: I was working full time. But at weekends the shopping had to be done, food had to be prepared for the week ahead, the children had to be entertained. Don't get me wrong, I'm not complaining – and I didn't complain then. I loved my weekends, I loved my job, and I was, still am, besotted by my children. I had wonderful help from Gilly and Quinny . . . But when I look back, as I have so much recently, I see much more clearly that although Don and I shared a home, we were living parallel lives.

We had been on those separate paths for some time and the distance between them increased in tiny increments, so small I didn't even notice the drift apart until it was too late. I did not have a bad marriage, Don was not a bad husband, but I had forged a life of my own and eventually we found ourselves in different places, wanting different things, and the bond between us was no longer strong enough to withstand the strain.

Of our three children, Caron was most like Don. She in- herited her wily Irish ways, her ability to debate and argue from her father. They both looked for the unusual side of any story, the quirkiest person in the crowd. You'd never get a standard answer from either of them. Don was always very considered – Michael says that if he ever had a problem he'd freely discuss it with his father. Later in life he'd call him up and ask his advice. There would be a big silence and Don would say, 'I'll call you back tomorrow.' But Michael would want an answer then and there. Don would simply reply that he needed to think about it. 'But I need to know now!' And Don would say, 'No, son, I'll call you back tomorrow.' When the advice finally came through, it was always better for the consideration. Like Don, Caron never opened her mouth before her brain engaged: it wasn't that she consciously considered everything she said, but she had this natural ability to listen, then be thoughtful, understanding and funny in her quick-fire response without ever being predictable. In a strange way, her what–goes–round–comes–round attitude, which often seemed barmy, was quite karmic and Buddhist.

Don was liked, well respected and admired in the business. Not bad for a man who, like me, had fallen into it virtually on the spin of a coin.

My father had gone for a cursory interview at the newly opened ABC studios in Manchester. They were looking for people who had experience working with cameras to become cameramen. He had none, but he did have a cousin in Cork who ran a pharmacy where they processed people's holiday snaps and a quiet confidence in his abilities – to bluff, if nothing else. Knowing the interview was coming up, he spent much of his annual summer trip to Ireland quizzing Brian Owen on the finer points of lenses, exposure, etc., and cheerfully regurgitated large chunks of information at his interview. He felt it had gone reasonably well and, anyway, it was a toss-up between that and going to sea. An extraordinary choice for a man who only had to set foot in a rowing-boat to feel seasick. He left it up to the gods: if ABC called him with the job before the day he was due to set sail, he'd take it. Otherwise he was off.

The day drew closer and closer. Nothing came through from the television company. Eventually his mother woke him up on the morning the ship was due to sail. He grunted from the depths of his bed, 'What's the weather like?'

Pulling the curtain aside, she surveyed the rain lashing against the pane.

'Terrible!' He rolled over and went back to sleep. The next day a letter arrived from ABC congratulating him on becoming one of their first cameramen . . .

Michael remembers his father teaching him how to play poker. According to Don, every boy needed to know how to gamble and they'd play with copper coins. Once Don took an IOU from his young son and when, later, Michael tried to go to bed, Don asked for repayment. Michael offered, not unreasonably, to pay his father in the morning, which Don wouldn't accept. After an argument Michael stormed off and got Don his 20p. The lesson, of course, was don't gamble what you can't afford and always pay your debts. Such was the measure of the man. A lesson that has stuck in Michael's mind and one which he now respects and appreciates.

So, yes, he was a big influence on the children, but when Caron was little Don wasn't around much. Nothing unusual about that: the division of parental roles back then was more rigid. But when she began in-depth self-analysis to find the root cause of her disease a particular memory surfaced:

In it I was four or five years old, wearing red T-bar shoes – this detail stuck out. I was standing in our lounge at home feeling very alone. 'What else is going on?' she [the therapist] asked. I continued, 'My dad is in the room watching TV – a book on his knee – but it feels like he won't do anything with me and that I'm not real in his life.' Now, in my adult self, I know that he absolutely adored me, but then, it felt as if he never made regular time for me, and from that period it had translated into the feeling that somehow I wasn't good enough. The answer was – at this very young age – I made a vow to myself to shut down my heart so I wouldn't get hurt by anyone else, so I would be safe, and wouldn't volunteer how I felt unless I was very sure of my feelings, and I'd pretty much stuck to it. It all felt very strange, like a sort of dream. I went home and slept.

Two days later I asked my mum if I'd ever had red shoes with a T-bar.

She confirmed I had, they were my favourites, and we talked about how much Dad had loved me but it was also true that he didn't do very much with us as children at the weekends because he regularly played golf, Saturday and Sunday. They were those macho times in Ireland when men did what they wanted to do and the rest of the family got on with it . . .

During her many analysis sessions, Don, like the rest of us, went under the microscope. She would ask me whether he had ever played with her. She would ask me why he was always sitting in his chair reading and not watching whatever she wanted him to watch. She asked me a lot, as she did all of us, and I fear that most of the time the answers I gave her were not satisfactory. Don was a family man, but he was not especially hands-on. As a parent, Paul, like Russ, is the reverse: both are extremely 'hands-on' with their sons – Paul would be a self-confessed emotional wreck if his went to boarding school. But Don's attitude to many things where the children were concerned was quite different from Paul's. Take the battle over the electricity bill. Don went mad if the kids left the lights on, to the point when there would be massive arguments about the price of electricity. Now occasionally Paul's boys will leave the whole of the top floor on, taps running, lights on, music blaring, and he finds himself wanting to shout but he doesn't: he stops himself because he doesn't want a repeat performance. He is also amazing with Gabriel and Charlie, which I know would have made Caron extremely proud. In a way I think he sees it as his promise to Caron, and he is fulfilling it beautifully. Even Michael admits that his affection and huge respect for his father came when he was older and understood the kind of man he was. As I've said, Paul received the lion's share of Don's discipline and there were times when communication between them was strained. He says nowadays that he misses his father more than ever. He would have loved to show him his children: Jake and Beau. He would have liked Don to witness what kind of man he has become and what he has achieved in business. I know that Don would have been immensely proud of them both. Boys need mothers. Men need fathers. And all women, irrespective of age, like to be Daddy's little girl.

I think that Caron's loyalty to Don, their true closeness, only really materialized when we separated. That was when she took up the mantle, when she began to feel responsible for him. In a way, fate played a big part in our separation. I was at the height of my career in Ireland. I was doing an hour-long show every night on Ulster television: the news was given the amount of time it was worth, ten minutes or fifty, and the rest was taken up with current affairs, lifestyle films and celebrity interviews. It was the perfect antidote to the Troubles. Audiences loved it. If we didn't get five programmes of *Good Evening Ulster* in the top-ten ratings every week we wanted to know why. I was happy: I had the world on a string. I wasn't looking for a change but then a strange thing happened. In July 1981 I was asked to go to England to stand in for the legendary Jimmy Young on BBC Radio 2 for two weeks. Excited, I rose to the challenge and naturally accepted. This was big network stuff. I'd always loved Radio 2 and had listened to it as a housewife. I did my homework, studied the programme, its style, the guests and subjects covered. I devoted myself not only to the task in hand but also to stoking the fires that fuelled the famous Wogan–Young on-air handover. In fact, I did as much research into Wogan's day-to-day life to tease him with as I did into world affairs for the Jimmy Young programme. I gave my 'grandfather', as I called him, as good as I got. It seemed to go well, and on the last day David Hatch, the Radio 2 controller, called me into his office. I thought he was going to offer me a cup of tea, but he floored me by offering me a daily programme. I thought it was a joke: making a jump like that, from regional to network, was a huge adventure and an enormous vote of confidence. I was so excited: all I had wanted was to do it well enough to be asked back as a stand-in again. That he thought I had done it well enough to do it every day was thrilling, tough and daunting. David changed my life.

However, I still had a daily television news programme to do at home and I couldn't let UTV down. I told the BBC that the earliest I could think of accepting their job offer was the end of the year. They said, 'Fine.'

Now I had to put it to the family. I went home and had a big round-the-table discussion, and this is where the irony begins. I am a great believer in fate: if they asked me a year earlier, with one child doing A levels, one doing O levels and one still at primary school, I couldn't have taken it on. But the timing was perfect. Caron had accepted a place at Bristol University to study English and Drama. Paul, whose academic record to that point by his own admission had left a lot to be desired, had thrilled us all by gaining a scholarship to the Guildford School of Drama to continue doing what he loved, which was stage management. Michael was still at primary school, but he was born unfazed by life and I knew he would land on his feet anywhere.

My family had shrunk to a movable feast. And that in itself was a big factor. In my heart of hearts I was devastated at the thought of Caron and Paul leaving home at the same time. Empty-nest syndrome had set in, and Radio 2 offered me a way out. They offered me a valid reason to move to England other than that of being a soppy mum who couldn't stomach the idea of suddenly seeing Caron and Paul only a few times a year. If I was working in London I could drive to see them or would happily have them to stay at the weekends, dirty washing and all. I wouldn't have to worry about plane journeys; there wouldn't be a sea between us.

The family, and especially Don, agreed that I'd be hell to live with if I didn't give it a go. Don, to his credit – he was a man who didn't like change – said that if I didn't try I'd always be wondering, 'What if . . . ?' and therefore we should make the move. Then another ironic thing happened: Don was offered a job in South Africa. Until that point, he and I hadn't been apart for more than twelve days at a time in our twenty years of married life. But we agreed it made sense: if I was going to London, he should take the job in South Africa. At the time it seemed fair and sensible. But the consequences were far-reaching.

So I came to London with ten-year-old Michael, got him into the senior school in Sevenoaks and began a whole new life. I didn't know a huge number of people, but it was an exciting time, meeting new colleagues, making new friends and being in a new city. I would come home and tell Michael all about it, and I suppose our deep friendship began then. I used to worry that I leant on him too much during that period and told him things I might not normally have told a ten-year-old. I used to worry that our relationship became too adult too quickly, but he assures me it was fine – better than that, it was fun. He says he certainly doesn't feel as if he was robbed of a childhood. In many ways, he had more experiences than most boys his age because I was effectively a single mum. I took him everywhere. Obviously he wasn't at cocktail parties every night but if there were things he was interested in, he came with me. It has made him into the socially capable man he is today. Like Caron and Paul in Ireland, the perks were considerable: what boy wouldn't have wanted to meet JR from *Dallas*, days after he'd been shot?

Don stayed six months in South Africa when he was supposed to stay four, and the blunt truth of the matter is that by the time he came back I'd moved on. He tried to live in London but it didn't work out: he had a comfortable life in Northern Ireland where he was director-producer of the BBC's six o'clock news programme and drifted in to work, an easy fourteen-minute drive from home, at one. In London, he was working on national TV at the imposing BBC Television Centre during the train strikes, and he didn't like it. In the end he decided to go back to Ireland. By then I knew I didn't want to. We had drifted too far apart. I have never believed that absence makes the heart grow fonder, and although I hope a happy marriage can't be broken up, it needs to be continually nurtured. Had my head been turned by the bright lights and the big city? Yes, with hindsight, I guess it had. I had discovered a part of me that had been dormant since the days I donned sequinned dresses and performed on stage. Glo was in her gladrags again. London was fun.

I don't think it came as a huge surprise to the children. Paul can still vividly remember Don telling them: why was Dad making such a fuss? Okay, he wouldn't be seeing much of them, but with Paul at Guildford and Caron at Bristol he didn't anyway, so things weren't going to change that much. If it had happened when we were all still ensconced in Hillsborough, it would have been a very different story. Paul was doing his own thing, living alone at sixteen but learning to do what he loved, and the separation almost got washed away.

Caron, I think, took it harder. She was always more analytical than Paul, who has a strong mind and a natural ability to forge forward and rarely look back. Paul believes there was an element of taking sides: Caron felt a strong loyalty to her dad while Paul was loyal to me, and Michael saw it as the best of both worlds – I made sure he visited his dad regularly at Hillsborough.

Caron felt the split on a deeper level. There is almost always a victim in divorce, and in this case it was Don. He remained in the family home until his death, and kept all of our furniture, including my portrait, although it was moved to the attic and faced the wall. He wouldn't let anyone have it. It does not make me feel good to write this, but I suppose a bit of Don never recovered, never moved on, and for that, of course, I am eternally sorry. When my day-to-day responsibility to Don ended, Caron took it upon herself to prop him up, and became maternal towards him. It was always she who went back to

Ireland for Christmas, usually taking Michael and later Russ, while Paul stayed with me.

Two years after the separation we were divorced. My lawyer gave me the best bit of advice: you cannot put a lid on twenty years of marriage because there will always be births, deaths and marriages. How right he was. I always tried to keep the communication line open. When Don used to visit London we were always able to sit down as a family, and I hope the children appreciated that. The family circle was still there. Occasionally Don and I met after work and caught up on our own. It was still a good relationship. I wrote letters to all of the children explaining that, although I was really sorry about the divorce, I couldn't live a lie. Caron kept hers, and I think then began to understand that it had never been my intention to get divorced: it was not the vision I'd had for my life, and when I'd married her father I'd truly believed it would be for ever. I apologized and asked them to accept my judgement. Of course, I know from general research that, clearly, children would rather their parents were together than apart, but parents are people, with all the human failings. I think when children look at their parents they just see togetherness – they don't think, Is she in love with him and he with her? They just see a unit that has looked after them, which is what they are used to. You don't think about your mother in terms of love and passion.

Caron was forging a new life of her own at Bristol University. I know she was sad about the break-up, and desperate for us still to be together, but Don and I didn't indulge in tantrums and tears, there were no terrible fights for her to endure, so it was all as gentle as possible. She talked to Shaun, her boyfriend, about it – he was part of the family at the time – but her other friends don't remember it as a time of schism. They knew she was upset about it but understood that our lives had simply drifted apart. Caron explained it thus: Mum has had a great surge in her career and Dad doesn't like England.

And while I was, temporarily, the bad guy, Caron at the same time was proud of my new job at Radio 2. When I started work there there was a picture of yours truly on the front of the *Radio Times*, which Caron was the first to show to anyone who was interested. And a few who weren't, I should think.

Caron quickly made many friends at Bristol. She always surrounded herself with a great crowd of people and from start to finish had a riot. Her greatest friend from there, a person who remained her friend to the end and not only knew about the cancer but visited Caron in Australia twice and Switzerland once, was Johnny Comerford, now a major television producer himself. He recalls meeting Caron for the first time. 'Caron was incredibly Irish when she came to Bristol, spoke with a much broader accent than she did in the end. The university was full of public-school boys, with all their airs and graces, preconceptions and judgements. But Caron was completely unaware of "class", nor did she care about it. She was always terribly interested in people irrespective of where they came from. That made her very accepting. If someone was a bit eccentric and had a good story to tell, then she thought that was great. She didn't give a monkeys about what school someone had or hadn't been to.'

I think Caron defined herself by her Irishness in those days. It allowed her to be the sociable wildcat, although the shyness was developing. Johnny and Caron lived with three other people, and I gather everyone asked about the girl with the amazing looks and figure, but she didn't see it herself. That is not to say she didn't have an element of vanity: Johnny tells me that they weren't allowed to go into her room unless she had her full makeup on, and if they did, she'd pull her duvet over her head. He says she'd look in the mirror, pull faces and play with her hair, but it wasn't a vanity that was about self-promotion: it was about wanting to look a certain way. What he knows for sure is that she never thought she was beautiful and, of course, that was part of her appeal. I can't imagine her being less than confident about her looks – she was always stunning to me, right up to the end – but she obviously was, and to this day, I don't know why. But again, there was a dichotomy to Caron: shy, yes, but a show-off too. No one who wore the sort of clothes she did could have been described as a wallflower. She dressed to be noticed. A very thrown-together look that was a cross between Madonna and Siouxsie Sioux of Siouxsie and the Banshees that kept her busy browsing through Bristol's many charity shops. She'd pick up a tutu and a pair of stiletto heels, which she'd paint green, then put them on with a big floppy hat and happily walk down the high street. A very striking, post-punk glamourpuss.

I put it down to Stephanie Bretherton, who awoke my more flamboyant tendencies. I met her the day I had my interview for Bristol, in the drama department – where else? Originally from Cheshire, she was the daughter of the then chief of police in the British Virgin Islands and, to my Northern Irish eyes, she looked amazing. Long chestnut hair, dyed blonde underneath, wearing gold harem-style trousers, wide sash, bright pink jumper and exotic shoes. I felt very plain beside her. Enthusiastic and friendly, she was into Germaine Greer, vegetarianism, yoga, and spent every Saturday night at a club in Liverpool devoted to David Bowie. We both got on, and became firm friends. She continued to be a free spirit and was always taking off at a moment's notice to cook on a boat sailing halfway around the world. As she said, 'When offered the chance of adventure or security, I always choose adventure.'

Maybe not just an influence in the wardrobe department, then.

I went to Bristol with three new pairs of jeans and a blue duffel coat and returned that Christmas term wearing black trousers covered with pink pompoms and matching streaks in my hair. Jeans and duffel coat would have made perfect candidates for the wardrobe inspection. By my second year, I'd moved into a flat with Stephanie and an art student called Diane Minnis. She lived on a farm in Northern Ireland and her mum would send emergency food parcels, worried that we wouldn't find enough proper food to eat in Bristol. She could have had a point: when the grant got low, given the choice between the supermarket or a good night out, Tesco was low on the list.

Diane was and remains a wonderfully eccentric, joyous character – not unlike her paintings, huge riots of colour and shape. Cars with faces, huge tulips, greengrocers' windows bursting with life, magical towers curling over. She dressed as she painted.

Together the three of us plundered the second-hand shops and markets of Bristol, pooling our finds and spending at least two hours every week getting ready for the ritual known as Saturday Night. Half the time the preparation was more fun than the actual event. In and out of each other's rooms and wardrobes, we would layer net and tulle under fabulous fifties dresses, little beaded cardigans, and often topped with a huge old Crombie coat. I remember Diane swanning around in my dad's old maroon and black striped satin dressing-gown as a sort of coat for months. He was most amused.

I had a pair of my mum's original winklepicker slingbacks. They were lime green and I was deeply attached to them. They achieved near-cult status and there was a picture of them on our kitchen noticeboard. Nearly impossible to walk in, I would opt for something a bit more sensible and put them in my bag, changing them just before I went into that evening's venue.

I generally wore them with a long pair of white cotton stockings from Vivienne Westwood. No trip to London was complete without a visit to her shop at World's End on the King's Road. I thought then and still do that she's one of Britain's most inventive designers. Back then, on a student grant, all I could afford were the stockings – ten pounds a pair. I thought they were fantastic. I wore them endlessly until they were grey and had holes in the feet. Mum called them my surgical stockings, was completely bewildered by them and surreptitiously cut the ends off when they became particularly ragged. Eventually they ended up as ankle socks.

She was a party girl too, which by all accounts didn't begin at Bristol. She had incredible stamina and was always one of the last to bed. She shared with her new English friends her desire to experience things, meet people and settle into a good long chat. In Ireland you call this getting together for a drink 'and a bit of *craic*', an expression closely associated with my daughter. It was always time for '*craic*'. She was a limited cook, but that didn't stop her asking an array of people back to dinner at their completely ill-equipped flat. She once rang me to ask how to do chicken for twenty people. Naturally I enquired as to how many chickens she had, to which the reply came, 'Just the one.' She went ahead with the dinner party, which, on the food front – like many after it – was a bit of a disaster, but always, always full of more than just a 'bit of *craic*'.

She didn't really know how to drink back then either, I gather. There seemed to be a fairly routine pattern to the evening. She'd have a drink, get very jolly, then quite quickly become argumentative, and soon after that she'd be in the bathroom. It was always three stages and always quite quick. Shaun went to surprise Caron one day, taking a train to London from Canterbury, then another to Bristol. When he got there she'd gone to a concert with her friend. At four a.m. he woke up and she still wasn't there. Suspecting the worst, he messed up her room and left. He got home, knackered and furious, at four o'clock in the afternoon. Caron rang him in tears and told him she'd just stayed over at her friend's flat. Somehow she convinced him to pick up the bag he'd just put down and get back on the train to London, back on the train to Bristol. When he got to the flat, he rang the bell, but there was no answer. She'd said she'd cook a big dinner, so he assumed she was doing some last-minute panic shopping and went to the pub to wait. When he went back he met someone at the door who was also there for the dinner party, but there was still no answer. So they both went back to the pub and got horribly pissed. Then they returned to Caron's flat and broke in. What had happened was that Caron's flatmate Diane had arrived back from holiday with a litre of gin.

He was not the only one paying surprise visits. I often beetled down to Bristol at weekends to see Caron. I would appear on the doorstep with flowers and food, and Shaun would have to get dressed, walk into the kitchen and pretend he'd just arrived. As if I didn't know. I suspect that he put up with a great deal from my daughter over the six years they were together. I know that on his twenty-first birthday, at a dinner in Covent Garden, Caron stormed off because Shaun, for once, was getting all the attention. He had to chase after her and talk her into coming back. He admits that he put up with a little more than he would have later because, back then, he didn't have a benchmark as to what was acceptable or unacceptable behaviour. Because she was so fantastically good at arguing, she could convince him and others that they really wanted to do what in fact they absolutely didn't want to do. It was a skill that remained with her. Russ, bless him, for a totally different reason gladly put up with her more demanding ways right up to the end and was forever doing things he didn't necessarily want to do.

Flatmate Johnny also had a girlfriend – a less demanding one, I think – called Cathy, who, like Shaun, visited regularly. Johnny and Cathy are still together, married with three children. Their eldest, Milo, was Caron's godson. Although initially Johnny and Caron were friends, over the years Caron and Cathy developed a friendship that was independent of him. Cathy says Caron never had any airs about her, so maybe her tantrums were reserved for members of the opposite sex and her brothers. She said you always knew where you stood with Caron. If Caron didn't like you, she didn't pretend she did, but if she did, she was the most loyal friend you could have, and that friendship was never doubted. So the spats and tantrums were forgiven – more likely laughed at, which was no bad thing.

So, overall it's gratifying when Paul says I was the hub of the family. I have striven to maintain a strong family bond, like most Irish mothers, and I believe that few things are as important as creating a core strength. I appreciate it when he and Michael tell me I got the balance between family and career right. I am glad they know that I maintained our family unit for as long as history allowed. More than that I am delighted that they weren't aware as children in Northern Ireland that they had a mum in the public eye. If their main memory is playing cricket in the BBC corridors, hiding behind the studio weatherboard and canteen chips and fried onions, perhaps I didn't do such a bad job and, like theirs, Caron's childhood was normal. I hope I was something of an inspiration to them.

I am sorry that Caron in the end felt responsible for Don. I am sorry she felt the need to protect him and make it all right for him. But I chose honesty. I believe, now more than ever, that you should live for today – not irresponsibly, but our time is finite. Don was always saving for the future, but he died young, with a bank account full of money and a million and one things he never did, although he could have done them all. We have one life and there are many things that can restrict us, but it shouldn't be ourselves. This is no rehearsal. This is it. I'd like to think that the experience of our divorce, although it was hard at the time, made Caron grow up a little. I hope it made her wiser and that some of the invaluable advice she gave her friends in later life came from that perspective.

5. Lights, Camera, Action . . .

When Caron left university in 1983 she thought she wanted to be a programme researcher. Then she decided maybe she wanted to present. So I said, 'Why don't you write to all the programmes you might want to work for and send a CV and a photo and ask them to hold your details on file, even if they aren't looking for anyone at the moment?' So that is what she did. She wrote to a lot of programmes, including, of course, *Blue Peter*.

I wasn't worrying too much about what she was going to do next: I was just happy that she was coming home to London without the pressure of study looming over her and that we would get to spend more time together. I knew a job would come her way. Caron was always very conscientious and, however late she stayed up in Bristol, she always worked. While exams didn't seem important to Paul, they always were to Caron. Maybe it's a boy-girl thing – maybe it was just Caron. I believe her intellect, which enabled her to gain good grades and a degree, also gave her the ability to question things, which she did with force to the end. Therefore when she became a presenter, it was only natural that Caron would be asking pertinent questions. She liked to dig deep. Be analytical. Sometimes presenting is more mundane than that. Not always, of course – you wouldn't say Jeremy Paxman or David Frost was mundane – but some of the 'lifestyle' television is. It isn't that she was too superior for it, but part of Caron went untapped, and much later, this became a source of deep-seated disquiet in her that she couldn't escape. Should she have concentrated on her artistic side and, if so, should it have been painting or writing? Did she make the wrong decision when she was twenty-one? It is impossible to know how far-reaching any decision may be when you are so young. I loved presenting so, naturally, I thought it was a good idea. I also thought she could be a great actress: she'd done plays at Bristol and the Arts Theatre in Belfast. Like Paul, I was fairly sure she couldn't be a singer, but there have been less able acts in the top ten, so who knows? Perhaps the problem stemmed from the fact that she could have done anything she turned her attention to. For right or wrong, that was television, front of camera, like me, not behind, like Don.

She had returned to Northern Ireland frequently throughout her time at Bristol, and out of the blue she got a call to say that a presenter on *Channel One*, a youth programme, had been tragically killed in a car crash: could she come across to present the programme? Literally overnight, Caron was off again, on another adventure. I was slightly disappointed in a way that she was going, just when I thought I'd got her back and she would be around for all those cups of tea and chats. She moved back into her old room in the family home, and took up with Don where they'd left off.

It was Caron's first taste of regular television: Don could steer her through the work, mentor her and give her tips. They often met up at the BBC club after work, then padded around the house in the evenings, had dinner together in the kitchen and put the world to rights. It was a very special time for her to be with Don on her own: they forged their adult relationship. I don't think Paul ever got that chance, having left home at sixteen and being very independent by nature, but Michael and his father had routinely spent time together because we had split when he was young, so seeing Don was an assumed part of his life and he spent many school holidays in Ireland with him. Caron and Don became very close and remained so. I imagine them sitting happily in the front room reading, as content to be silent as to chew the fat over a bottle of wine. I'd like to think that that is exactly what they are doing now, when Caron isn't popping over to check on us and let me know she hasn't gone. Not completely.

Caron had a ball working on *Channel One*. She would hare off around the countryside in her little Mini doing regional stories, then inevitably end up going out in the evening with whichever bizarre character she'd met during the interview and having a laugh. It was a good period in her life and wonderful for her future career. She was on a steep learning curve. Regional television provides exceptional foundations for anyone considering a career in television. She had to do everything. She had to master every aspect of putting together a piece – find her own story, do her own research, plan her own questions and write her own scripts. Later, as you move on to bigger shows, the budgets increase and suddenly there is a production team to carry the burden of responsibility. Her time in Northern Ireland fed an already inquisitive mind and gave her the freedom and confidence to develop a nose for a story. Generally she relished being back home where her personality fitted. She was never happier than when she was sitting at a dinner-table, or in the pub, with a drink and a cigarette, which seemed to go along with the drink, chatting. She loved all the chat. Something you always get a lot of in Northern Ireland is 'chat'.

In 1986, because of that letter she'd sent off earlier, the producer of *Blue Peter* rang up and asked Caron to come to London for an audition. You never know what life's going to throw at you, do you? She'd just been over for the weekend to see me and some friends, and had basically spent her travelling budget for that month. She rang me on the Monday and asked me what she should do. Was there a snowball's chance in hell she'd get the job? Was she up against hundreds of others? Was it worth taking time off work? I had to go on air 'live' so couldn't really chat, but she continued talking to David Jacobs, who was passing through the studio. He said, 'Listen, any of us will lend you the money. Just come across. If you don't try you'll never know.' A bit like me and Radio 2.

She came over and got the job. On 13 November 1986, Caron Keating took over from Peter Duncan, joining Janet Ellis and Mark Curry as a presenter of the number-one, flagship, legendary children's programme, *Blue Peter*, and became a national pin-up overnight.

Almost from the start Caron was unfairly accused of having got the job through nepotism. But that is to underestimate the producer, Biddy Baxter: if you think she would have hired anyone for any reason other than that they were right for the job, you're wrong. The name Keating did not link Caron to me in England. No one knew who she was, except that she'd been working on Northern Ireland television. *Blue Peter* was Biddy Baxter's life, and the other presenters never doubted for a minute that Caron had been chosen for any reason other than that she fitted into the mix. It had to work. Caron was by no means a given. Her accent was incredibly thick, really strong, which Janet says would have been a mark against her had she not been perfect for the job. In fact, Janet's only concern was whether the dynamic of going from two men and one woman to two women and one man would work. I asked her what her first impression of Caron was, but she can't remember ever not knowing her, or having to work in with her or find out what she was like, because Biddy Baxter had got it right. Caron fitted straight in. Janet thinks the nature of the show meant that if it suited your personality you could do it. You couldn't make someone good at it. It was a team show, not a one-man band, and the essential quality Biddy Baxter looked for was whether each presenter had an intrinsic understanding of the spirit of the show.

Caron's profile sky-rocketed overnight: that she was taking over from Peter Duncan and was linked to me saw to that, especially when it was combined with her overall appeal. Since her death I have received letters from women who were girls at the time, telling me that Caron epitomized everything they wanted to be. It wasn't that she was iconic, rather that she was an inspiration to a generation. She dared to be her own person even on a show as tightly scripted as *Blue Peter*. And it wasn't just the girls who liked her: boys all over Britain fell in love with Caron in droves. I have their letters too.

Janet and Caron loved doing *Blue Peter*. It was hard work. They had to learn scripts twice a week and there was always filming in between. There was never 'autocue', everything was done from memory. I had been the main purchaser of pipe-cleaners and sticky-back plastic for Caron when she was growing up – like so many children, she was a *Blue Peter* addict so we had to make everything that they made on the show. If, for some reason, I hadn't got the stuff that was required, I was in the doghouse for the day and made to feel a complete failure. My children grew up watching *Blue Peter*. Because the pro-gramme was such an institution, and still is, the fact that Caron was presenting it seemed unreal to me.

I still felt as if I'd only been over from Northern Ireland for a minute and was very much enamoured with London. I loved the access it gave me to the theatre, the Royal Variety Shows, the Chelsea Flower Show, Wimbledon and so on. Now that Caron was back, we could do so much together. I was so proud and so excited for her because I knew that the jump from Northern Ireland to England is huge. Not only was she taking on national TV, she was taking on a British institution.

At that time I was doing an ITV chat show called *Sunday Sunday*. Naturally, at the London Weekend Television (LWT) headquarters all the monitors were switched to ITV, but on Caron's first day I had everything switched to BBC. We stopped rehearsals and turned on *Blue Peter* and, of course, I wept buckets, I was so proud. Biddy Baxter pushed them all hard, but she trained them well too. Once you've done *Blue Peter*, which is live, you can do anything – you can work on the hoof, remem-ber words, cope with unexpected or dangerous turns. Although *I* didn't cope so well watching my little girl doing them.

Caron sort of took over Peter Duncan's role as the dare-devil. I remember her swimming with sharks off the coast of California. I knew she had had to learn to deep-sea dive, which, quite frankly, to someone who never learnt to swim, was terrifying enough. I was watching that episode with her, and I had my hands clasped over my mouth, shouting, 'Oh, no, my daughter,' and she'd give me a little nudge and say, 'Mum, I did that two months ago. Don't worry. I'm right next to you, nothing's going to happen to me.' Then I would feel really stupid. Sometimes I can still feel that little nudge. I can hear her whisper into my ear, 'Don't worry, Mum, I'm still next to you.' I wish, I wish, I wish that were so.

At the beginning, Caron's 'look' caused a great deal of complaint:

When I started work on *Blue Peter*, I'd come straight from a job presenting yoof programmes for BBC Northern Ireland. I didn't get paid very much, so flamboyant second-hand clothes made for an interesting look. On the odd occasion when I've looked back at old tapes, I appear to be wearing my entire wardrobe at once. Endless layers of stuff, bits of lace tied on, cotton stockings over tights, wild polka-dot skirts with wide sashes, net petticoats, all topped with a bowler hat at a rakish angle. The effect was often startling and divided the viewers neatly into those who loved the look and those who clearly didn't. The latter proved to be much more vocal in their opinions and were particularly keen to have their views heard. They wrote in to the programme and, indeed, the national press in droves. In my Filofax is a clipping from the *Daily Mirror*:

Blue Peter

The producers should do something about Caron Keating's dress sense. She would be better employed in the Blue Peter garden – keeping the birds away!

J. G. Crawshaw
Ramsbottom, Lancs

I don't know whether J. G. Crawshaw thought his letter would have me rushing to the racks of suitable TV outfits (after all, my mother had been trying for years) – but I like to think it had the opposite effect and made me even more determined to retain my own unique sense of style. It probably had a lot to do with expressing myself. On a show like *Blue Peter* which is very tightly scripted, it often felt as if we were mouthpieces for someone else's thoughts, and could easily be replaced by any number of previous presenters. The scripts in the main could not be altered: time was tight, it was live and in the early days there was no autocue – so we tended to stick to what was there. Wearing something outlandish was my way of demonstrating that although I might be saying something similar to what Valerie Singleton had said, I wasn't her.

Viewers seemed terrified that their children would start to dress (or, worse still, talk) like me. The programme's editor, Biddy Baxter, got endless complaints. I don't think she ever quite got the hang of my 'look'. She generally liked the presenters to be in something bright and colourful so she could tell us apart from the more sombrely attired production crew. Strange dressing was not encouraged. I remember hearing that one of the former presenters – Michael Sunder, who famously danced half naked at the Hammersmith Apollo with a snake – had emerged from his dressing room one day clad from head to toe in black leather. He was unceremoniously shoved back in by one of the producers – Alex Le Gere – a wonderfully eccentric, ex-army man, who was heard muttering in his very English tones, 'No, no, no, not the thing at all, dear boy.'

Biddy would often appear in the makeup room minutes before we went on air and eye me suspiciously. 'Is that what you're wearing, darling?' Mild disapproval permeating her every word. And at the merest hint of black – 'You look like you're going to a funeral.' By then it was usually too late for her to do anything about it – we were almost on. However, when I decided to leave the show after three years, they had a design-an-outfit for me competition. Ninety-seven thousand children entered, making it one of the biggest responses ever. There were the most incredible designs and I eventually chose a short red velvet dress, with a sticking-out lace underskirt, with butterflies, attached by piano wire, floating around it, a beautiful hat swathed in roses and green tights with yet more roses winding their way up my legs. It was gorgeous – the programme had it made up for me and I wore it on my final show . . . It still hangs in my wardrobe somewhere.

Janet's response to this is as dry as ever: 'You'd think we'd all been walking around in sludge-coloured 1950s clothing . . .' Obviously they weren't, but Caron's idiosyncratic style was legendary. These days, some of those eccentric clothes hang in my wardrobe. When Russ moved out of their house, Menlo, in Cornwall, he gave me the unenviable task of sorting out Caron's clothes. She was shopping three days before she died and there was a mountain of stuff to go through. Anyone who has been through that traumatic black bin-liner ordeal will know how distressing and emotional it is. Some things had to be given away, but each item I dispensed with broke my heart again. Some went to her friends. A few of the stranger pieces may even have found their way into the odd dressing-up box. I hope they have. I kept a lot. Hooped dresses, shawls with long tassels, embroidered wraps, T-shirts with Caron-like emblems – each piece smacks of her personality and I couldn't bear to part with them. Maybe one day Caron's sons will have daughters, and who knows what maverick streak will appear down the line? Maybe they'll enjoy the hooped skirts and brightly coloured shoes. I certainly love wearing some of them. I use her handbags, I wear her shoes. I've even had some of her clothes altered to fit me. I find a strange comfort from it, as if Caron comes with me when I wear them out. There is a particular jacket that I treasure. It is the blue sleeveless one she wore on that long journey home the day before she died. I have never washed it and it still smells of her. Sometimes I lie on my bed, clutching it to me. Beau, Paul's son, has a blue comfort blanket that he sometimes hangs on to for dear life. I watch him and think, I have one of those . . .

If you read what Caron wrote about her time on *Blue Peter*

carefully, you may see, as I do, an element of the writing being on the wall in her dissatisfaction with her career. The germ of frustration had been planted. She wasn't just a mouthpiece. Maybe Shaun is right: her TV ambition got in the way of her true talent. She never really bought into the industry terribly well, that whole celebrity lifestyle. Perhaps because she didn't find it fulfilling. In no way do I mean to bite the hand that feeds me: I love my job and have found it incredibly rewarding, but television is fickle and can be shallow. A producer once said to Caron, 'Darling, presenters are just commodities.' Well, Caron was many things, but she wasn't fickle or shallow, and was determined never to be a commodity. Why did she stick at it then, after *Blue Peter* ended? Well, she was successful and it's difficult to turn your back on that, especially if you don't know what you'd really like to do. And there were the trappings and perks, as there always had been. It was JR and fried onions all over again, but this time it was her own achievements, not mine, that got her into the Green Room. We as a family and her friends still meet people who had pictures of her on the wall. Girls aspired to be like her, she was Blu-tacked on to teenage boys' bedroom walls. She turned heads.

Caron and her university friend Johnny had moved into a flat in Lavender Hill, Battersea. It had two bedrooms, although the second was literally a cupboard under the stairs. The idea was that Caron would start with the large bedroom and then they would swap. Frankly, Johnny should have known better. If anyone was under no illusion about Caron and her little ways, it was him. Needless to say, the large bedroom barely held her clothes, let alone her makeup and hairspray. She was never, ever going to live in a cupboard under the stairs. And I'm afraid she was congenitally untidy. But she was a joy to be with and they had a lot of happy times at that flat. Happy times, and late nights. Janet Ellis is six years older than Caron and had just met John, who is now her husband; soon after she met Caron she became pregnant with her son. I think she was quite a stabilizing character, a grown-up for Caron to talk to who wasn't me – Caron probably told me about a hundredth of the things she got up to at that time!

She was young, free and single, but also well financed and famous. She spent many nights in the VIP room at Brown's nightclub, a particularly salubrious establishment. I think she had a dalliance with a pop star, whose name I've chosen to forget. Apparently she even got Michael – who, to me, was still about three – into Brown's. He remembers hanging out with footballers and Mandy Smith, and being introduced to the owner, Jake. Exciting times? Yes, but I'm glad I didn't know the details. Michael remembers that after leaving Brown's one night, they parked the car on Battersea Bridge and watched the sunrise. Up all night is one thing, up all night and driving makes the hairs on the back of my neck stand up. By the way, Battersea is now Michael's favourite bridge in London and ironically his home is half a mile away in Fulham, where Caron was born.

When Caron was living in Johnny's cousin's rather more immaculate flat, she decided it was time to do something about what she considered a pretentious piece of art that hung in the sitting room, a drawing of a torso. It was late. She had been out. She took a thick pen and, on the wall beneath it, drew the torso some legs, complete with a hefty pair of platform shoes. The cousin eventually came to like the addition, and there the legs remained until he sold the flat. Much, much later, when Caron was ill and everything was under the microscope, she agonized that she had partied too hard. She feared she was paying for the 'good times'. Janet says it was not uncommon for Caron to stay up all night, then go into work and do a live show. Did she party harder than anyone else at the time? I don't think so. She was young, she'd just come to London and she was having a ball. All of her friends told her that it was pointless, stupid and damaging to blame herself for her illness. She didn't bring cancer on herself because she had fun in her twenties. If that were the case there wouldn't be such a thing as an ageing rocker. Party giants are still going strong and Caron was an ant compared to them. Cancer was not her fault, but we couldn't convince her of it. It took a Buddhist monk to release her from that particular demon.

Caron appreciated the stunning opportunities that *Blue Peter* offered her. Among the hundreds of things she did – motor-cycle-sidecar racing, abseiling down skyscrapers (dressed as Snow White, complete with Seven Dwarfs), strapping herself to aerobatic aircraft – I think the highlight was taking *Blue Peter* to Russia for six weeks when *perestroika* was in its infancy. The team spent as much time looking for food as they did for stories, and when Caron arrived home I was waiting at the airport with a hamper full of the goodies they had missed over the weeks they were away. During the trip Caron had appeared with the Moscow State Circus and done all the high-wire stuff. Years later, on New Year's Eve in 1998 we took Charlie to see the Moscow State Circus in Dublin. I remember telling him, 'Mummy did that,' when the high-wire walker came on. Of course, he didn't believe me but in the interval a tall, broad-shouldered, moustached man came over to us and said to Caron, 'I remember when you came with *Blue Peter*. You appeared with our circus.' Caron was thrilled, and Charlie was deeply impressed.

Caron said of *Blue Peter*: 'It is so successful because it caters for all those children who are not desperately trendy. It is such a constant. It has always been there in our living rooms twice a week. And no matter what is happening in a child's life – disasters at school or parents splitting up – their three favourite presenters and the dog will be there to say hello to them . . .' She never regretted being a part of that.

But *Blue Peter* spits you out after a while. She'd done three and a half years of flying around the country doing dangerous things, standing out in cold weather, throwing herself off cliffs. If Russia had been her *Blue Peter* highlight, then standing under a waterfall in Wales one New Year's Day was the opposite. She said it was the coldest thing that had ever happened to her. She went blue, and it took her days to thaw. There were other things she didn't like. Once she had to sing a solo on a Christmas special, some terrible Irish song: she felt exposed and silly being separated from everyone else – singing in a group was one thing, but singing alone was something else. As was being made to dress up as Mrs Santa Claus in a tiny skating skirt.

The break came naturally, I think. She was twenty-six, and there comes a time when you want to move away from children's television, a transition that is notoriously hard to make. It even took Philip Schofield a while to make a name for himself in mainstream television. A lot of people get stuck in the mould. Valerie Singleton was always associated with *Blue Peter*, no matter what else she did, and Caron was wary of that. So, it was time to make a move. And she knew exactly whom she wanted to implement it for her. Enter one Russ Lindsay of James Grant Management – the other hero of this story.

6. A Knight in a Tesco Trolley

There wasn't a lot that Russ hadn't done before he set up his business with Peter Powell twenty-one years ago. He'd been managing bands, done a stint as a croupier in France, been a courier and, all the way along, he'd had a ball. Peter Powell, meanwhile, was a DJ on Radio 1. By a curious chain of events Russ ended up as his A&R (artist and repertoire) guy. He'd been DJ-ing on the south coast when he met Peter and offered himself as a roadie. Peter told him to come to the studio and they'd talk some more. So, Russ went to the *Top of the Pops* studio, where it soon became clear that the two men had a natural affinity and admiration for each other. Russ knew the music Peter was playing, because he, too, had been a DJ, and was offered the job.

A week later he arrived at the Radio 1 studio. Peter threw him the keys of his Porsche and sent him on an errand. Poor Russ, it must have been terrible. But from those humble beginnings, he and Peter created James Grant Management, a highly successful stable of talent, which, over the years, has managed the cream of the crop. I would like to say now that not many business partners would have allowed their partner to pack up and move four hundred miles away to Cornwall. The twelve thousand mile move to Australia was even more of an ask, but Peter gave Russ his blessing, knowing by then that Russ had enough on his plate without having to worry about whether he'd have a desk to come back to. That may not seem as magnanimous as it was: after all, Caron had a terminal illness so the time Russ had to spend at home with his wife was finite. But that isn't right: we never thought like that. Caron was going to beat it – people had conquered worse. Their move to Australia was open-ended. No one knew, least of all Russ, when they would be back or if they'd ever be back. Their plans were as changeable as the Cornish sky.

I found their decision to move incredibly hard to understand and, as a mother, I am programmed to forgive and accommodate. But Peter has proved that the waters of friendship can thicken to become more like blood than blood. On behalf of Charlie and Gabriel, I will always be grateful to him for his continued support of their dad. He knew that Caron was unpredictable, both professionally and personally: he'd had to weather the occasional tantrum and smooth over the ruffles caused by Caron storming out of the odd television studio. He would have witnessed her more abrupt handling of domestic situations, yet his support for Russ never wavered. If you think I'm being harsh about Caron's professional stroppiness, I have it on good authority that in some circles she had something of a reputation for it. Yet others say they never ever saw that side. Most of the time she was the consummate professional, but she could be moody and wouldn't click into what she had to do. On one occasion she had taken umbrage with a particular film crew, I don't know when, who or where, but she stormed out of the studio and slammed the door behind her. A fabulous exit, except she found herself in an annexe with no way out. She stubbornly waited there for two hours, texting her co-presenter, until the crew had left. Silly girl, you might say, but that was Caron: it wasn't all roses – some sharp Irish thorns came with the package. Peter Powell was under no illusions, unlike Russ and me, I suppose, who were blinded by love.

From the moment Caron met Russ she talked about him. His name came up a lot, even though they started out as friends. Russ was going out with a lovely girl and apparently they were close to an engagement. His best friend was Philip Schofield, who had recently come back from New Zealand. As Philip's manager, Russ did what he does best, and got him into children's television where he quickly became a huge name. Always checking out the competition, Philip and Russ used to watch *Blue Peter*, and were particularly enamoured of the 'goddess', as Russ put it, on the screen. Like so many people, Russ immediately fancied Caron and developed a safe, on-screen crush. She was beautiful then, no doubt, but now he says he found her at her most beautiful in the last few months of her life. She had changed, of course: the cancer and the treatments had ravaged her body. But he was right: she radiated something from inside that was mesmerizing, absolutely mesmerizing, and I think it was true beauty. Anyway, Russ said to Philip that he should ask Caron out. He was on *In the Broom Cupboard*, a children's continuity programme, at the time, and eventually he did. They all became great friends. For about two years Philip, Caron, Lesley, Russ's girlfriend, and Russ went out together as a foursome. As a result, Caron and Russ became really good friends. He says he never thought then of Caron as anything other than a friend: first, he was in love with someone else, and second, she was his mate's girlfriend. Later, it became even more unlikely that the two would be anything other than platonic friends because Russ managed her. I know that he's chivalrous, but can any man be so pure of thought?

Friends of hers knew long before Russ and Peter that Caron was determined that James Grant would be her agents. They weren't quite so sure. But, in true Caron Keating fashion, she wouldn't take no for an answer and simply kept going back for meetings until they changed their minds. I am not sure how secure Philip and Caron's relationship was: I know she wasn't always happy with the way things were, and this alone would have made it difficult for Russ to manage her. Philip was the rooster in their yard and Russ's best mate, and Russ's loyalty, professionally and personally, quite rightly lay with him.

This proved no obstacle to my daughter. After one raucous

night out Caron pushed Russ home in a Tesco trolley – apologies to Tesco – and supposedly, during this uncomfortable trip, he agreed to manage her. Maybe she wouldn't let him out, maybe she threatened to tip him into a bush, maybe she just spun him round until he was giddy, I don't know, and neither does Russ: to this day he has no recollection of saying they would manage her and still doesn't quite believe that he did. But that didn't stop Caron calling him early the following morning to ensure that he kept his word. He went into work, awash with Resolve and tea, and had to admit to Peter the mess he'd got himself into. Caron had done it, she was on the books, whether their number-one star Philip Schofield liked it or not. Caron wasn't going to take no for an answer. It was just another example of my daughter's formidable tenacity, stubbornness and wilfulness. I thought those traits were simply facets of her fun-loving personality, which made me adore her more. Little did I know that her zest for life would keep her alive long after the doctors had closed her file.

Part of Russ's job in those early days was to take the talent out on the road. As well as Philip, there was Andi Peters, Zoe Ball, Emma Forbes and most of the other Saturday-morning crowd. Between them they did a lot of gigs so Russ was out most nights driving them to the middle of nowhere to do 'children's discos'. They got paid good money to play music, throw free records at the kids, missing their eyes by millimetres, and sign a few autographs. No wonder Russ's girlfriend finally got fed up and left him.

Caron hated those live performances: as with singing and acting, the idea was one thing, the reality of doing it on your own another. She was scared of the stage, the crowd, the reception, and she wouldn't let anyone be her roadie but Russ. They would arrive at Great Yarmouth, for instance, to find two and a half thousand under-eighteens, inebriated with cider and excitement. Caron, the goddess from *Blue Peter*, would be introduced, but instead of stepping on to the stage she would push Russ on instead. He was left with no alternative but to fill in for her for fifty-five minutes, doing his DJ act. With five minutes to go, Caron would finally come on smiling sweetly and do her bit. Most managers would have been furious, but I think Russ probably enjoyed his stint at the turntables, and when Caron did come out, she made the most of her five minutes and no one complained or asked for their money back. The pair spent a lot of time together, drove around the country, listened to music and chatted endlessly. During that time they developed a deep friendship that forged an unbreakable bond. When Caron was ill and could only rage at Russ about the enormity of what she was facing, that bond held fast and true.

Russ's memory of Caron at that time is of a complete and utter maverick, with her wily Irish ways, her big hair, mad clothes and sparkling eyes. She must have cast some spell over him, platonic or otherwise, because, as the story of the road trips shows, from the beginning he let her get away with murder. Russ is quite philosophical about Caron's trickier side. He worked out a long time ago that you do not get a woman who is as bright and intelligent as she was on one side without her being slightly difficult on the other. He says, though I'm not sure I agree, that if he had that sort of charm he'd be tricky too. How did she get away with it? Because she inherited from her father that amazing repartee of the south, the lilt, the song. She was beguiling. She weaved the magic. She was simply so charming that you didn't mind doing what she wanted to do, or doing something for her that you wouldn't ordinarily do. You just didn't mind. She was charming – but that wasn't it. She was wild, and her wildness was contagious – but that wasn't it either. It was the combination of all her traits, that magic concoction of spirit, humour, intelligence, childishness, wide-eyed wonder, beauty, sweetness and spike that allowed her to behave as she did and made others behave differently too. On top of all those things there was something else, something unquantifiable, that even I can't put my finger on. Maybe her special something was as ethereal as the magic of the spirit of Ireland.

By the time Caron was twenty-five, it was clear to everyone that her relationship with Philip had fizzled out. In the meantime it was reasonably obvious that Russ and Caron had become more than friends, although nothing had actually happened. Caron's great pal Yasmin Pacha, whom she worked with daily on the show *After 5*, reckons that a pair of swimming-trunks was responsible for what developed: the story goes that Russ appeared in some fancy shorts and Caron suddenly saw him through different eyes. I think it was more likely a mixture of their deepening friendship, finding themselves single at the same time, and that in the weeks leading up to 'the event' they'd spent a lot of time together. Then again maybe it was as simple as Caron seeing Russ in those shorts and thinking, Hello, Tiger. Love works in mysterious ways, that's for sure. Whatever the catalyst, some time soon afterwards Caron and Russ were at a birthday party together. Russ had been talking to a girl with whom he thought things were going quite well, when suddenly he was grabbed, swung round and snogged passionately. Then Caron grabbed his tie and said, 'You're coming with me.' Needless to say, Russ did not refuse. Once again, my daughter had acted in her own idiosyncratic, decisive way, leaving no room for doubt. You could say that Russ didn't have a chance – or alternatively that, despite his claims to the contrary, he'd been plotting it for years. He has said on the record that he wanted to marry Caron from almost the moment they met, but circumstances did not allow it. Maybe for him it was a matter of biding his time. They locked themselves away for the next three days, 'In a place of complete bliss,' says Russ, where they fell hard and fast in love. Then the press found out.

'GLORIA'S GIRL GETS PHIL'S BOSS', went the headline, or something equally trite, recalls Russ, which to his mind couldn't have been further from 'Caron and Russ are madly in love, over the moon, ecstatically happy, and flying high'. There were photos to beef up the story – one of Philip Schofield and one of me. Caron and Russ laughed about that. Thankfully, Philip was man enough and true enough to himself to know that Russ hadn't crossed any line, overstepped the mark or stolen his girl. He hadn't really made Caron his girl, so everyone was happy.

Once she started going out with Russ, that was it. I always knew that he would look after and cherish her, and I was right. He was exemplary throughout their married life. And I mean exemplary. As a parent you always wonder who they will marry, if that person will augment your family structure or fracture it. I could not have been happier when they got together. I have loved Russ like a third son from those early days and I still do.

All her friends will agree that she married the right man. They say that when you know, you know. And Caron did. For a short time, life gets very simple and easy because you know you're doing the right thing. There is no shoehorning, no quiet doubts, no cold feet, no change of heart. That all came later. We don't like to admit to Caron's dissection of our relationships, but both Russ and I had to endure them. Cancer gave her her sharpest thorn: she was capable of slicing her relationships wide open and cutting the heart out of them, even though all we ever did was love her. Deeply and unconditionally.

It was obvious to us all that their relationship was serious, and things moved pretty fast. Within weeks they were living together and from then on they were a unit. It was just a matter of time before they announced their engagement. And, boy, what a romantic proposal it was. Russ planned it all. First Caron was picked up from the studio by motorbike and whisked off to the airport. They flew to the South of France and drove to Château Éze, a stunning hotel that sits on the edge of a medieval village overlooking Monte Carlo. I can hear Caron recall the day he proposed. They were sitting in a romantic restaurant from where they could see all the way along the coastline to Cap Ferrat. As the sun went down, the lights on the shore started to twinkle below them. Russ was unusually quiet and withdrawn and Caron couldn't understand why he had suddenly become moody – here of all places. Finally all was revealed. He took her out on to the balcony, bent down on one knee and asked her to become his wife.

Back at home I waited for the happy phone call. Russ had let me into the secret and I had no doubt that the answer to his question would be an unreserved yes. It was, they called, and he has been an integral part of our family ever since. I know there have been times when I've been the archetypal mother-in-law, but I cannot reiterate often enough that Russ has been exemplary, loved my daughter endlessly and cared for her extraordinarily.

Russ and Caron were married at St Peter's Church near Hever Castle in Kent in 1991, when Caron was twenty-nine. We all stayed in the castle over the wedding period. The night before the wedding itself we had a wonderful girly dinner during which Caron presented me with a hinged silver photo frame. One side of it had me tying her hair in bunches with the words 'from pigtails' engraved on it. The other side was left blank for a wedding picture but with the words 'to wedding veils' etched underneath, a Val Doonican song that could always bring tears to my eyes.

Their wedding day was one of the best days of my life. My beautiful daughter pulled up at the church in a horse-drawn carriage sitting beside her incredibly proud father. People were hanging out of windows, the pub was packed, onlookers lined the church wall: they had all come to see the arrival of this princess bride. I will never forget how she looked as she walked down the aisle. All brides bloom on their wedding day and Caron was no exception. She was bursting with joy and it radiated out of her. She looked absolutely breathtaking and Russ like a young Rob Roy, with his long hair and Lindsay tartan.

They made their traditional vows and when finally they turned
to their friends and family as a married couple we all burst into
applause. The atmosphere was vibrant, joyous and full of love.
The applause kept up until they were back outside the church,
Mr and Mrs R. Lindsay.

At the reception, a stunning affair at Hever Castle, the
speeches were made. Of course, Don had been rehearsing his
for months and was word-perfect. But Cathy Comerford, who
was then still Cathy Clark, the bridesmaid, remembers listening
to Russ's speech with something close to envy. She had never
heard one from a man so in love with his bride. 'I have married
the most charming, intelligent, elegant and beautiful woman
possible. I look forward to a long, long time with you, Caron.
It is a dream come true for me. I love you enormously – you're
the best thing that has ever happened in my life.' His eulogy to
Caron at her funeral, when he stood in the same spot in the
same church as he had to be married, was full of the same
feelings. As he said at the time, 'My wedding was the best day
of my life. How ironic that I should be standing here again on
the worst day of my life.' It was agony and heartbreaking to
listen to it, but for a few seconds, here and there, you could
almost believe you were listening to the speech he had made at
their wedding: it was so full of love, pride and admiration for
Caron. He talked, with no notes, for fifty minutes. He said he'd
just ramble on a bit, but his words were perfect, as they had
been on their wedding day, because they were spoken from the
heart. 'Caron was everything a man could wish for in a woman.
She was beautiful, intelligent, witty, fun-loving, caring, honest,
loyal, loving and, latterly, a most wonderful mother. I was the
luckiest man in the world, because for sixteen and a half years,
I was the one walking the path with her.'

They didn't get that 'long, long' time together. Sixteen and
a half years was not long enough. But he still counts his blessings.
The best thing, he says, in all of this dreadful illness, is the time

he had with Caron. If she'd been taken in a road crash, or by a really quick disease, they would never have had that time to spend together loving each other, getting to know each other. Their relationship grew, there is no doubt about it, and I understand when he says that after the cancer set in they lived the last forty or fifty years of their lives in seven. Their unison, lives, marriage, friendship became faster, bigger, deeper, wider. Somewhere subconsciously Russ must have known that they didn't have much time left and therefore was determined to make whatever they had work. Everyone who has ever been married or had a long-term partnership will tell you that the relationship is cyclical. It has ups and downs. There are times when you don't need any other human being, and others when you can't be in the same room as your partner. Like anyone else, they had their spats, and when they did they never hid it. You knew if Russ and Caron had had an argument. All of that is normal, of course, in any marriage, unless it's played out against the threat of death. They coped in just seven years with the ups and downs that people normally deal with over decades, and with the unimaginable twists and turns of fighting a life-threatening battle. Every aspect of their lives was intensified. Russ feels that in many ways they were stuck on fast-forward, that they condensed their lives to a highly concentrated mix. The only thing they couldn't do was fast-forward the boys: Charlie and Gabriel didn't grow up at seven times the usual speed.

Russ acknowledges that to have time with someone you love is a reward. He thinks back to the world wars when millions of men were slaughtered and one day you got a letter through the post that told you your child, your husband, your father was dead. No goodbye, nothing. He thinks he and Caron were lucky. I think they were robbed of many years together. He feels honoured to have been given that time with Caron. I feel empty that they have no more. But he is right: he had an amazing chance to truly understand and love his wife.

I hated Caron being twelve thousand miles away from us, but Australia gave us all some incredible times with her that I look back on now with awe and gratitude. Russ is right: you do love someone completely differently when they are dying. Let me try to explain what I think those seven years gave Russ and Caron. As a mother you love your children no matter what. Mothers stand by their murderous children. A mother wouldn't think twice about donating an organ. A mother's love is infinite. Russ loved Caron like that. It was unconditional, the way a parent loves their child. I used to get so angry with him for agreeing to let her stay in Australia: I would plead with him to put his foot down and just come home – I'd suggest he had to come back and work, that he couldn't just follow her on her latest whim. But he wouldn't. She tested him to the limit, but he held fast. To me the move to Australia would have been bad enough without cancer. With the threat of cancer, it was devastating. At times I resented the whole thing, Australia, Russ, the people who told her she could cure herself, yet rock-steady Russ just went along with all of it. Not because he loved it there too: in the beginning he didn't – he certainly didn't take to the dubious characters who turned up on their doorstep clutching yet another life-saving elixir – but he allowed Caron her adventure. It was not his place to take away her endless hope to self-heal, her quest for a miracle. And in the end they were on the adventure together: as he saw it, if they could give Caron another day, week, month with the boys, the healers, gurus and shamans could stay. He'd buy their elixirs, put them up in his house, because every extra minute beyond what she had was worth it. He wanted to keep Caron alive as long as possible for the boys. And ultimately that was what got her through those final years.

We didn't talk about death, only about life, but she did say to me more than once, 'I don't care about me but I don't want my boys to grow up without their mum.' Well, on that she and I were as one. Despite all my initial resentment of why she chose

Australia, I now believe it gave her extra time, that she lived as long as she did because of the freedom and hope Byron Bay gave her, and I will be grateful for ever for the depth of Russ's love for my daughter. I honestly don't know many men who would have done what he has and made the sacrifices he made.

As Russ says, if your partner is ill, you don't expect them to be washing and cleaning. You may love your partner now, but if you were told tomorrow that they were dying, how much more would you love them? How much greater would your understanding be of their moods and habits? They were dealing with something of such grave magnitude that there was little room for minor irritations. When the pain was bad and Caron couldn't sleep, when she was overtired, angry, desperate and her moods were filthy, Russ accepted it and gave her room to rage. Even now he doesn't consider that he had any other option but to follow his wife on her search for life to whatever end. He thinks everyone would have done what he did, and I love him for that too.

Cathy Comerford recalls one of the many nights that she and Caron got quite drunk. The reason for their frequent inebriation, apparently, was that neither thought the other drank much. Therefore they mistakenly used each other as a benchmark for how much to drink. Obviously that was a disaster, because they both thought the second – nay, the third bottle of wine was always a really good idea. Anyway, this particular drunken night they dissected their respective marriages. Bottle one: Russ and Johnny were heroes. Bottle two: they lamented having married men they hadn't thought they'd marry. Cathy comes from a sporty family: no one speaks on Saturday because everyone is listening to the results. Johnny, Cathy sighed, was from a different species of mankind, more cerebral, less competitive. (On hearing about this discussion Johnny refuted his lack of sporty manliness and quickly turned the conversation to football.) Caron said she'd always thought she'd marry a poet, a maverick like her, happy to dance on the winds of chance and live chaotically. Bottle three: they came to the strangely insightful conclusion that two similar people attempting unity would never work. Two ethereal beings or two fighting over the sports channels didn't have the *yin* and *yang* that make for a good partnership. They had married the right men. Without a doubt, and if Caron were here, she would agree. She always said that Russ was her anchor.

Although Caron could be quite hard work for Russ, she was strong too. She brought out in him many qualities that had hitherto lain dormant. While he grounded her, she brought out his deeper, artistic side, his own quieter maverick side. I don't think he much wanted to move to Cornwall, but in the end he loved the sea and messing around in boats. I know he didn't want to go to Byron Bay, but in the end he was as barefoot as the rest of them. Caron enabled him to stop and see angels. Before they met, it was work, fast cars and boys' toys for him. I hope he holds on to that spiritual side now that she is no longer here to fuel it, and that he passes it on to their boys. I sense that Gabriel is a miniature Caron in many ways – there is something of the leprechaun about him, so maybe he will lead his father, showing him the angels, reminding him that there is a fourth dimension. He certainly has the right name.

So, maybe Russ was right in his wedding speech. Maybe, even after all that has happened, he is still one of the luckiest men in the world because he lived for a long time with that intensity and depth of emotion. He loved *in extremis*, and it must have been amazing in parts. During the seven years of cancer Caron was not ill all the time. There were days when they could jump in the surf, walk on the beach, sing to the moon, incredible times of respite from pain that they shared, appreciated and held on to under the umbrella of unconditional love. We are all capable of it but often, in the hurly-burly of life, we forget. Russ and Caron weren't allowed to forget. Worse, just as they did forget, the cancer would spread, and they'd be reminded of the sword of Damocles hanging over their heads once more.

Caron was very conscious of the fact that facing a terminal disease was the last thing either of them ever expected. 'Till death us do part' sounds quaint in a sixteenth-century church, producing images of geriatrics sitting in a rose garden, being cared for by their children – an acceptable vision of the end. Age has downsides that a healthy young person can't imagine, and if they do it's in a controlled environment, a home maybe, a nurse coming to help. You don't imagine your partner will become your carer while you're still in your thirties. Being carefree is supposed to be an entitlement of youth. If Caron and Russ were aware of anything at their wedding, it was that their lives were ahead of them, that children lay ahead in the future and there was an expectancy of life unfurling. It was all about beginnings, not endings.

Caron was a private person: she didn't want outside assistance when things got rough, not even from me or her brothers. The only person who was allowed to help her on that intrusive, personal level was Russ. By the end Caron knew that their relationship had moved into yet another dimension, in many ways deeper again. Although she remained very independent, there were things she couldn't do. Sometimes that meant Russ fetching her shoes, looking up something on the web, driving the boys to school, cooking. At others it was more serious. By the end Caron depended on Russ for everything. In the last six hours of her life, she was saying, 'Where's Russ? Where's Russ?' He was vital to her and she panicked if he was out of her sight. I have talked of how I felt at the beginning of Caron's life when it was she and I against the world. At the end, it was the two of them, with the rest of us offering whatever support we could.

GET REAL DAY – recognize who you have in your life and how much they love you. It seems like for so much of my life I've looked outside myself for something else – something more. When I first realized that, it was like a confusion of what I wanted – more love, more attention – I couldn't even really see what I already had. I don't want to forget this morning or yesterday in the realization of where I am – it's like 'what are you doing?' I have an amazing family that truly love me and I'm away from them and that feeling is here and very strong. I am surrounded by people who care for me here, though in a different way to my mum and brothers and really close friends. I somehow haven't appreciated what I actually have and have always had and I want to fully appreciate Russ in particular. He's been so fantastic – everyone has.

It feels like it's time to give up the fanciful notions and ideas and get real about what's going on in my life and get stuck in.

Concentrate on life with the children, Russ – living – doing what I love and to start trusting my instincts and really listening. Not talking to others and taking on their stories. Sometimes I allow myself to act irresponsibly, do things that will ultimately cause pain and right now I'm stopping that particular waste as it can very likely explode in my face and actually cut me off from some of the things I really like doing here.

'Should I be here or at home?' Byron is still the place for me to be, I feel. It will be different when they are all back tomorrow and we have that family life going on. I can't wait to see them, just so gorgeous to hold them and be with them.

Remember this is what your being is longing for – example of when the mind starts checking up and urging you to do this and that, remember this feeling today. *Life can* be family, painting and looking after yourself and them obviously, bit of writing etc. etc.

Also, felt I really want to get my health sorted – some sort of treatment – whatever is appropriate. Unless a miracle happens and it all collapses and disappears by Thursday, I give in to whatever is highest and best for my health.

What an amazing teacher it has been and such a learning process about love, reality, being real, perception, sight and seeing my needs – voicing what needs to be said. It seems at times in lieu of really saying what's needed, I developed a naughty side that is still mucking around and I love that bit, though it now has to be in context. 'Princess and naughty side' are great though it would be more useful to be outspoken in truth with herself the woman to appear. The princess is going for ever – maturing – let her go, grow up and be responsible – not expecting others to do it for you.

Take the initiative.

Love and power within me

Wonderful to be me

Accept – celebrate spark of light to illuminate my life.

I say Caron tested him to the limit, and she did, in many ways, many times. For Russ some of her questioning must have been heartbreaking to bear. But she knew she'd been with someone special. She knew, too, that no one else would have done what he did. The questioning eased off towards the end, and with that came a growing sense of spirituality and serenity, and the realization that Russ had been there for her all along. As a result there was greater calm and peace between them. They complemented each other in so many ways. I think that was why Caron and Russ made such an impact wherever they went.

They were two good-looking, vibrant, interesting people with a lot going for them. Whether they were living in Barnes, Cornwall or Byron Bay, the gatherings, parties and action were at their house, around their kitchen table. Towards the end, that was partly for practical reasons, because Caron couldn't be out at restaurants, but mostly it was just how they were: they invited people in as they always had.

But that open-house policy caused problems too: if your door is always open, you can't control who walks through it. Throughout Russ and Caron's married life they attracted some wonderful people, but during the last seven years they attracted others too. Some were just there to accept their renowned generosity, others more dubious than that. The more vulnerable Caron was, the less wonderful some of these people became.

Again, Russ held steady, but it must have been hard to watch
her fall for the promises of another guru, harder still to let her
go, hoping that her inherent wisdom would bring her back.
Whoever turned up, wherever the searching took her, she
always had her anchor to come back to. Thank God, because
some of the paths on which she found herself could and did lead
to dark places.

7. The Reluctant Star

If some people are born in a trunk –
I was born with a microphone stuck in the back pocket
of my Babygro . . .

So Caron chose a career in television. But after *Blue Peter* came to an end, she found it hard to attach herself to the right vehicle. She lurched about for a while, presenting *Top of the Pops* occasionally and some current-affairs programmes. Then came *Fourth Dimension* on Channel Four, a scientifically based environmental programme, which appealed to the discoverer in her. *Summer Scene* was next, the BBC's rival to ITV's extremely successful *This Morning*. It was a daily outside broadcast from The Garden Festival near Abergavenny in Wales. Caron loved being out in the fresh air: it got her away from the city and back to her rural roots.

Michael had just left Bristol University, with the same degree as Caron, and was lured towards broadcasting. She told him to apply for a job as a runner, which he got. Caron, of course, had paid a visit to the executive producer, claiming that she was lonely living in a remote Welsh cottage on her own. He obviously didn't know her very well: 'Caron' and 'lonely' are two words I would never put together. It was nepotism at its best, and benefited them both. Quite rightly, Michael was put on the lowliest jobs – driving and a bit of research.

He and Caron had three great months together, playing house in the Welsh cottage. They worked fairly hard during the day, then had raucous evenings in the pub or dinner with the crew at the cottage, which inevitably ended up with a sing-song and a few jars. Paul was a visitor, as was Don, the ever-present male figure in Caron's life.

What was so amazing about Caron was that although she was in this cut-throat business, underlined by vanity and full of people desperate to progress in their own career, it was never that way with her. From early on, she only did things she wanted to do. She was always more interested in the people and the stories she covered than she was in her own career. That was why she loved doing *This Morning* so much. It wasn't the presenting she loved, it was the opportunity to meet such a diverse range of people. The topics and guests on *This Morning* always had an interesting angle. The fact that she was so good at presenting and looked great on camera was almost incidental.

In a strange way, her reticence drew programme-makers to her: they were intrigued by the reluctant star. And that she was so discerning meant that she was always in demand. She could probably have had any job she wanted – it was almost a coup to get her.

Paul remembers paying her a visit on *Summer Scene* and being amazed at how relaxed she was. As the producer shouted, 'two minutes' – remember, this was live television – he'd watch Caron pick up the script, glance through it, then ask him what they were going to do for lunch. She would go back to the script only when she was counted down to zero, then cut to camera and do her piece without a stutter. Totally unfazed.

She always did have an amazing ability to multi-task, and Janet Ellis will testify that this is the *Blue Peter* grounding. On top of that, she also had an unusual degree of mental dexterity and swiftness – it was simply how her mind worked. I am the complete reverse: I have to lock into whatever I am doing and give it my full attention. Paul remembers many times when he and Caron would be racing around my dressing room at BBC Northern Ireland, jumping over the sofas in some life-and-death chase, when I would suddenly say, 'Right, you two, out.' I had to focus on the programme ahead. It is still the same today: whether I'm reading research, writing a letter or working on the cancer foundation we have set up in Caron's name, I need quiet space to do it.

Maybe because I came from a relatively poor background, I had to work harder to become as good as I needed to be in order to change the course of my life. Caron didn't have that particular drive, but she was different from many of her peers: although she wanted to be good at her job, she wasn't ambitious to the point of forsaking all else. She certainly wasn't looking for a profile. I know it bored her senseless doing the 'my favourite colour' or 'what's in my fridge' interviews that often accompanied a new show. She even got a bit annoyed if it impinged on her social life. You could say that was because she was spoilt or you could say it was because she was more interesting than that, and did not want her life to become superficial. I think she was just more interested in the quality and happiness of her life. She went to showbiz parties and press nights under duress. She wasn't interested in networking, or sucking up to the bosses – she didn't like to play that game because she wasn't interested in status. Of course, she liked to be comfortable – she'd been comfortable for a long time – but she wouldn't notice the type of car she was being driven in, and certainly wasn't impressed by a personalized number-plate.

We have all worked with many presenters, a fair few of whom aren't a patch on her in terms of talent but phenomenal in terms of ego. Caron's friends think she had little ego – none for a business awash in it – but I'm not sure about that. I have to agree with Russ that everyone in the business has an ego, but some are bigger than others. If you don't have an ego you don't survive. And Caron survived. *This Morning* was the last regular programme she worked on, a much-coveted position. She didn't have to resort to using her sexuality to advance her career either, which quite frankly she could have. She was a girl's girl from the beginning. She could wrap you around her little finger, yes, but boys and girls alike succumbed because of her agile mind and charm. There was no 'cleavage and slit skirts' about Caron. She certainly possessed all the attributes, but it just wasn't her thing. Despite a stunning figure, she never even wore tight clothes. Nor was she ever desperate enough to do it.

During the years after *Blue Peter*, Cathy Comerford worked for James Grant and was often on the road with Caron. They shared a lot of hotel rooms, and Cathy noticed her intense need for privacy: Caron would get dressed in the bathroom, or in a corner of the room with the lights off. As Cathy says, 'If I looked like she did I would be dressing in the corridor.' In many ways I'm glad she did not walk around thinking she was gorgeous, although she was. Vanity is ugly on even the most beautiful faces. But there is a part of me, as her mother, which finds it sad that she had such insecurities and lacked confidence because Caron had more star quality than most.

The one thing I will never know is what it's like to have a so-called 'famous' parent. I don't know if I partially caused her introversion. I'm not stupid – I know that escaping that particular shadow isn't easy, even harder if the business you choose to work in is the same. Early on, it didn't bother her to be Gloria's girl. I know she had a huge amount of love and respect for me and my career. But as she got older it was irritating to be constantly associated with me, almost a burden. Unfortunately it was inevitable that we would be compared and contrasted. For my part I loved working with her. Competition between us, imagined or otherwise, never crossed my mind. I just loved her company, admired her talent and would have happily worked alongside her until they wheeled me out of a studio. But Caron felt that people were always trying to put us together, that it was hard for her to have separate opinions. She wanted very much to be considered her own person. I understand that while I was celebrating our similarities, she might have been wanting to prove our differences. And we were different – as the way we worked showed. She wanted to do things away from me but at times producers liked us to be together, and I can see why: we were a nice mother-daughter package. Finally she agreed, and in the early nineties we did *Family Affairs*.

Family Affairs was a BBC production and covered topics like how to bring up children, and other aspects of family life and in one year, gave us the opportunity of including Michael as a presenter, dealing with young issues like do kids spend too much time on computers. Because it came under the education banner, we had to work to a strict format; accuracy, and getting across certain messages were of paramount importance. It was not a comfortable experience for Caron. For a start it was too restrict- ive – too many interviews had to be almost rehearsed to make sure we got those educational messages to the viewer, and I think she decided then that we weren't going to do that again despite the fact that it had been running for four years. If she was going to present, it would be in her own right. Some years later we were asked to do *Open House* for Channel Five together and she said to Alan Boyd, the programme executive, in front of me, 'Mum has her career and she's very strong and very popular, and although I have my career she will always be senior to me, not only because she is my mother but because she has had more experience than me and that will always be the case. She is always going to be the stronger player in authority to me and I don't always want to be playing second fiddle.' In other words, don't lump me with my mum. For my part there was never any question that I was competing with Caron. She was my beautiful, extremely talented daughter. I was so proud of her achievements and only wanted the best for her. So being compared to her wasn't even a consideration. Yes, we were in the same business, but how many sons follow their fathers into the building profession, how many children of doctors or lawyers become doctors or lawyers? So far my part there was never a question of competing with Caron.

I know that when Radio 2 asked Caron to present a couple of programmes, she declined. By then I was doing other things, but she didn't want to step into my shoes. That says a lot about her too. Neither she nor the boys have ever coasted along on my coat-tails, as some children of other well-known parents in the industry have been known to do. Caron once worked alongside the daughter of a particularly well-known man in the business, and was genuinely surprised that she didn't write her own scripts, do any of her own research or go out and find stories. Caron couldn't understand why not – it was the bit she enjoyed most. She always had a good instinct for a story. The direct consequence of this was that Caron quickly became popular among the hacks, while the other girl never won their respect. I tell you, those old-school journalists are the hardest people in the business to win over. Bubbly blondes from *Blue Peter* are not usually their favourite sort.

Caron always prepared, and I'd like to think that that was something I'd been able to pass on: I taught her to do her homework. I always stressed to her that with interviews you must do your research – you've got to know the person before you interview them. She put this into practice and never tried to 'get away with it'. Professionally, and privately, when she was with you she was locked in one on one. She had this knack of making you feel special – she wasn't one for looking over your shoulder searching out the next person. A friend told me Caron always saw the inner person. One of the things I miss most of all is the one-to-oneness that I, and all her friends, had with her. She was always the girl I loved talking to most in the world, about life, business, family or anything else. The mere fact that she was my daughter was a huge bonus and a gift. I loved her reactions, she had a very interesting take on everything. If I ever had a problem, whether it was serious or otherwise, she had an off-the-wall but logical way of looking at it. It was a weird mix, had us both roaring with laughter but with a result. The reason why spending time with her was so rewarding was that, whether we were laughing, crying or mulling things over, she always made you feel like you were the only person in the world. We used to call it that 'Caron feel-good-factor' – it felt good to be around her.

Once again, my paradox of a daughter appeared to be breezing through life, with a career that others would have given their eye teeth for. Here was someone almost fighting off success even though she was very good at what she did. If she didn't care about the work she was doing, she wouldn't even bother doing the prep. Cathy remembers picking her up in a car to go on location and she'd have no idea where they were going. She'd still charm the pants off everyone when they got there. However, if there was something that interested here she was fantastic. They'd go up on the train reading about whatever subject was being covered and come back on a high.

She was a clever girl, an instinctive journalist and quite bold with her questioning. I can understand where her dissatisfaction with presenting came from: she wanted to report. As Paul says, and he has seen the underbelly of the entertainment business in all its forms, if you go into the industry looking for enlightenment you will be dissatisfied. He thinks television never gave her the vehicle of satisfaction and fulfilment she needed. Although Caron always had a strong sense of what she thought she wanted to do, she was a Libran and sometimes couldn't make up her mind about what that was. It was the love–hate syndrome that naturally leads to questioning, oscillating, doubting and doubling back, as Paul says, quoting the old U2 song, 'You still haven't found what you're looking for . . .' When we watch old footage, which we do now sometimes though it is a bitter-sweet exercise, we can see that what she really loved was getting beneath the skin, getting to that inner person. A piece about a broken washing-machine isn't very satisfying. Her interview with Ike Turner was a great example of what she was capable of: she launched straight into the subject of domestic violence and gave him a really hard time about how he'd justified hitting a woman. Suddenly she went up ten gears. She was underachieving and I bet she knew it. She was so talented at writing and art, but television rarely gave her a way to express her creativity.

We always talked about business, but Russ was the one advising her. In latter years, when our interviewees crossed over, she would often call up and say, 'Mum, have you done Sean Connery?' and I could steer her towards the subjects I knew he'd respond to. And vice versa. We compared notes a lot and had a real belly laugh about things when they went wrong, or when we came across intolerable people. I remember when Raquel Welch came to be interviewed for *Sunday Sunday*: she asked for a salad and was wholly unimpressed by the soggy lettuce leaf, sliced tomato and boiled egg that the production assistant brought her. She picked up the egg and threw it across the makeup room, screaming, 'What's this?' Oh, yes, we laughed about those things.

Caron had the most wonderful wicked sense of humour and a delicious sense of fun. Yes, she was quick to blow up, but most of the time she was laughing. I don't blow up often but, my God, when I do, it's time to duck. As my mother always said, 'You don't miss anyone and hit the wall. It just goes bosh.' Maybe it's that Northern Irish thing again, of dealing with things in a very direct way: we have to get these things off our chest. Or maybe it's just a fiery temper. In our defence, I say that because we were mostly doing live telly, we didn't always have time for the softly-softly approach. I can't speak for Caron, but I know that if I lost my temper at work it was because the show was live and there was no time for niceties. I had to get it right. We were the ones on screen, the ones who'd look the fool. I used to say, 'Look, it's nothing personal, it's just the beast of live TV.'

In 1992 Caron got the job of entertainment correspondent on *London Tonight* – the showbiz desk of London News Network, part of ITN. Yasmin Pacha, one of the few friends Caron told about her illness, remembers when she joined. Their boss at the time was a producer called Bob Massey, slightly brusque but a good man, who'd been in charge of interviewing for the position. He had interviewed a couple of quite well-known people, but they were so full-on compared to Caron, who just breezed in, was so natural, warm and friendly – such a relief from the 'ambition on legs' type – that he hired her. Little did he know that, just as Don had bluffed his way into ABC, Caron had played him:

We'd just moved house that morning, and Russ, helpfully, was feeling terrible and lying face down on our bedroom floor while men shifted wardrobes and boxes around his groaning form. Eventually I headed off to Mum's house in Fulham to wash off the cobwebs and dust from the move and make myself reasonably presentable for the meeting. It is really unlike me to be early but that day I found myself sitting outside LWT with about twenty minutes to spare. Idly I flicked through the radio stations eventually settling on Radio 4's arts programme *Front Row*. It had a piece on a new controversial Irish play that had opened in Islington, the latest movie reviews and a music piece. I half listened to the programme, nervous about what they were going to ask me.

Finally I went in. 'What story would you put in tonight's show?' the editor inquired. I thanked the gods and Radio 4, and launched into hastily recalled details of the play. Later they asked if I could produce and edit my own films. It was one of those moments when I knew the absolute truth would lose me the gig – but there was a strong possibility that it was merely a previously untested talent. I made my choice. 'Yes,' I replied.

'Could we see one?'

This proved slightly trickier – but a film-producer friend allowed me to pass off one of his as my own and I got the job. The first film I made had to be edited about six times. I would sit in the darkened editing suite, willing the list of shots on the page in front of me to weave themselves magically into some kind of cohesive, entertaining story. 'What shot do you want next?' the editor would call. In the first few sessions I was overcome at this point with an overwhelming desire to go to the loo, get some chocolate, tea – anything rather than have to make a decision. I prayed they would have sorted it out by the time I returned and, more often than not, they had. I must have spent the first six months subtly bribing editors with snacks and warm drinks until the glorious day when one turned round and said: 'You're one of the better reporters at putting pieces together.' The bluff had paid off.

We ran close to the wire, though. Often you would be editing a story with the programme already on air and slamming it into the machine with a minute to spare. On one such occasion I bumped into the editor having just made my time slot. 'Better than sex, isn't it?' he quipped. Well, I'm not sure I was ever enthralled to quite that degree.

Yes, the bluff paid off. In more ways than one. Caron went into what was a very tough news environment from what was rather derogatively considered a background of children's television. Yasmin was an investigative journalist and admits that they slightly dismissed the showbiz desk to some extent even when you hadn't the added burden of having come from the children's sector. But despite Caron's feeling of inadequacy it soon became clear to Yasmin that Caron was good at her job. Live TV and pieces to camera, she did brilliantly. At first the technicians thought, Here comes another pretty blonde to add to the pile, but when they watched her at work, saw how ultra-focused she was, they quickly re-evaluated her. As Paul says, she could look at a script, then turn to the camera and deliver the words. Her concentration and overview were phenomenal. Yasmin agrees that Caron probably never thought she was as good as she was. To deliver words with warmth, accuracy and passion to an inanimate object like a lens is a great talent. She could do it.

Yasmin says she was not only natural but unaffected and unassuming. She says people liked being interviewed by her, whether they were stars or members of the general public, because she was a bright girl and had a natural curiosity that disregarded rank. When Caron was doing the showbiz stuff her intelligence and quirkiness stood her in good stead: she wouldn't insult the big stars – who, remember, do press junkets back to back – by asking the same old questions. She would find a new, bizarre angle and get them talking. The result was that people liked coming on the show. They were comfortable with her. Yasmin admits to the fiery side of Caron and her microphone. Once Caron was interviewing Tony Curtis, the actor, at his art exhibition. It was like getting blood out of a stone. She tried everything, deviating wildly from the norm to get his attention. It didn't work. He was obviously tired, and bored, and had had enough of the circus. So Caron pulled off her mike, threw it down and walked away, hands up, saying loudly, 'What's the point?' For a while, a bemused Tony Curtis went on discussing his paintings without her. In the end he was incredibly apologetic, coaxed her back and, together, they delivered a perfect interview.

In my darkest days since Caron died, one of the most comforting things Yasmin has assured me of is that Caron was proud of our extremely close mother and daughter relationship and proud of my career achievements. Perhaps I did help her more than I realized. Apparently she would study me objectively as a professional, see my strong points, my weaknesses, and mentally make notes of things that worked and things that didn't. She'd do it with other presenters, but I'm told mostly with me. Assuming that was the case, I am flattered. I hope it means she thought I was a bit of an inspiration, rather than a threat. I hope I was someone she wanted to live up to. I know from the conversations I've had that she would often say to her colleagues, 'I was listening to Mum on the radio and thought, That's a clever way of doing it.' Or 'Mum says if you do it like this, it might work . . .' Yasmin also said Caron had told her many other things over the years, hints and advice I had given her, which Caron liked to spread around. I think the professional link augmented our mother–daughter bond. It certainly gave us common ground and always something to talk about. And as far as having a mum in the public eye went, again Yasmin says it was never an issue. Pure and simple. But this was long before Caron's dark days of questioning and searching.

Caron had been having a ball, but the best was yet to come. In 1993 when she discovered she was pregnant, Russ and she were over the moon. I will never forget when they made their announcement to all the family. We were in the New Forest spending Christmas and New Year with our great friends John and Michelle Carlton-Smith – all having a Christmas Eve drink around the fire, when Caron and Russ delivered their fantastic and exciting news. They had lost one pregnancy very early on in their marriage when they weren't really ready, but now they were, and the birth of their first child was eagerly anticipated. Caron enjoyed the whole process of being pregnant. I do remember, in the height of summer on an exceptionally hot day, Stephen and I came home and found her, weeks away from giving birth, lying on the sofa literally panting in the heat. Next to her Che, our Labrador, was lying prostrate in much the same manner.

One of the most marvellous things Caron gave me, maybe the ultimate gift, which I never would have even dreamt of asking for, was the privilege of being at Charlie's birth. One day she said, 'Would you like to be with me and Russ at the birth?' What a phenomenal gesture. It was so generous, something I will always treasure. Caron had a long labour and we were there all day, in and out, getting bottles of water. When it got quite close to the actual birth, I felt I couldn't stay in the room because they had to use forceps and I thought it was getting too personal. Outside the door I could hear a woman in the next room screaming, and I paced up and down, praying that Caron wasn't going through that sort of pain. Then Charlie was born, and they called me back in literally as they cut the cord. I saw him being placed on the scales, still covered with blood, having his Apgar test completed and they made sure everything was working as it should. It was. Indescribable joy. It was one of the most emotional experiences of my life. When they put him on Caron's chest, she just looked at him and, with her big wide smile, said, 'Hello, baby.' It was very very special, a second I'll never forget.

Gabriel's birth of course took place in very different circumstances. Don had just died and Caron had to have the baby induced. But it was just as magical and I felt the same surge of being so fortunate to be there again through the labour. This time I stayed in the room, saw Gabriel being born and the cord being cut. Now I look back and wonder whether in the great scheme of things, I was there for a reason: there is no question about it, the bond is even stronger and more immediate when you see a baby being born. A gift from God – an extra layer of attachment, an extra layer of understanding. Often when we are celebrating the children's birthdays, I quietly reflect on the joy and privilege of being right there at their births.

I was present at Paul's son Jake's birth for an unexpected reason and saw him seconds after he was delivered. It was Christmas night, I'd slaved over the turkey and trimmings, had a wonderful time with the family that evening and fallen into bed completely shattered. Because Sandy, my daughter-in-law, was so pregnant I'd given her our bed and Stephen and I were on the fold-out in the study. It felt like I'd been asleep for just seconds when I felt a gentle tug on my arm and Paul said, 'Mum, Sandy's gone into labour.'

The whole house was buzzing. Caron was timing Sandy's contractions, Paul was ill with a fever, Russ was scraping ice off the cars – it was mayhem. Michael was asleep and didn't know anything about it until the next morning. I was doing panto in Bromley at the time and was due to be on stage on Boxing Day so took a separate car. Paul who was suffering from flu and no doubt nerves was lying in the back of the car which Stephen was driving. Sandy was holding Stephen's hand while he drove, saying, 'I never thought I'd be holding your hand.' We got to the hospital and, because Paul was sick and Sandy's mother was away in Switzerland, I obviously stayed with her. Missed the performance but saw Jake born. Fortunately, Paul recovered enough to get into theatre gown and mask. It was an honour to be with Sandy while she was in labour, to be around during the Caesarean and see Jake in Paul's green-gowned arms. I had never seen Paul look so proud.

Beau was born on the night before Stephen's and my wedding day. Naturally we just had to see him. I simply couldn't walk down the aisle with seven grandchildren and not have seen the eighth – Stephen's sons, Dominic and Matthew, have four children between them. At six o'clock in the morning, I laid eyes on the best wedding present anyone could wish for and was an exceedingly happy bride. Of course, I would have wanted Sandy and Beau there on the day but, as I know from Caron's birth, childbirth is something you can't completely plan for.

With Charlie's birth I became a grandmother for the first time. Journalists had asked me before how I felt about becoming a grandmother and I would say, 'Hugely excited, but I don't really want to be called Granny, thank you very much.' But when the baby is born you realize you couldn't care less what you're called because it's deep unconditional love all over again. It's almost better than having your own children because all you have to do is love grandchildren: the discipline and routine are no longer your immediate concern. It was such a joyous time.

Each grandchild is a gift and I love them all to distraction. Now they give me my best and most rewarding times.

In those early days of parenthood, Caron and Russ were living in Barnes, West London, and I was able to spend a lot of time with mother and baby. I was always in and out of the house, pushing the pram proudly around the 'village' and the pond. Now I find the weight of responsibility for our grandchildren even greater but completely joyous and rewarding at the same time. When they stay with us in Sevenoaks on their own, at times I'm quite nervous. When it's your own children you know you're doing your best – but heaven forbid that anything should happen to a grandchild when they're with us because maybe Paul and Sandy, or Russ would think we hadn't been taking enough care of them or paying enough attention. As it was for Caron, Sevenoaks is a mainstay in Charlie and Gabriel, Jake and Beau's lives. Charlie came here as a baby, and the tea-set he played with is still here, as are many of the children's other toys. They know where everything is, the books and paints are still kept in the same cupboard, and they adore Stephen, who is the perfect grandfather. He is always making things with them – wooden planes, swords and shields – or 'fixing', as Charlie used to call it.

They are always drawing and painting pictures for us that I stick up all over the kitchen. One of my favourites is a Nana's Day card that I received on that first ghastly Mother's Day without my daughter. It was a day I thought I wouldn't survive, and the reason to go on came in the post. If the truth were told, my grandchildren have truly helped me through the past year. At my bleakest, when I could see nothing ahead but crippling sadness, the children would remind me that Caron is still here for her spirit is in them. When loss is at its deepest, it is a huge beam of light to watch my grandchildren because I see them as a symbol of the future and that life does and has to go on. If I ever feel glum when they're not here, all I have to do is look at the holes in my hedge where their football has gone through to be reminded of their inexhaustible zest for life. Just like Caron's. They're always up to something. One of the few things Caron asked me to do was this. She said, 'Promise me you'll always look after the boys.' And as long as I have breath in my body, I will.

8. Working Mother After Five

25 July

Today is Charlie's birthday – it feels like yesterday that he was born and I feel so blessed to have had this wonderful boy born into our family. Joyful, kind, gentle, fun-loving, loyal, sensitive, patient, laughing, singing, honourable, artistic, home-loving, gorgeous – our son.

Eagerly on this day nine years ago we wanted to meet you. You'd played football in my tummy for the last few months, your heel would suddenly cross the stretched landscape of my belly as you stretched and rolled in your water chamber – safe, secure, loved and sheltered. It was hard to persuade you to leave – desperate to know you, I was induced. 'Tell me when you're fed up reading *Vogue* and the womb goes squiggly and we'll know something is happening,' said the doctor. It was a gentle day – looking at your tiny clothes, little nappies and Babygros, that I could only dream about putting on you. And then towards the end of the day, my baby began to unfurl, getting ready to present this miracle – it's been growing for nine months. Hello, baby.

12 May

Just read a book Charlie gave me, *The Dream*, about a boy who is asked by the animals to help clean up the planet and keep it that way. Charlie wants to do it too – save animals and the environment. I feel as if my beautiful, sensitive son has entrusted me with his own dream. Recently he has been composing songs about talking to and helping animals survive. It seems to be quite a calling to him and he is certainly wonderful with them. Both he and Gabriel are enjoying and being fabulous with Pippin, our little mongrel puppy, who's been a truly inspired addition to our family and very, very loved.

Caron was totally elated after Charlie's birth in July but she was back at work in October. She appeared to take everything in her stride. Physically she bounced back quite quickly – I don't recall any stretchmarks or hard-to-shift pregnancy weight. She just got on with it, as she did everything else. Going back to work after childbirth wasn't unusual in our family. I went back ten days after Michael was born – madness, maybe, but it had seemed a good idea at the time. Fern Britton, the presenter of *After 5*, had given birth to twins and couldn't get back to work as quickly as she'd anticipated so Caron was asked to take over full time. I think in many ways the two years that followed Charlie's birth were the halcyon days of Russ and Caron's marriage. They were a glorious couple, young, handsome and blessed with their firstborn. Work was good for both of them; they could afford child-care and back-up, and had a lovely house. It was a carefree, happy time with no serious worries. They were exceedingly lucky in that Russ didn't work the conventional seventy hours a week in the City: he was his own boss. From the very beginning he took to fatherhood like a duck to water and loved spending time with Charlie.

A lot of men, my first husband included, do not change their ways when children are born, but with Caron and Russ it was a fifty-fifty split. Caron made sure he was a new man and had strong views on sharing parental responsibility, which stands Russ in good stead now that she has gone. From the beginning he changed his fair share of nappies and could do a bottle as well as any maternity nurse. They were equals in everything. In business Russ was flourishing and so was Caron, so not only were they balanced in terms of their allocation of responsibility but in terms of their income. It was an even-pegged, happy relationship on all fronts. They both completely and utterly adored Charlie from day one. Many fathers take a while to bond with their children – babies are scary to the uninitiated – but not Russ. Maybe Caron going back to work so soon allowed father and son to create a bond independent of her. Russ didn't have Caron peering over his shoulder all the time, making sure that the nappy was on the right way. Like a lot of modern men, Russ learnt early to fend for himself and the boys in the kitchen. Strange, isn't it? It's almost as if he has been in training since the day Charlie was born. I don't know, but it makes me think: is it all written in the stars? Is it all part of that big picture?

After 5 turned out to be the perfect job for Caron. She could be at home in the morning with Charlie, have a social life with all the other Barnes mummies, go in to work in the afternoon, and still be home in time to put Charlie to bed and have the evening with her husband. And she loved her job. She interviewed a lot of people for *After 5*, did a lot of great reporting and honed her skills. There was no superiority on set, and Yasmin can't recall any tantrums either − in any case, she wouldn't have put up with any nonsense. Yasmin has on her kitchen wall a photo-montage of all the people who worked on *After 5* at that time, from the presenters to the researchers, the producers to the news editor. Not every show you do has such a family feel. Caron worked with this great gang for three years and made some solid, long-lasting friendships. The Soho House Mafia, they were: central London − the 'in place'. Endless girly dinners were had there. They sat around chatting late into the night about anything and everything, drinking champagne and poncing fags. Those get-togethers made Caron happy: her wild streak had retreated by then. Friends knew that she'd partied harder in her twenties, but once children are on the scene, you go through a portal and there's no going back.

Even I made it on to *After 5*. It was their Christmas special and I brought Charlie on as a big surprise. You should have seen Caron − the pride just beamed out of her, stronger than all the studio lights. They had set up a living room, with a fireplace and tree, and there were cameras everywhere. It was a big deal for what was effectively a small-budget show, and as always

Caron was word-perfect. They didn't have autocue, so, like *Blue Peter*, she learnt her script, like the professional she was. Honestly, you see so many people who are supposed to be professional, and they stop endlessly: Yasmin says they never stopped because of Caron, only because something technical had gone wrong.

The Christmas special wasn't the only time I went on the show. I brought out a cookery book of my mother's old Irish recipes and Caron, never one to miss an opportunity, teased me live on air that she couldn't recall me ever cooking any of the dishes. In fact, all she could remember was endless fish fingers. I should have told them the boiled-egg story and got my own back. And what a case of the pot calling the kettle black. Although she improved hugely and was more eager when she became interested in vegetarian cooking and healthy organic food, she was not what I would call a natural or enthusiastic cook. Janet Ellis remembers being at the house in Barnes for a dinner party. Caron was looking angelic in an apron (I think perhaps Janet was drunk – I'm not sure Caron possessed such an item), standing at the stove stirring a simmering pot. Peter Powell walked in and said, 'What a picture – a beautiful woman, in a beautiful house, a wonderful mother, a glorious wife, a great presenter and here she is cooking a fabulous meal . . .' What a load of baloney! Caron had many talents, but a domestic goddess she was not.

Yasmin puts another slant on Caron's lack of culinary skills. She says they were all as bad as each other at that time. Dinner at any of their houses was pasta, sauce out of a jar, and if you were at Caron's a Sarah Lee Apple Danish with ice-cream for pudding. No wonder they took up residency at Soho House for their dietary requirements. Cooking came later, as the children grew up and Caron became more interested in a much more healthy diet for them. But by then, of course, Caron had other things on her mind.

Perhaps the only serious blight on that blissful time was Caron's next miscarriage. It was worse than the first because she and Russ really wanted a second child. But again, her positivity gave her the ability to look at it philosophically. She believed, since it had happened early on, that it wasn't meant to be and bounced back pretty quickly after a couple of days off work. After mourning her loss, she made herself believe it was for the best. Generally she was very practical – but not when she became pregnant again, this time with Gabriel. She was at work very early editing a piece. An editor told Yasmin that she was a bit worried about Caron: apparently she'd had a car accident and 'looked a bit wobbly'. So Yasmin went in to her and asked if she was okay. She clearly wasn't: her neck was hurting and she had a severe headache but, conscientious as ever, she felt she had to finish the work. She wouldn't allow herself to go home until Yasmin told her it was mad to stay, reminded her she was pregnant, and pushed her out the door. Turned out she had major whiplash.

Another trait that Caron's colleagues recall was that she liked to send naughty little messages around the office, always maintaining the butter-wouldn't-melt expression on her face. Or while she and Yasmin were making small-talk to someone, Caron would whisper something rude in her ear and watch Yasmin struggle to keep a straight face. I think Caron enjoyed being naughty like that because it was unexpected, because she didn't look the type, because she liked to be re-evaluated. She liked to shock:

There is something magical about live TV. Knowing that as the words leave your lips they are simultaneously being heard in living rooms all over the country. The thought that I literally could say whatever I wanted and no one could stop me used to make me feel giddy at times. *After 5* started with a long, sweeping shot round the studio as the opening music played and frequently I would sit there, overcome with a sort of mild Tourette's, thinking up phrases packed with swear words to start the show. I never quite plucked up the courage.

The closest I got was telling a couple of reporters to 'F*** off'. They happened to work for the *Mirror* and for some reason it ended up on the front page – as though they were shocked that a *Blue Peter* presenter could possibly know such a phrase. A surprising number of my peers congratulated me afterwards – I can only think that more of us are tempted to turn the air blue than we let on. Though I did once introduce a particularly flirtatious guest who happened to be on after a film about fairgrounds with the words, 'You look like a fella who's had a fair few rides in your time.' Both of us snorted with laughter, which, of course, grew the more we tried to control it.

Once Yasmin and Caron were talking to the boys from East 17, and they were doing the angelic-boy act – anti-drugs, how Elvis had influenced them. After they had walked off Caron said, 'They're talking to us as if we're their aunties. We're rock chicks, can't they see that?' Oh, yes, Caron was always up for a laugh. A strange mix of whimsical and practical. And always very positive.

The gang at *After 5* always worried about work, but I gather Caron always gave logical and thoughtful advice, without being 'nice'. Yasmin remembers being terribly upset when the press called her and her female colleagues 'journo-babes'. But Caron said, 'Ooh, I wouldn't mind being called a journo-babe. We are thirty-four, after all.' After a moment's thought, Yasmin agreed.

Caron was also very kind to her peers. When Fiona Foster got bad news at work, she retreated to her dressing room. Caron appeared with a pen and paper and, before Fiona could sink too low, had written a list of all the people she had to phone and what she should do about the situation. Another time one of the researchers, a girl called Elka, was tearing around the studio in a panic having decided to get married at the last minute. She didn't have any shoes. Caron came in the next day with her own wedding shoes and said, 'You'll need something borrowed, so take these.' Another colleague remembers not being able to afford maternity clothes when she was heavily pregnant, but the next day Caron duly appeared with hers saying, 'You need these more than I do at the moment!' She was an extremely caring person, always thinking about and sensitive to others, acutely so. Yasmin says she can hear Caron saying, 'God, I wasn't that nice,' but she was. She just didn't make a big deal about it. When Yasmin and her husband were going skiing, Yasmin had mentioned in passing that they didn't have any of the kit. Caron turned up the day after with a huge bag of skiing stuff for her, and Russ's stuff for her husband.

Apparently she was always lending Russ's stuff – Russ too, if she thought he could help. When Yasmin went for a new job, Caron immediately offered Russ's help with the contract. I doubt she even asked him. I'm sure he didn't mind – she would have done it out of respect for him: she always admired his business acumen. Again, it demonstrates how complementary their relationship was. Caron was bright, but not business-savvy; Russ was the focused one – he covered the angles. Mind you, that didn't stop the girls ganging up against him on those oestrogen-heavy, booze-fuelled evenings in Barnes when the Sarah Lee was overcooking in the oven. Poor Russ! I know what those girly dinners were like – they'd end up screaming with laughter, loud, bawdy and blue. I'm sure there were moments when Russ wanted to run from the kitchen-table witches.

At lunchtime it was generally assumed that Caron would make a mad dash to the shops. With her determined stride, she could be in Covent Garden in six minutes flat. Boy, could that girl shop! She was professional, a career shopper. If it were an Olympic sport, she'd have won consecutive golds. If there was ever a problem, retail therapy was the answer. Another of

Caron's mottoes: If the going gets tough, the tough go shopping.
She wasn't shy about it: if it was a case of the green or the blue
top, she'd get both. Among all the thousands of things I miss
about Caron, those wonderful shopping trips we shared are one
of the things I miss the most. It wasn't what we bought that
made them fun, it was being together and laughing. I would
come out of the dressing room and Caron would cock her head
to one side and say, 'Far too mumsy. Try this.' Or she would
pick out a scarf that went perfectly with the jacket I was looking
at. Sometimes when I'm out and about alone, I see mothers and
daughters doing the same thing. I am consumed with envy when
I see them sit down for a glass of wine and lunch together.
Sometimes I feel like going up to them and saying, 'Treasure
this moment. Do you know how precious it is?' I would give
anything for just one of the glorious days we spent together, out
on the town with my beautiful daughter, sharing private jokes,
treating ourselves to lunch, talking about everything and
nothing. I would give everything.

Her colleagues agree that it is only now that they realize quite
how beautiful she was. Although she shopped like an addict,
she wasn't one of those immaculate women who are constantly
co-ordinated. (No guessing why not: Caron always used to say,
'Mum can't talk without her lipstick on.' I certainly never tapped
into the grunge look that she perfected.) But at the time, her
looks weren't a big deal: she'd go to work in one of Russ's
shirts, a pair of jeans and Doc Martens, often no makeup and
hair up in a pencil. It was a far cry from the days of hiding under
the duvet in Bristol: presumably she'd got more comfortable
with her appearance and was happy to be scruffy. By then she
knew she could glam up if she had to. However, Yasmin was
always aware that she wasn't confident about her figure, and
though she shopped for England and would try on quite daring
outfits, they weren't the ones that made it to the till. Again,
there is that Caron Keating dichotomy: vain but shy, confident

but unsure, outgoing but understated. Yasmin keeps it simpler: 'More often than not she was looking as rough as the next person.' She never changed.

When I presented *This Morning*, I would go in bleary-eyed, in whatever happened to be handy and clean. An hour later, after some intensive input from the makeup and wardrobe department, the wonderful Lee Din, who did makeup, would stand back, look at me and pronounce, 'Thank God you're back. We'll send your sister to the attic for another day.'

She had enormous style, and a fantastic eye for clothes and art. In all her houses the kitchens looked the same. She had so much stuff, teapots, Victorian china, wooden cherubs, you name it, and all her friends have items in their houses that she made them buy. I can pretty much pick them out. It was all very distinctive: little sayings on the walls, heart-shaped mirrors, candles, fairy-lights – she created a lovely environment. Poor old Russ – it's a man's nightmare, I should think, especially since his taste is minimalist. Somehow he and Caron agreed early on that Caron wouldn't be irritated by his neatness and he wouldn't be annoyed by her clutter. Since every one of their houses was filled with Caron's bits and pieces, I suspect my daughter got her own way again.

But apart from a bit of mess, I don't think Caron gave Russ much to worry about: when she'd got her man that was that. She was off the market. The only threat he might have had, if he had been around at the time, was David Essex. Sorry, Russ, but there's no point in pretending that Caron had anything other than a massive crush on the man. I'm fairly sure it was public knowledge. The *After 5* gang used to give her so much stick about it. Somehow they managed to make him a regular on the show – they even got him for Caron's birthday and the last show she did. Of course he knew why, and it became a standing joke between them all. He was really sweet about it and didn't seem to mind a doe-eyed presenter asking him questions on subjects he knew nothing about.

Of course, what the gang at *After 5* didn't know was that Caron had known David for several years. They had met for the first time in the early eighties. I was singing on *The Val Doonican Show*, and Caron had always idolized David, he had adorned her bedroom walls for years. So when she discovered he was appearing too, she was over the moon. While I was out on set strutting my stuff, David went to my dressing room and asked Caron if she would like to go with him and watch my performance in the studio. He didn't have to ask twice: she was in seventh heaven. Some time later he was to play in Bristol. As Caron was still at university he said he'd send her some tickets and took her phone number. It was getting better and better. But instead of ringing her about the tickets, he asked her out to dinner in London. How could she refuse? Her boyfriend at the time, Shaun, accompanied her to the station and she waved him off, dressed head to foot in the student grunge uniform, and pretended to leave for Bristol. What she actually did was go to the toilets, change into her finery and set off for Broadcasting House. There he was – David Essex in reception, surrounded by adoring fans, when Caron turned up dragging an ancient carpet bag behind her. David prised himself away from the crowd, hoisted her dirty laundry into the boot of his blue Rolls-Royce and whisked her off to the Elephant on the River for a night to remember. What went on during the filming of *After 5* was child's play compared to that. See what I mean about Caron appearing to do one thing, then doing something completely different? I should make it clear that nothing happened at the time – all a bit of fun.

So, David Essex could turn her head, but generally Caron saw showbiz for what it was: she was impressed by talent, not celebrity for the sake of it. Her mistrust of and distaste for phoney people increased with age. Unfortunately the business has its fair share so Caron probably came across more than most. When she did, she didn't waste time pretending to think otherwise. Consequently, while she had great friends and was loyal to the end, she also made some enemies. She wasn't going to waste a precious evening talking to someone just because they could help her up the ladder, and some of the people she brushed aside did not take kindly to it. Caron didn't care. She knew who her friends were, and equally they knew they could always depend on her.

For two and a half years Caron presented *After 5* live, had a great social life, an adoring husband, a beautiful boy, money, a great career, a lovely house, a supportive and spoiling family, her looks and her health. Yes, Caron had it all. Then the cherry on the cake. A second pregnancy that stayed the course. However, to return to Don, Caron didn't see as much of her father as she would have liked during her pregnancy. And she wasn't only pregnant: she had a toddler and was working full time. Don had been retired since the age of forty-nine. Until now Caron and Russ had gone to Ireland to see him. It was easier that way because Don was just a bit stuck in his ways by then. Now, though, Caron wanted him to come to her. Not as easy as you'd think. For one thing, Don was always pleading poverty. He would never just buy a ticket. He'd always go on stand-by and wait for the cheaper seats, which often never came up. He would send the children cards saying, 'See you soon,' but a visit took weeks to plan. As Paul says, it would have been easier to plan a world tour with the Royal Family than get Don to England. Perhaps the situation was made slightly more complicated by the fact that Don now had a third son, Patrick. Even though they didn't live together, Don saw Patrick every day and was very close to him. In the end Russ provided the solution: he bought the tickets for Don. Even that wasn't straightforward. Don would faff about and miss three days of the holiday. Maybe changing his routine had become a hurdle as he got older. We all travelled relentlessly: Paul was off all over the world setting up sound systems for concerts and the like, Caron and I travelled for work and Michael rarely keeps still. But Don was not impetuous like us in that respect. So no, they sometimes didn't understand it.

That's not to say that when Don finally arrived he and Caron didn't have a fantastic time. They did. In the end the children were simply amused by his quirky habits, like never turning on the heating or sitting in a pitch black house with just one light and the television on. One of their endearing memories is of when Caron and Paul went over to Don's for a weekend. They put Sunday lunch on to cook slowly while they were at the pub. Unbeknown to them, just before they left, Don turned everything off so they ended up having lunch at seven p.m.

Caron had noticed that Don was slowing down a bit. When he came to stay with her they were supposed to be going to an exhibition together, but he said he was too tired, so she took Yasmin instead. His earlier trips had been busy and full. But all of the children were busy – life was fast-paced – so it was hard to spot the warning signs. Although I always considered my relationship with Caron as close and bonded as any mother and daughter could be, I would say that Don was a safe place for her. He was there all the time in the same house. Paul didn't quite see it like that: he thought Don should move on, that it was odd for him to be stuck in the house that represented their childhood. But Caron found it reassuring. She took a lot of responsibility for her dad, was naturally protective of him and wanted to look after him. Every Saturday they had their 'Don chats', so even though they didn't see each other much, they were still exceedingly close.

So here was Caron, heavily pregnant with Gabriel, just about coping with juggling her life. One weekend Yasmin and she drove home to Brighton for a hen night. Yasmin remembers it vividly because they were talking about pensions. Caron told

Yasmin that she didn't have one, and Yasmin was shocked at her lack of forward planning. Caron, game as ever, took her bump shopping in the Lanes, and together they bought up Brighton. Then Caron wanted to go and get a bag of chips and a cup of tea, even though they were due to go to the hen-night dinner an hour later. Yasmin agreed, so off they went and sat on the beach eating chips. Again, Yasmin remembers it because Caron talked about 'white noise', communicating with the dead, the spirit world and life after death. Perversely, or maybe reassuringly, she'd always been fascinated by 'other-worldly' subjects and was always quite spiritually aware. But it was objective. Apart from losing my mother, to whom she had been exceptionally close, Caron had never come face to face with death, and although the loss of a grandparent is sad, it isn't traumatic. It is the order of things, and when things are in order, there is less need to question them. That was all about to change.

On the following Monday night, Yasmin threw a baby shower for Caron and another girl called Claire. It was a really lovely evening. Although she was cross that Don hadn't made it over to see her, Russ and Charlie at Christmas, Caron was looking forward to a trip they had planned to Florida in February, with him and the new baby. It was turning into quite a gathering as Yasmin and her husband John, Fiona Foster and her husband were also going to be there at the same time. They planned to meet up for one of Don's famous barbecues. Everyone has vivid memories of what happened next. Yasmin had to go to hospital for a major operation. When she came out of surgery John told her that, out of the blue, Caron's father had died. Her first thought was concern for Caron. She knew how precarious the last weeks of a pregnancy can be. She was right to worry.

On 24 January 1997, I got a message to call my father in Ireland, only to be told by a stranger on the other end – a policeman, as it turned out, plus the son of a neighbour – that Dad had died of a heart-attack. I was nine months pregnant at the time with my second son Gabriel and it was just the last thing I was expecting.

Life has never been the same since. There are certain events which come along and just turn what you remember as your life totally inside out. Things continue to shift and move in a way that astounds, intrigues and often terrifies me. But it was the start of the most extraordinary journey which continues to career along in the most unusual way.

I was thirty-four at the time, working in TV, about to give birth any day and totally unprepared for this event. My first reaction was to get on a plane to Ireland and just be at his home to see where he was, to smell his smell – that slightly stale odour of cigarettes.

I travelled in a large man's coat and managed to get on the plane without anyone noticing my very large bump. We'd already arranged for an obstetrician friend of the family to get me into hospital if I went into labour.

I don't remember much about the flight, except the relief of getting to the house, falling into my mother's arms and just sobbing and sobbing. She had been in Belfast the night before, doing a live TV show, and there had been many calls trying to resolve whether to tell her beforehand or not. In the end we decided to let her do the show without having the knowledge that Dad had died.

He died sitting at the end of our kitchen table, a long rectangle where we'd had endless conversations deep into the night – countless family meals – meals where there had been just him and me. Then, after the divorce, many meals by himself.

He'd been eating nuts and cheese, drinking a glass of red wine, and been found with a really peaceful expression on his face, the most peaceful the coroner had ever seen. Apparently his head had just dropped on to his chest as if he were asleep.

Later, a friend told me that he and Dad had discussed death and decided that when the time came, the best thing was 'to get the fuck out'. In that respect, it was pretty perfect – just a bit too soon.

On Saturday mornings we'd both listen to *Loose Ends* on Radio 4, and afterwards in what we'd call my 'Don time' we'd share our thoughts and lives on the phone. When I rang the house that Friday night after the urgent messages on the answerphone, an unfamiliar country accent answered and I knew then what had happened. While I'd been out shopping that day, feeling slightly strange, as though part of me already knew what my ears had yet to hear, your spirit was soaring off to some other planet. Your body was propped up in your usual spot at the end of the kitchen table, where you so often peacefully saw the evenings away, but your spirit had moved on in the next great adventure.

The hours we spent around that table – eating, drinking, smoking but always talking. Spirited talks, drunken talks, great long talks, talks that reached far into the night and were continued the next morning. So much so you often had to put your hand up just to get a word in edgeways. Now that table sits in my home but it isn't the same without you. If I sit there and talk to you – will you still hear me and listen like you did so well all my life? Would I ever have known about so many things in my life if you hadn't told me? The magic world of books, books we both escaped into and delightfully shared with each other. When you died, I was reading one that had a photo of a little dark-haired boy on the cover. It reminded me, from those old family photographs, of how you looked as a kid. I was keeping it for you.

Then there were all those journeys back from Fermanagh where we spent so many of our weekends, when we played *Simon and Garfunkel's Greatest Hits*. It was the only tape you had in the car – I still know all the words.

Who's going to try and stop me spending my money now – buying dresses I don't need, trying to bargain with the girls in M&S when you used to say, 'It's only a bargain if you need it'?

It was a shocking day for all of us. I'd thought Don would go on and on. I knew something was up while I waited to go on air, but never linked everyone's strange behaviour to him. I can remember it as if it were yesterday. There was no buzz in the studio, no exuberance. It was as if people were avoiding me, and of course they were. It was a big starry programme with David Soul, Caprice and Val Doonican, and although I thought I'd done a good job, still no one said anything to me. The next thing I knew Stephen skimmed me off into a dressing room and told me that Don had died at home of a massive heart-attack. It was such a shock: he had been a man who took things easy, played golf, read books – it had seemed there was no stress in his life.

Paul was on a work trip in Thailand, a seven-hour drive south of Bangkok. He says that getting home was an out-of-body experience he'll never forget. Michael rang him at two a.m. and he spent the whole night not knowing what to do. He still had to rig the show he was working on, and until a replacement arrived he had to carry on. People kept coming up to him and saying, 'So sorry about your father, but where do you want the RF mics placed?' Finally he boarded a flight to London, then another to Belfast. It felt like it took him a year to get back. And when he did, we were all there. Including, amazingly, his sister. Overdue and ready to give birth at any time.

Russ was there when Caron was called with the news late on the Friday night. The expression on her face said it all. Utter disbelief. It could not have come at a worse time, because during the latter weeks of pregnancy she hadn't wanted to fly. Don had kept promising to come over, but never did. The fact that he hadn't been there at Christmas, a time of tradition that Caron particularly adored, had really upset her. It wasn't as if there'd been animosity between them, but there had been a little friction there never had been before. When the news came she was tired and hormonal, so it floored her. Johnny Comerford, knowing how close Caron was to Don, went straight round to her house. He says she was in a very bad way, terribly shocked and upset, and it was in that state that she made the decision to go to Ireland.

When we look back now, what she did seems mad. On the

plane she actually started having contractions so when they arrived she and Russ had a choice of going straight to the hospital or to see her father. She managed to calm down and decided she wanted to see her father, so they went to the funeral parlour, which, again with hindsight, was not a good idea. It was not the place for a heavily pregnant woman, unbalanced by hormones, exhaustion and grief. It was awful: when they walked in, they found Don strapped to a gurney that had been pushed against a wall. It was a family-run funeral home, and things are done very differently in Ireland: the Irish are much more relaxed than the English about death and corpses. In the old days, there was much truth about the coffin being propped up in the corner while all around had a bit of a hooley. In fact, Paul distinctly remembers as a kid playing with his grandfather while he lay in his coffin, laid out in the bedroom. There was a lot of eye-poking, arm-lifting, and getting his mates over for a look. Open coffins are the norm in Ireland, and dead bodies are not unseen. The funeral director probably thought that Caron knew what to expect. Paul and Michael might have coped; Caron did not. 'Your father's over there,' he said, as if he was pointing out a delivery. Caron couldn't get the image out of her head. She didn't like Don being alone in that room, left in a corner. She didn't like that he'd died alone. She didn't like that he'd lived alone. She didn't like any of it.

Paul still has the magazine Don had been looking at when he died. He'd circled that evening's programmes. He also has the monkey nuts on which Don had been drawing faces. It was one of the quirky things he liked to do: draw faces with a lead pencil on the shells, then crack them open and eat them. It had been a peaceful end to a peaceful life. But Caron couldn't see it like that. She saw it as a lonely death and, once again, felt the burden of responsibility.

Until then, life had been carefree – there were a few ups and downs, naturally, but they were termite hills, not the mountains that Caron faced from this point on. So far, she had had a charmed life. Something she said over and over again. I would imagine that a lot of thoughts went through her head in that funeral parlour: if Mum had stayed with Dad would she have spotted something, sent him to the doctor, taken better care of him? If Mum had stayed with Dad, would he have eaten better, drunk less, lived longer? If Mum had stayed with Dad, would he still be alive? No one could have foreseen how potentially fatal that time was for my daughter. Caron travelled the world trying to find out why she'd got cancer, and the answer, as always, lay much closer to home. If there was any reason, and I still don't know that there was, but if there was a catalyst for Caron's illness, this was it. The chain of events started with Don's death. Caron was a ticking time-bomb. Overdue, over-wrought and overtired. The fuse had been lit.

9. A Matter of Life and Death

Russ and Caron flew back to England the next day, Sunday. As ever, trying to be practical, she decided on the Monday to have the baby induced. She said to me, 'I want you to be there,' so I flew back too. I desperately needed to be by her side – be with her at this deeply traumatic crossroads. Gabriel was born twenty-four hours later. I will never forget the image of that beautiful baby lying in Caron's arms. She didn't know whether to laugh or cry. Of course there was huge joy in seeing Gabriel for the first time, but there was overwhelming grief that her father had died. It was another long and tiring labour and Caron was pretty beaten up. She and Russ agreed further down the line that, with hindsight, they would have done it all differently. It is Irish tradition to bury the dead quickly, but why didn't we just delay the funeral? She could have had Gabriel in Ireland, rather than fly backwards and forwards. At the time, though, she felt she wanted the familiarity of Queen Charlotte's Hospital, where Charlie was born. Drastic as it appears now, it seemed like the best solution at the time. Anyway, none of us was thinking clearly.

Gabriel's birth made Don's death even more poignant to Caron: her father would never see this precious little boy because her father, who was so important to her, had gone. She didn't think for one minute that Don's soul had arrived back in Gabriel, but his middle name is Don so he is irrevocably entwined with the grandfather he never met.

When Gabriel was six days old, Russ, Caron, Charlie and he flew back to Northern Ireland. When I think about all that time I spent alone with Caron in London because I didn't want to fly home with a newborn, and yet here was Caron, making the same journey back with this tiny creature for her dad's funeral. It was and still feels surreal. I cannot express how symbolic it was to watch my daughter walk down the aisle of the church to take her place in front of her father's coffin, with this week-old baby in her arms. It was a heart-wrenching moment.

While we had been in London for Gabriel's birth, my sons had remained in Ireland to sort out the logistics of the funeral. The eccentric people of our old village regaled them with some of the funny things that had happened during the week – in times of crisis, black humour is often the only way to cope.

One small example was when Don was in the coffin in the house, his brother came in, looked at Don, then turned to the boys and said, 'Your dad's looking awfully well. He's lost a lot of weight since I last saw him.' As Paul says, 'Very *Little Britain* before *Little Britain* had been invented.'

While we had been back in England overseeing Gabriel's birth, Paul and Michael had spent a bit of time with Don. I think it gave them the edge in coming to terms with losing their father. But it was by no means uncomplicated – for Paul especially. He hadn't seen very much of Don in recent years. When he was over Don had tended to stay with Caron and sometimes when Paul and he met up the atmosphere was slightly strained. Paul was a successful businessman in his own right and Don's little ways had started to feel unfairly like chastisements. Once Don had lectured him about spending too much money on a car – he said it was disgraceful. An argument followed. He was doing well, why couldn't Don just say, 'Well done, son'? After such occasions they wouldn't see each other for a while. So, no, it wasn't uncomplicated for Paul to lose his father at that point in his life.

Michael had always maintained a strong link with his father and our old home. He visited as regularly as he had since our separation. As much as I hated being without him, I made sure

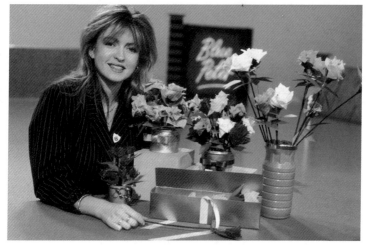

All those years of practising with sticky-backed plastic and pipe cleaners paid off

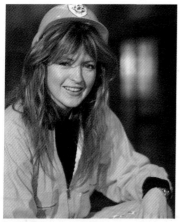

A *Blue Peter* escapade – one of hundreds of thrills and spills

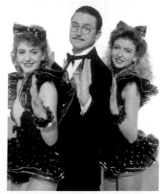

Christmas entertainment on *Blue Peter*: another snazzy song-and-dance routine. *From left to right:* Yvette Fielding, Mark Curry and Caron

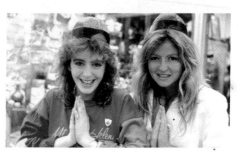

Blue Peter trip to Russia. No food, but lots of shopping

Dear Gloria,

I was very saddened and shocked to hear of Caron's death, as we had worked together when we were both at the BBC, Caron in Children's Department working on Blue Peter, and I in the Health and Safety Department.

Our paths crossed quite a lot when Caron was doing something of a hazardous nature and it was my job to make sure that she had received proper training for the task and that the people she was working with were fully competent, and if necessary to check them out.

Over the period we were together I managed to photograph Caron in some unusual places and situations, some of which I have included here for you. I do have others, and at the moment I am trying to re-organise my negative and slide library. It has grown quite a bit and has tended to get out of hand, but any other slides or negatives I have of Caron, I will gladly send them to you.

I recently saw Caron's story on television and one thing that still came across was that she always got on with the job, regardless of how difficult, and never ever complained. I would often ask her if she was ok and her reply was always the same "Yes." If I thought she was in difficulty, I had the authority to step in and stop the production. I never had to. In some ways the decision she took not to have the second operation was typical of her attitude when we were working together. Even though she was very ill her eyes were still shining bright and that was the main thing I noticed about her when we worked together, and you can see it in some of the enclosed photographs.

I was privileged to have met her and worked with her for a number of years and will always remember her for the true professional she was.

Kind Regards

Stewart

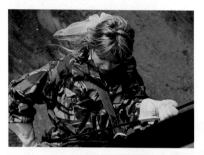

Abseil training with the Royal Marines. Caron was to abseil down the two-hundred-foot-high Bristol and West building, dressed as Snow White, to turn on the Christmas lights. The marines were playing the seven dwarfs!

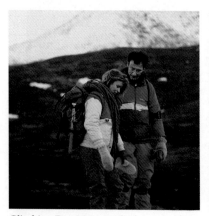

Climbing Ben Nevis with Stephen Venables

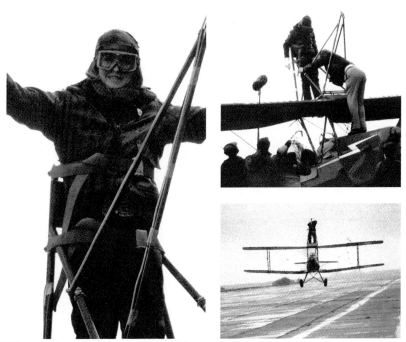

Wing walking at Cranfield Institute of Aeronautical Engineering, during the open day and air show

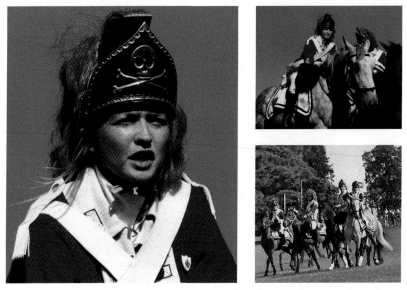

Re-enactment of the American War of Independence

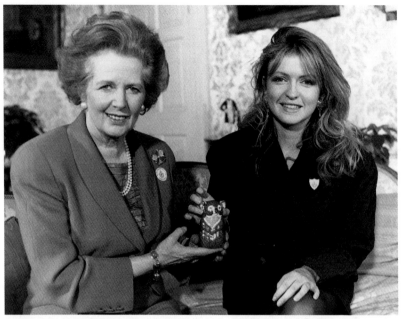

A visit to Downing Street. Caron adored the opportunity to show her journalistic edge

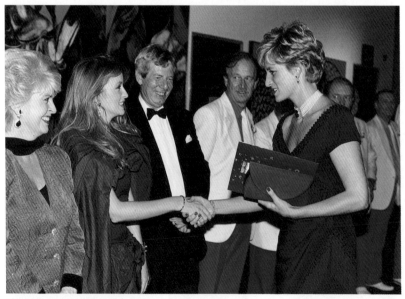

One of many royal occasions. It is incredible that both of these beautiful young mothers have been taken from us

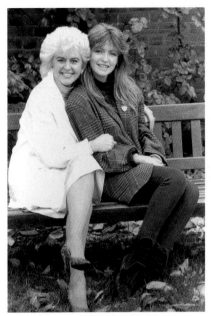

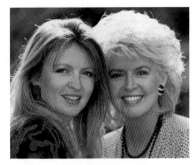

Early *Blue Peter* days: a shot taken in the back garden of Caron's first flat, which she shared with Johnny Comerford

A press launch in the *Blue Peter* garden at BBC Television Centre. Proud mother and excited daughter with another fine example of Caron's charity-shop dress sense.

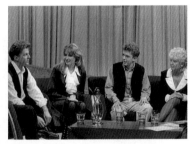

A rare family television appearance together on the Gerry Kelly programme in Northern Ireland

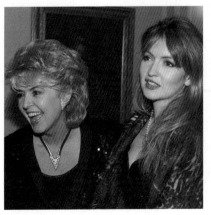

The girls out on the town at a first night in London

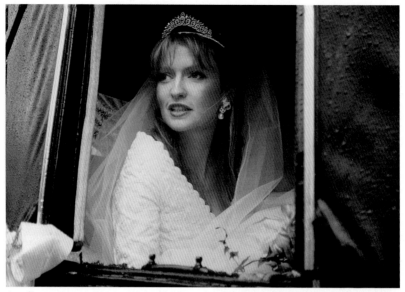

A radiant princess. Caron arriving for her wedding at Hever Church, in a horse-drawn carriage

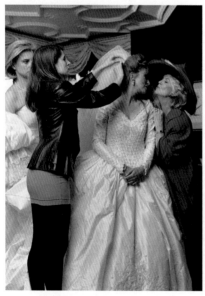

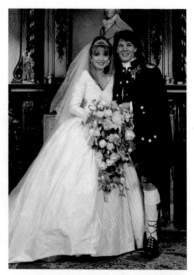

Caron and Russ on their wedding day, Hever Castle, Kent

From pigtails to wedding veils.
To the left of Caron: Cathy Comerford (bridesmaid) and Jane (hairdresser)

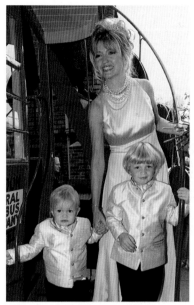

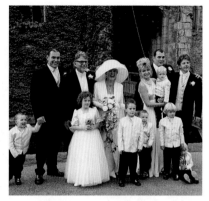

Family album time at the drawbridge of Hever Castle with seven of our eight grandchildren and Stephen's sons Dominic and Matthew

Gabriel and Charlie, two of the best-turned-out page boys. All set to walk down the aisle

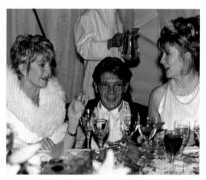

'Caught in the middle'

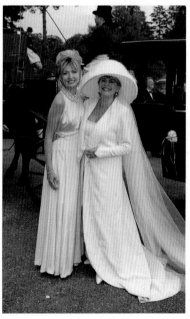

Hever Church again.
This time, my wedding, 1998

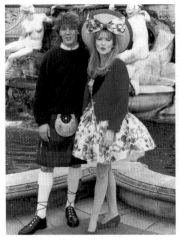

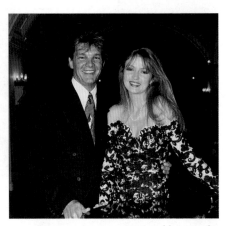

Caron and Russ in their honeymoon outfits. She looked as delicious as her strawberry dress

A golden couple. Handsome, exquisite and vibrant

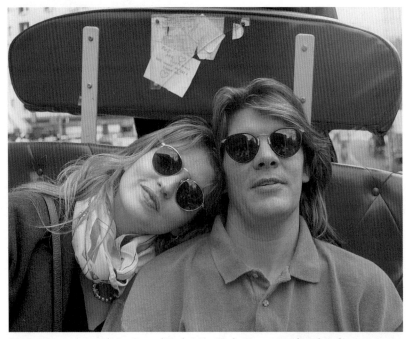

Romantic carriage ride in Central Park, New York. Happy, carefree days for Caron and Russ

that he went back to Northern Ireland to be with his father at Christmas and holidays. If I had to be away, Don would come and stay in Sevenoaks to look after Michael who was at school there. They shared an easy closeness. However, both Paul and Michael have a lot of love and respect for their dad and I see many of Don's finer character traits in both.

Paul and Michael got some kind of closure during that week before the funeral, and they did it on their own, because from the moment Gabriel was born to when Caron died, she was the focus of our attention. She needed to be supported and nurtured because she was the most vulnerable. However, the boys may say that that had always been the case.

We planted a silver birch tree in our garden, the same colour as your hair, and in a suitcase I have your old green jumper and it still smells of you. When I was little I used to love it when you and Mum returned home after a night out and came into my bedroom to kiss me goodnight, your coat smelling of the atmosphere you'd been in – again that stale smoke – and Mum a heady mixture of lipstick and perfume. All was well in my world.

In the months after you left my mind was turned into turmoil. Anxious, nervous days followed by sleepless nights, wondering if I would ever get back to any sort of normal life again. Maybe my perception of 'normality' has changed. I have often tried to analyse why Dad dying affected me in such a huge, huge way. Someone once said that the world is divided by those who have lost their parents and those who haven't. Now, I'm not sure I agree, but at times it seems valid.

For me, it was as if I'd lost my anchor – my safe haven – the one spot where I could totally be myself and with my connection with who I was. The world seems a terrifying unpredictable place and I have now been cast adrift – thrust into the wind – my ship battling across a stormy sea.

At the same time, life marches on relentlessly. I gave birth to my glorious son Gabriel – induced early so I could go to my dad's funeral, afraid to leave it in case I went into labour over there in Ireland. I still have a photo of myself, my husband and my mum – all totally exhausted and wrung out, with a wonderful bundle of life and joy in my arms. I suppose the eternal picture of life and death. Somehow I wasn't in a place to see it. Having lost you, I had been given another life – this tiny baby whom I didn't know, and at this stage was not really in a fit state to properly look after. Now I realize I was staring back at the past rather than addressing the present. It's a strange thing how the prospect of a tiny baby can be totally overwhelming and make one feel so helpless.

There was a great deal of anxiety. Caron wrestled over not having brought Don to England for Christmas. She blamed herself. I know what that feels like: I went to Australia seven times in two years. Now I am consumed with anxiety: should I have gone over, rented a house and stayed. Should I? Should I? If I'd known what I know now, maybe I would have. Then again, perhaps Stephen is right: maybe she needed space to heal. We couldn't uproot our lives. But maybe we should have. You see how it sends you mad? And how it doesn't bring them back? And you want the madness to stop, but then you're afraid they really will be gone and you don't want them to go. You go round in circles because your brain doesn't know how or where to stop.

Caron behaved as though she was the only one who'd lost a loved one. There it is again, in black and white: a brutal reminder of how I feel today. My sons had lost their father too, but it was Caron we worried about. My sons have lost their sister, but I am their major concern. I feel I want to be stronger for them – I try to be – but losing a child is all-consuming. I cannot comprehend the unbelievable depth of my grief. I can't seem to get over the terrible loss from my life. Is it selfish? Sometimes I feel it is. When I think about Michael I can't imagine what he's going through. Caron was his sister, and in many respects a second mother to him. He loved her over and above the obvious. No doubt there have been times when they've wanted to scream, 'What about me, Mum? What about me?' For eight years Paul and Michael played second fiddle to grief, depression, then cancer and that really saddens me too. I want to pay tribute to Paul and Michael, who at all times during my life, but particularly in the last eight years, have been the most incredible tower of support and strength for me and have selflessly coped in their own way with their own grief. Their understanding and appreciation of the loss that a parent suffers, that I'm suffering, when a child is taken away from them has been limitless. I thank them from the bottom of my heart, for that and for the million and one things they do for me every day.

After Caron died, I lived in terror of the first anniversary of everything: her first birthday, the first Christmas, Valentine's Day, Mother's Day – a particularly hard one – my birthday, Easter . . . The list goes on and on. Every single date sent me straight back to 13 April 2004. The wound tore open again. Any semblance of healing vanished. I compare it to being steam-rollered, completely flattened: you feel you will never lift your head again. Then, just as you begin those tiny moves towards rejoining the world, just as you raise yourself marginally off the ground, back comes another steam-roller, another date, and reverses over you until you are so flattened and so exhausted that you can't even imagine raising your head, it's so far beyond you.

I spent my last Mother's Day in a cocoon with Caron. We were in Switzerland where she was having treatment. It was the day she gave me the painting of the tulips, the painting which she did specially in Australia and brought over in her suitcase. It was the day we came as close as we ever did to discussing her death. All Caron's life she had presented me with something on Mother's Day, those yellow primroses she wrote about, something she'd made, a surprise lunch. So, yes, I knew the first one without her would hurt deeply. I was dreading it. The day arrived and who should appear on my doorstep in Kent, laden with bags of goodies, but my two precious sons. I was not allowed to lift a finger from that moment onwards. They cooked me a sumptuous Mother's Day lunch, complete with Paul's Pavlova, which he hadn't made since we all lived in Northern Ireland. It was something I had taught him to do, and now my sons were teaching me the limitless depth of family love and support. I cannot thank them enough for that.

As they do for me now, we stepped up to help Caron in whatever way we could so that she was better able to cope with what was happening to her. Only a few days earlier Caron had been a happy, excited girl with a baby on the way and everything to live for. Then birth and death crashed in on her like a huge wave. There is only so much anyone can take. Birth, with all the joyous emotions it evokes, is exhausting. Death is exhausting too. But within three or four days of coming home Caron found herself incapable of sleeping. From then on the exhaustion became overwhelming. As I've said, Caron told her friends over and over again that she had had a charmed life. She'd been on a pedestal since birth. She'd never been forced to do anything, and everything had fallen into place for her and she hadn't really had to 'grow up'. We all looked after her. Caron was a needy person. Personally I felt I had given her a great deal of time. But if I hadn't gone to Barnes whenever I could, Caron wanted to know why. She was my best everything and I always loved being in her company so I didn't mind, but in truth there was a pressure from her to be there. It wasn't one-way traffic: I leant on her too – she was the one I turned to many times when I was troubled. When Don died, Caron knew she'd reached a watershed of sorts. As she said, she'd read that you don't really grow up until you lose a parent. And I think she thought, Now I must be a grown-up. I must make this okay. And in trying to pick herself up, in trying to be the grown-up, she didn't let herself mend. Above everything, she wanted to get back on track for Gabriel's sake.

When Yasmin called her a few weeks later, she had a strange, disconnected conversation with Caron.

'Are you getting by?' asked Yasmin.

'Getting by.'

'What are you going to do?'

'Well, I've got some work to do . . .'

Work? Surely it was too soon for work? Yasmin said.

For some, including myself, work provides a focus, which is a kind of therapy in itself. On top of that, Caron was brought up, like the rest of us, with a strong Ulster work ethic. There was subliminal pressure to get back out there. It was accepted that you had maternity leave and then you went back to work. But in hindsight after Gabriel was born she shouldn't have gone back: she simply wasn't fit – physically or mentally. For me, work has been my saviour: it gives me something to get up for, and maybe I'm able to think about something other than Caron's death. Sometimes, though, when bad things happen you just fall from one thing to the next without ever analysing 'Is this the best thing to do?' Perhaps in a couple of years' time I shall be thinking I was mad to work in the first year after Caron's death: I should have taken myself off to Dublin, relaxed, read and built myself up. But at the moment work seems to be the thing to do: I want to keep myself busy and it gets me by. Hence this book – a kind of therapy in itself. But how do I know? Was I mad after I broke my shoulder in fifteen places to put myself back to work after ten days? Probably. Then again, that kind of tenacity gives you strength to fight in the face of adversity. That kind of tenacity means that when you're faced with a life-threatening illness, you say, 'I'll beat it.'

But going back to work after Don's death and Gabriel's birth exacerbated Caron's problems. Looking back now we all knew that, from the day we all came home, she couldn't cope. Although it was never formally diagnosed, Russ thinks she had pretty severe postnatal depression for about six months, if not a year. They'd just bought a new home: they were both doing so well at work that they jumped four rungs on the property ladder, going from a Victorian terrace to a serious six-bedroomed house with a massive garden, for Barnes, and a driveway. But it was not home. More than that, Don would never see it. Caron was completely wired, couldn't sleep and couldn't concentrate. She also found breastfeeding difficult. (Who knows? Perhaps the cancer was already performing its *danse macabre*.) She'd express milk, mix it with formula and let Russ do the night shift with Gabriel, but it didn't help: she still wasn't sleeping. Seeing someone you love lose their ability to cope is hard, especially since Caron had always been the driving force in that family. Russ thinks we all have the ability to ping out, and I agree. Lives are lived on such a tightrope these days, people are pushed, work is tough and competitive, and most people are more highly strung than they should be. So, just a small tilt of the pendulum and *ping*!

We had had no direct experience of depression, so we didn't know what we were looking for or at, but now we are pretty convinced she was suffering from it. She said the exhaustion affected her eyesight, saying it was like seeing through a prism. In the end her body shut down. She needed to regroup. She needed to fight.

But she didn't do any of that. Instead she got back to work and was soon travelling round the UK, doing entertainment interviews for *This Morning* and consumer programmes. One evening she went to see Janet and was telling her about what she was doing and just started to cry. Mid-sentence the tears were flowing down her cheeks, and she went on talking and crying, unable to stop either. Janet told her to go home and tell everyone that she wasn't going to do it any more. I don't think she did. That pressure again, to be something, someone.

So there she was, trying to cope, absolutely exhausted and unable to sleep. She was in a spin. She didn't know whether to laugh or cry, she didn't know whether to be joyous or distraught, and in the end it got too much for her. She could barely nurture herself, let alone Gabriel. She didn't know where she was and eventually the depression took hold. It wasn't simply the amalgam of death and birth as we had assumed, though that had been the trigger. By now, it was clinical. She struggled on without sleep – now that I don't sleep I know how her mind went round and round in circles about her dad.

Stephen and I went to Barbados for a break. Caron hadn't been terribly well before we went, but we didn't see it for what it was. Soon after we arrived, Michael called me and said, 'You probably don't want to hear this but Caron wants you to come home.' Categorically. She was in bad shape. We got on the next available flight out and were home by ten thirty in the morning. Russ arrived with Caron half an hour later. That day Caron looked worse than I had ever seen her. She got out of the car, supported by Russ, looking as if she was in a trance. Her skin appeared to have gone black and purple around her mouth and she was limp like a rag doll. The depression tablets she had been put on seemed to have lobotomized her. I wanted to scream, 'Oh, my god, what have they done to you?' but, of course, instead I said, 'Hello, darling, come in, let's get you to bed . . .' The screaming went on silently in my head. She went to her room, the room where she died, and the network took over.

Russ went home to look after the boys, while Stephen and I bunkered down in Sevenoaks to care for her. Because we were still supposed to be on holiday, the phone didn't ring, no one came in and, apart from getting food, nobody went out. It was beautiful weather. Caron painted and rested. They were like stolen days. Stephen was building a new boardwalk round the swimming-pool, Caron did mosaics, and I cooked three meals a day to get her strength up. I brought Jan de Vries, the homeopathic specialist, over to Sevenoaks and he started to build up her immune system. We got her off the depression tablets and she started to mend, a little. But she had to go home at some point: she had two little boys who needed her and a husband, who was doing brilliantly but needed her back.

As soon as she got home the sleep problem started again. She kept thinking she'd die because she couldn't sleep. The solution? She went into the attic of that huge house, put cardboard over the windows and slept there, in the pitch black among the clothes rails. She was very ill and started to grab for cures and explanations. Yasmin had done a report on the healer Jack Temple, and Caron interpreted a phone call from her as a sign to call him, that he could cure the madness that was eating away at her as she lay awake night after night in the attic.

Luckily Russ and Caron had a great Southern Irish nanny to help them: nothing fazed her. She was a salve for all. But she couldn't stop Caron's tears: she was weepy because of her dad, weepy because she wasn't coping, weepy because she was hormonal, weepy because she couldn't work. Finally a friend recommended a therapist who was part reflexologist and part healer. She was a slightly older woman, whom Caron really liked talking to. She was very soothing, massaged the pressure points on her feet and gave her a homeopathic remedy to bring out suppressed emotions. The emotion provoked in Caron was anger. She started thrashing around: why had this happened? Why? Whose fault was it? All the feelings she'd been trying to rationalize up to that point went haywire. And maybe they needed to.

I wanted to understand what Caron was doing, what the woman did and said, so I went to see her myself. I only had the reflexology and maybe I just had a bad experience – but I didn't like it at all. My heartbeat appeared to change the day I saw her. I felt that the whole balance in my body had altered and I never went back because I was afraid. Honestly, it took months to go back to normal. So, I wasn't particularly keen. Even Michael went to see her. Contrary to me, he found her ineffective and questioned her about what the 'essences' she administered were made from. She told him, 'What is important is that it's all made with love,' which was not nearly satisfactory enough for him.

But he was careful not to ridicule it because, as he says, one person's quack is another's saviour, and although reflexology might not work for him, that didn't mean it wouldn't on others. (Indeed, carried out by the right practitioner, it is a very good and helpful treatment.)

Yasmin says Caron learnt a lot about herself during this period, things she needed to learn, so despite my reservations, I have to accept that in the end it helped her. But my suspicions have never been entirely allayed. I accept that maybe some deconstruction was necessary to put the building blocks back in order, but there was a personal consequence to all of this that I found incredibly hard: Caron felt she had to step back from me. She felt she had to handle the depression by herself. So, for a short time, she pulled away. She wouldn't talk to me on the phone or see me. I understand that she needed to be angry, I understood that it was cathartic, but I didn't understand the silent treatment.

I think part of the problem was, that Caron was hearing loose suggestions that were open to wide interpretation. It was the first time I had heard the saying that 'You come into this world alone, you leave it alone.' I fundamentally didn't agree with it. Caron took it to mean that she had to be more of her own person and be responsible for herself. Her knee-jerk reaction was to separate herself from me. As Janet says, the solutions were only ever passive actions, but they planted seeds in her mind. As far as I could surmise, the seeds that the therapist sowed were that the 'intensity' of our relationship was damaging her personal development. In not having to grow up, she hadn't reached a level of maturity to cope with her own children.

I was already suspicious of the woman, but even I have to accept that her reading of the situation wasn't as far-fetched as it sounds. I remember Russ complaining that at weekends Caron wanted to get everyone in the car and come over to Sevenoaks when all he wanted to do was collapse in a heap after a long week. But, no, over they would come, which I loved, of course, but maybe part of the reason Caron wanted to come was because once the nanny had gone home she couldn't cope. When she came to Sevenoaks the network could take over. Meals were cooked, the boys were worshipped and adored, and a little of Caron's burden of responsibility reallocated itself to us. Whatever the reason, we were always thrilled to see them.

Up to the point when she saw the therapist barely a day went by when we didn't speak. If two days went by it was a question mark. If three days went by it was an exclamation mark. Suddenly she didn't turn up for Sunday lunch and I couldn't get hold of her to find out why. I knew something was wrong when Russ made poor excuses on the phone. There was no, 'Look, Mum, I need a little space to get my head in order.' Her quest at that point was largely undefined. So it was withdrawal by cold turkey with no explanation. Naturally I was confused and terrified. I thought the woman had said, 'Cut yourself off from your family,' and I didn't know when it would end.

It wasn't only me. Russ got it too: she'd chuck things around the kitchen in a rage. Maybe all of it was a natural response to grief, exacerbated by the suggestions of someone else. But it was an anger that came from grief – not towards me, Russ or the boys. Just grief. Grief alone can send you mad.

I was so scared that I went to Jan de Vries and asked him whether a practitioner could do this. Why would Caron be distancing herself? Bless him, he went to see Caron on my behalf and pointed out to her that at this time, more than ever, Caron needed her family who could surround her in love. Shortly afterwards I received this letter:

Sunday

Dear Mum,
Having spoken to Jan de Vries last night – I just wanted to try and put your mind at rest – everything is fine – you mustn't worry, because you are putting yourself through unnecessary suffering.

As I tried to explain to you before – I just need a bit of space in my life at this precise moment in time to get to grips and discover who I really am and what I really believe in, myself. Our lives are constantly changing and it is important from time to time to closely examine our beliefs and ideas about things and make sure that they still fit the person we've become.

A lot has happened in my life in the last few months and it has been very frightening for me at times and I have got to make sure that it never happens again. The only way I can do that is to really know myself and find my own inner strength to rely on, because at the end of the day, as we all said time and time again, no one can take away your pain, or live your life for you, and if you don't have that inner strength to get you through then you could be very lost.

And I have discovered a lot in recent weeks and will be a much healthier person for having looked at and shed some of my outdated and redundant ideas and emotions. The therapist who I'm going to knows what she's doing – she is completely qualified – has a medical background and I have total faith in her and I'm not usually a bad judge of character.

The family is not being ripped asunder as Jan de Vries put it – all I'm doing is giving myself time to sort things out and heal. Now the fact that I'm not seeing you at the moment is not a personal slight on you, although if you choose to look at it that way that's your choice – you know I love you very, very much. Nothing has changed on that front – our relationship will continue to be as good as ever, but you have got to let me have this space – it's only another week or so. I am not a child any more, I'm 34 with 2 children myself and have to lead my own life in whatever way I see fit – it may not be what you would do – but then there are things you've done in your life, which I wouldn't have chosen. That's what life is, we're all separate people.

But I promise you, it will be even better than before. I am feeling a daily improvement which I know is what you want – try to look on it as if I'm away on holiday and there are no phones but I'll be back in just one more week. You are putting yourself through needless worry – trust me, you're not losing me, you're getting the improved version.

If you love somebody you've got to let them go free and they'll come back.

I love you and want to see you v. soon.

HAVE FAITH, NOT FEAR

Caron xx

Oddly prophetic, isn't it? She was saying that if you want to find out whether you can cope, you have to stand on your own two feet. You alone have to find the strength to deal with what life throws at you. Which, of course, is true. But where do you get that strength? I am damned sure you get it from love, and when push comes to shove, no one loves you as much as your family. We all know too well the damage that unhappy, unloved childhoods cause. So, the love of your family is the best backstop you have. Do what you have to do, but do it with them by your side.

But perhaps when a dependency is pointed out to you, you can't ignore it. Much later in Australia she was still battling and questioning that dependency. She used to talk to her great friend Melinda about why she was still so dependent on me. Why does Mum give me so much strength? Why do I want her here so much? Why does it make me feel better when she's here? Doesn't everyone need their mother when they're sick, no matter what age? Is it not simply a return to childhood patterns? Who administered the care back then, if not Mum?

Overall during those pivotal few months Caron discovered that she had to pull away in order to give herself the chance to work things out in her head. She had to discover why she wasn't coping, then learn to cope. She did that over and over again during the following seven years. She had to find that inner strength because things were about to get a great deal tougher.

Moreover, she learnt that life is based on love. And I think at the end, after all her searching, that was the conclusion she came to. And that was the knowledge she died with. She had loved and she had been loved, and that was what had given her the strength to fight. The pulling away was all over in weeks. By the time Gabriel was christened that summer, Caron was newly alive.

She dyed her hair red and had it cut into a short bob. It was a way of marking that she was a different person. She was also becoming slightly hippier. She'd say to us, 'I am learning to say no. I am learning not to do the things I don't want to do,' which of course didn't cut much slack with us, as we knew she'd spent her whole life not doing things she didn't want to do and getting away with it. Who cared? She was happy again.

The christening was a new start, the garden was lovely and all the kids were running around. Everyone remembers it because it was such a lovely day. Russ said a few wonderful words, as always, as did Caron. Everyone admired her for that because they all knew she'd had a dreadful time.

Yasmin remembers me just looking at Caron, listening intently as Caron talked about me. Then she held out her arms and we walked towards each other with tears in our eyes. Yasmin thought, Wow, what a bond. We did love and care about each other so deeply and I was so happy to be back in that place, together again. But it was such a happy moment most of all because little Gabriel, who'd been born into all the turmoil of Don's death, could now be fully celebrated.

It was a definitive and healing moment between Caron and myself, but it was Gabriel's day. As Caron was to write, later in Australia:

To Gabriel.
I'm in the summerhouse writing at my new table – it is an overall gorgeous space. I feel very blessed to have it – quiet solitude – I could

really write here and I don't have to write anything, other than what is in me.

GABRIEL – I have always loved you. I was just so scared and frightened when you were born. Scared of not coping with a new baby – I couldn't even look after myself. How I wish you and I had just snuggled up in bed together and done nothing. However, we can do that now – heal each other. I pray that I get to see you grow up – you and Charlie have been such a huge pull for me. I feel like I'm being given another chance – slim as it may seem – to be with you. I had planned for us to spend Mondays together, though my back has been sore all this year. I guess we have still had good times together.

All I can do is love you the best I know and forgive myself. What is the 'perfect Ma' anyway? I suppose on some level, I am perfect for you.

Know you are the most gorgeous, sensitive, loving and loved boy and you are perfect as you are. Funny, bright, charming, great dresser, clever serious thinker. Don't think others are out to get you or attack you – they're not – just be you.

Yes, you're slightly different and outspoken. If you have your own mind, it is a huge gift. Don't lose it ever, to be 'good' or 'fit in' and never think that there's anything you HAVE TO DO, to belong or be loved.

You are very much loved – allow others to see you and let them in. You are a perfect child of GOD – beautiful and holy, fiery, honest, direct qualities that are so wonderful. Never think otherwise, my beautiful angel boy. XXX

The thing that everyone feels so sad about, the overwhelming cruelty, is that Caron who really had taken a major hit, got herself together: she got her head round things she needed to get her head round. During those dark days and nights in the attic she had been to hell and back, but was out the other side and much calmer in her view of the world. Before Don's death, she had always been a manic planner. Now she started to relax a little. The only clue to what lay ahead was something she mentioned to Yasmin: she'd said she'd put on a bit of weight, not that she was bothered by it but that it was unusual for her. Apart from that, the horizon looked clear. The bad times were over. In Gabriel's name there was a great deal of celebrating to do. Naturally a lot of champagne was drunk and the last of the godparents drifted home in the early hours of the morning.

Gabriel's christening turned out to be a very significant day for quite another reason: it was the last time I saw five-year-old Gabriella, who at that time was fighting neuroblastoma. Gabriella was one of Caron's goddaughters, the daughter of Sonia and Steven Lynch. Sonia (then Baillie) was her great friend from those Methody days in Belfast. In fact, it was ironic that Sonia – as her longest-standing friend – ended up living two roads away from Caron in Barnes. In those final weeks and months of Gabriella's life, Caron and Russ were amongst very few friends who were allowed to visit and spend special time with Sonia and Steven and their exquisite little girl.

One of my lasting impressions of Caron's time with Gabriella was her account of how the little one talked all the time about being surrounded by angels.

10. Introduction to Oncology

The girl with the red hair didn't last long; the clouds passed, the sun came out, the mourning was finally over. The only difference was that we were pushing two prams proudly round the pond. The dye and the questioning were washed away. It wasn't that life returned to normal, it was better. Caron and Russ, Charlie and Gabriel were a happy unit. Eager to let the good times roll.

I distinctly remember Caron calling me and casually mentioning that she could feel a little lump in her breast. Neither she nor I, nor indeed her doctor, put too much emphasis on it, presuming it to be something as innocuous as a swollen milk duct. In view of the previous six months it would hardly have been surprising. He told her not to worry but to come back if it hadn't gone in a few weeks. The last thing I ever thought was that my beautiful, vibrant young daughter had cancer. And, anyway, she said she knew it was nothing. She felt fine – better than fine: she was back on track, enjoying Gabriel enormously, and had succeeded in putting the anguish behind her.

However, after six weeks had passed, the lump had not gone away and the doctor said there was no merit in leaving it uninvestigated. Caron agreed to have a needle biopsy, which proved inconclusive. The doctor wanted to be sure, and have the lump taken out. She didn't want that, but we coaxed and cajoled and finally said, 'Why don't you find out once and for all so you can at least put your mind at rest?' So, on 15 September 1997, Caron and Russ went to Parkside, a small hospital in Wimbledon, for a core biopsy that bordered on a lumpectomy. Even then, she was petrified that someone would find out.

I was with them that day – as always: we were a well-matched tag team. Caron looked at both of us from the first of her hospital beds and said, 'I just want you to know that this is not the way I chose to spend my day, and I'm only in here because you've nagged me. I am here under resistance.' Talk about laying the foundations of what was to come. She was really quite pissed off that she was having to waste her time like that. Afterwards Russ ran her down to Sevenoaks, then went home to look after the boys. We all assumed it would be fine. No real alarm bells were sounding.

Russ and I remember the day the result came through as though it was yesterday. He and I agree that, of all the days to come until her death, it was one of the worst. Russ had been enjoying a good day at work when he had the call. The oncologist simply said, 'Bad news, I'm afraid. I'd really like you and Caron, if she's up to it, to come and see me at six tonight.' Russ sat completely still for a second or two. He wanted to put the phone down, delay the inevitable, but he knew his wife too well: he told the oncologist that he would have to explain to her why she had to make that journey. So the doctor told Russ: Caron has breast cancer.

Wham. Bam. Breast cancer.

Stephen and I were in the garden, it was a Thursday, I think, we knew the result came that day and my stomach was upside-down. I was all over the place. Caron had said she knew it would be all right and I believed her. But the closer it got to diagnosis, the more worried I became. Finally the telephone rang. It was Russ. He said, 'I'm coming down, the news is not good.'

Even now I can distinctly remember feeling that my stomach had left my body completely. 'What do you mean?' I asked, putting off the inevitable. Wanting to keep the news at bay. Away from me. Away from my baby.

'It's come up positive,' he said.

Positive? What a bloody awful word that is. What was positive about this? Take back those words. Take them back.

The hour and a half before Russ arrived was indescribably disturbing. Outside it was a beautiful day and inside my beautiful girl was lying upstairs, relaxing, reading and enjoying herself, convinced that she was going to be all right. Stephen was trying to keep me calm, but I couldn't be calm. I was in utter turmoil. I stayed outside in the garden weeping silently, terrified that she would hear me. I had done enough interviews about cancer to know that people were cured. But I also knew that life would never be the same. Even if what followed was straightforward and it had been caught in time, I would spend the rest of my life worrying that it might come back. Watching, waiting. There would always be a nagging, doubting voice inside Caron too, 'Should I get another check?'

I knew that nagging voice would never leave me. I used to be a very carefree, upbeat person, who felt that everything was in its rightful place. I had beautiful children, a lovely house to live in, I was happy and fulfilled. Now her life, our lives as I had known them, had changed with that word 'positive'. My daughter had cancer. Cancer. It was a devastating blow. You carry your children, you give birth to them, and from that day you're petrified of anything happening to them. You want to nurse them, protect them, nurture them, do everything you can to feed them the right food, to look after them, to prevent accidents – to prevent *anything* happening to them *ever*. You want them to have the right company, to have lovely friends, so that they don't take drugs or fall by the wayside. You protect them in every way you can from day one. As a parent, that is what you do. How could I deal with this if I couldn't make it better?

So, Russ is right: apart from the day that Caron died, that was probably the worst day of our lives. I was numb, shocked and petrified all at the same time. I was angry, disbelieving and empty. There was a black hole in my stomach and an unintelligible buzzing in my head. All we could do was wait. Stephen and I had no idea what any of it meant. We didn't know anyone of Caron's age who'd been through it. We didn't know anything. We certainly didn't know how fightable it was, that there were variations, grades of invasiveness. We knew nothing.

Russ thought his wife might die there and then. Driving over to our house, he imagined himself alone with his two babies. He couldn't begin to imagine how he'd cope. With time you gain information and knowledge, which give you possibilities, which give you hope, and hope helps you survive. Yes, it's a roulette table – but at least you're playing. You're in the game. That day, as the sun shone in a glorious blue sky, it felt like the game was over.

Meanwhile Caron was upstairs reading a magazine, unaware of the drama going on below. The news had an effect on my entire system. From that moment on, it was as if I was outside my body. It was a movie I was watching, someone else's story. It wasn't, couldn't possibly be happening to my daughter. It's not real – and yet it's so real that it crushes you completely. You are steam-rollered by it. Hit. Flattened. Devastated.

I couldn't stay in the garden for ever: Caron would have wondered why I wasn't popping in to find out if she wanted anything. I put on some makeup to cover the damage and went upstairs. I realize now it was the first time I donned a mask that I would wear time and time again over the next seven years. I would put it on when the doctors gave us bad news. I would put it on for the camera, or for friends who knew nothing of Caron's illness. I put it on now. Caron was happy in bed, taking it easy. I brought her tea and some cake and I remember forcing myself to smile, but in my heart and soul I was mesmerized: she had no idea of how her life was about to change, no idea what

she was about to be hit with. No idea that she had been handed
a life sentence. No idea at all.

Russ and I wept outside when he arrived. We were in shock,
but I could hear Russ saying, 'It's small, we've caught it early,
the doctor is going for cure, they will remove it, it might involve
radiation, we're going back to find out.' I wanted to keep Russ
in the garden. I didn't want him to walk up the stairs to Caron's
room. I didn't want him to tell her. I wanted to protect her
from the awful information that was now raging in my head. I
wanted her to stay happily cosseted in bed whiling away the
afternoon in blissful ignorance. But I couldn't. I watched him
go in to tell her.

Caron was reading about Caroline Aherne's infamous question to Debbie McGee: 'So, Debbie, what first attracted you to
multimillionaire magician Paul Daniels?' She would later write
how odd it was that she was engaged in something so trivial
when Russ came in to tell her something so profound and
life-changing.

Naturally your partner in life is the person you fall back on,
but after a while I went into the room. We wept together,
hugging one another. But we had a similar conversation to the
one Russ and Caron would have in the car on the way back to
the hospital. The lump was small, so small they couldn't find it
the first time. It had been caught early – I had done endless
interviews with cancer patients so I was aware that made a
considerable difference. I knew the drill. But even though I was
saying all those words, trying to make it better, I also knew that,
for the first time in my life, I was not in control: I couldn't
make it go away. I couldn't put on a plaster and kiss it better.
The cameras weren't rolling. This was real. This was actually
happening to us. I had no idea what I was supposed to do; I
couldn't get rid of the cancer. With all the will in the world,
I could not make it better for my child. That makes any life-
threatening disease an excruciatingly lonely journey: lonely for

the person who has it and lonely for those watching. I felt a helplessness the like of which I'd never experienced before. I was used to doing things, having contact numbers of people, asking questions and getting answers, and suddenly I couldn't elicit the right answer. In the space of a few seconds my world had fallen apart. I tried in vain to piece things back together again, saying, 'Thank God you went today, I'm so glad you went, they've caught it early, it's small . . .' I was making it up as I went along – we all were. I suppose that went on for seven years in one form or another, depending on what stage we were at. It came like a whirlwind, forcing a million balls into the air, whirling dervishes – where do we go for the best treatment, who is the right doctor, the what, how, when? Not why. At that point, no one asked why.

The pair of them left Sevenoaks and drove to Wimbledon to see the cancer specialist. During that car journey there was a mixture of silence, disbelief, then suddenly they would be talking to each other in the same mad, positive way, although they had no knowledge of what they were talking about. Russ says that if you were to play back that conversation now, 99 per cent of it was fiction. It came from nowhere, gobbledegook – You're young, you'll be fine, young people don't die of cancer, you'll be fine, you're healthy, you'll be fine, you're seeing the best people, you'll be fine, you're not feeling ill, you'll be fine. You're only thirty-three, for goodness' sake, of course you'll be fine . . . It was bad news, but we'd all heard the miraculous survival stories, we knew there were encouraging treatments, people lived, thank God, more in 2005 than when she was diagnosed, but they lived, so Russ and Caron convinced themselves during that journey that she would too.

Left at home, I was a mess. Nothing Stephen could say or do consoled me. I took it extremely hard, not just because of the threat of death but, as I said, because I knew that life would never be the same. Even if the cure that the doctor was aiming for came, we'd always be worried: what if it returned? I had that *déjà vu* feeling. After all, I had already been through it with my mum. What if this lumpectomy doesn't work? What if she has to have a mastectomy? What if that doesn't work? The what-if syndrome. I was like that for the first few months. Caron was, and still is, the last person I think of at night. She was, and still is, the first person I think of in the morning and in the middle of the night. All during that period I would wake with a knot in my stomach, a knot in my throat: is this really happening? What is the outcome going to be? I was driving myself crazy. I can see only too well why people become mentally disturbed, I can see why people die of a broken heart, because the grief and worry can drive you insane.

One day I thought, I'm worrying about five, seven, ten years down the line. Whichever way this goes, Caron's life will never be the same – her longevity won't be as predictable. It just won't. We don't know what it will be. I was sitting on the edge of my bed and realized that I could be dead long before the cancer ever got a grip – if it got a grip. I could be under a bus myself. I could have a heart-attack, like Don. I held my head in my hands and forced myself to acknowledge that there was no point in worrying about things that might or might not happen ten years down the line. If I continued, I wasn't going to be of any use to Caron. If I didn't harness the downward spiral I would be a hindrance to her and she didn't need that. What she needed was all the support she could get. So, I did a head job on myself. I had consciously to teach myself to plan for today, each day, day by day. I would do whatever I could to help, and be there. I would support whatever complementary medicine Caron could find – I would even help her find it. I could take care of today. I couldn't take care of tomorrow.

The head job I performed on myself was because of Caron. If she could be positive, I had to be. From the beginning she set the tone and I forced myself to follow. She was being so positive about it that I had to talk myself into being positive as well. So later, I was saying, 'If the doctor says this operation should deal with it all, then it will.' Then subsequently, when it didn't work: 'The mastectomy will get it all out and you'll be free of it.' And then, 'You cleanse everything else and your body will cope.' When she knew the doctors were no longer going for a cure, when she knew she wouldn't be free of it and that all we could hope for was 'management', I said, 'Look, we'll manage it. There are new drugs being developed all the time. The success rates are really good.' Yes, you talk like that because you're trying to be positive and bolster your child, and in doing so somehow you talk yourself into it as well. In the end you believe it. It's the only way to get by. So, that was what we did from that first day in Sevenoaks. From the moment of diagnosis we donned the mask and dressed up the facts. A bewitching disguise for an imaginary story that we could throw ourselves into. For most of the time we convinced ourselves we would be granted our fairy-tale ending. Happy. Ever. After. Caron would survive.

Caron had to go for more tests at the Royal Marsden in central London. I didn't accompany her because she thought it would attract too much attention. She had decided by then that 'no one' was to know of her diagnosis so I had to stay away from such a specialist hospital. You bump into someone in the corridor and it's not going to be anything other than bad news. I arranged to meet Caron and Russ afterwards at The Brasserie on the Fulham Road. I think her intense hatred of hospitals started that day: when she finally arrived at the table she was agitated and disturbed. She was angry that this was happening. In that hospital it doesn't matter if you keep your eyes glued to the floor, there are patients all around you who are obviously really sick. There are people with growths, holes in their throats, tubes hanging out from under their robes, children with no hair from chemotherapy.

Now Caron knew what having cancer really meant. And how seriously it had to be taken.

Later that afternoon she was rewarded, however, for subjecting herself to the tests and screening with wonderful news. The cancer was confined to her breast: it hadn't, thank God, spread anywhere else in her body. When she went back for a further lumpectomy, which they performed because the cancer had been growing quite close to the breastbone and they wanted to make sure that they'd got it all out, she was much happier. With this last little operation, she'd be free of cancer. An intensive course of radiotherapy followed, which she coped with really well. Either Russ, their next-door neighbour Katie, Cathy or Michael would drive her to South Kensington and she'd sneak in through the back door of the hospital. Radiotherapy obviously takes its toll, but as a process it appeared quite easy. It is the meticulous measuring that takes time, marking the spot where the 'invisible rays of energy' would work their black magic. She'd go in, then we'd meet up and go shopping or for lunch. Caron was offered Tamoxifen, a gold-star cancer-suppressing drug, but after a great deal of consideration, she decided not to take it. Just to put it in context, she was extremely low risk, they had got the cancer out, it hadn't materialized anywhere else in her body and she had responded well to radiotherapy. Tamoxifen has side-effects, one being that it can bring on early menopause. Caron couldn't face that and, anyway, taking it seemed an unnecessary precaution. Now, who knows whether that was the right decision.

Our ordeal was over. Now it was just a question of making sure it didn't come back. Not such an outrageous wish since Caron had decided early on that it was in her power to do so. She said, 'Don't tell me this is genetic, that I inherited it from my grandmother, because that means it's outside my control. I have to believe it isn't. I have to believe it's within my power to stop it spreading, to cleanse and self-heal.' She gave us hope.

Confidence. If there is no hope, how can you go on? If there is anything helpful that I can pass on, it would be to acknowledge the power of positive thinking and living each day as fully as you can. It is hard sometimes but it is amazing how you can do it, especially when the patient, in this case Caron, was so positive: you have to be positive for them and subsequently for yourself.

From then on Caron was on a constant search for a cure, like many of the 750 people who are diagnosed with some form of cancer in the UK every day. Before her diagnosis, she had dabbled in the mind, body and spirit arena. Even before she saw her therapist in Surrey, she'd been interested in complementary health care. Perhaps the exploration into the 'self' had started more as a New Age California thing: she had a lovely husband, a lovely child (this was before Gabriel was born), a great job, enough money, loads of friends, so what was missing from her life? Why aren't I fulfilled? she had wondered. So, she'd had a little look at 'me', first quite lightly, and then, after Don died and Gabriel was born, she went a bit deeper. It was in keeping with the times: in the latter nineties people became increasingly interested in self-analysis, and Caron absorbed articles, programmes and enlightening books in her own inimitable style. With interest and humour. Of course, her initial search had been vague but, post-diagnosis she had a vital aim and purpose. Caron went on to explore every avenue open to her. What started as a curiosity in the mind, body and spirit arena became a quest. Some of her friends think that quest kept her alive, others that her strength of character did that, but no one will ever know. I like complementary therapies because of the additional hope and practical help they give you. They are the most wonderful extra crutch, and as long as they don't do any harm and you find the right practitioners, why shouldn't you use them in times when you need more support? Have the operations and whatever orthodox treatment is available, but if someone else can help keep a balance with natural and homeopathic remedies, then use them. If I were in that position it's exactly what I would do.

I ought to preface all of this by saying that these are simply my observations of Caron's complementary treatments, not recommendations. Having said that, I truly believe, as did she, that some helped to extend her life. We have always been a complementary-medicine family. I have been something of a vitamin freak most of my life. We would try a homeopathic remedy, for instance, and if it didn't work, we would follow up with orthodox treatment. When I smashed my shoulder playing tennis, four years of operations followed. But in one area the bone was not knitting together as it should. My surgeon recommended a bone graft, which would have to come from my hip. I couldn't bear to think of another joint being invaded and out of action so I looked around for alternatives. My doctor was in convulsions of laughter when I asked him whether my arm would drop off if I didn't have the operation. He assured me it wouldn't and gave me six months to try some specifically designed homeopathic remedies. Jan de Vries, the homeopath and naturopath, who had now become a family friend and a well-known practitioner of complementary medicine, gave me a remedy that targeted bone density and tissue replacement. It worked. Maybe it was coincidence, who knows?, but I believe it saved me from that final operation. I still take those supplements: Urticalcin, for maintenance and OsteoPrime to stop the onset of osteoporosis.

So Caron had grown up with that kind of philosophy, knowing that it wasn't bizarre, wacky or weird to examine alternatives to orthodox medicine. Naturally, I brought Jan in very early on in Caron's case, and we were intensely involved with his homeopathic practice throughout her illness. Also at that time, she met one of his colleagues, Hans Muller. He lives outside Amsterdam and is one of the most famous complementary specialists on cancer in the world. As soon as we saw him he put Caron on to a new regime; he warned her it would be tough but Caron was determined. She was prepared to do anything – everything. Even so, she was shocked at the strict regime he proposed: no coffee, no tea, no carbonated or caffeinated drinks, no wheat, no sugar, no processed food, no dairy. At first she used soya milk instead of cow's, but later rice milk. She was to eat a large amount of fruit and vegetables, organic where possible, and take up to forty enzyme tablets each day. At one point she was waking in the middle of the night simply to maintain the recommended dose. She was also on a high dosage of vitamin C and much more besides to boost her energy and general well-being. That wasn't all:

I was on a diet that would make a chocoholic like myself weep – oh, and I began each day by shooting coffee up my bottom.

This was suggested to me by a cancer expert in Amsterdam. A tall thin Dutchman whose Spartan waiting room and severe assistant should have alerted me to the possible austerities that lay ahead.

No wheat, sugar, dairy, 'white' [processed] food of any kind, chicken occasionally, monthly fasts and daily enemas were his recommendations for a healthy body.

As my shocked brain and even more devastated tastebuds struggled to take in the dietary recommendations, he went on to describe the coffee-enema procedure and how he thought it could become the kind of thing my husband and I could do together. Now, I don't know about you but coffee enemas have never struck me as a spectator sport – the thought of my long-suffering husband holding a bag of coffee and molasses while I tried to manoeuvre a small pipe up my rear end, slosh in some liquid and retain it for fifteen minutes at a time, was not a happy one. There are some activities that are best attempted solo – this was definitely one of them. When I say enemas had never struck me as a spectator sport, the truth is they'd never actually occurred to me at all, but they turned out to be a strangely pleasant thing. I have since discovered that people pursue all kinds of activities whilst the coffee does its thing – reading *War and Peace*, meditating, chatting on the phone (thank God videophones never caught on) . . .

Before cancer Caron always knew if something was a bit too bonkers. She wasn't stupid. But that was before she needed the practitioners more than they needed her, before she was vulnerable. There are some fabulous people in the mind, body and spirit business, and alternative therapies that are older and as powerful as penicillin, but if you open the door to them all, you will expose yourself to them all, and not all of them are good. The travelling salesman with his promised elixir of life is as old as prayer. We pray for the miracle and when we are desperate, we buy the bottle for the same reason that millions of people buy a lottery ticket at overwhelming odds: it could be the winning ticket, and that treatment could be the miracle cure.

She became worried about electricity waves so she took the TV out of her bedroom. She became nervous of the studios she worked in. She feared the multitude of power lines that criss-crossed overhead. She had a feng-shui expert over to her house who told her that one problem was that the house was situated at the end of a T-junction and the road came directly up to it. Now this unnerved her: she moved the furniture around so that she wasn't sleeping opposite the road. She took everything on board in terms of her well-being – sight, sound, smell, light, everything. It was Caron doing what Caron did: being practical and taking action.

My mother had always said to me as a child, and repeated it to her grandchildren, that if they were upset because they'd broken or lost something, or fallen out with someone, 'Ask yourself, is there anything you can do about this? Can you fix it, apologize, get another, talk to someone? If there's something you can do, do it. But if there isn't, if it's outside your control let it go. It's negative energy.' My father's maxim was even simpler: 'one day at a time'. So, we were taught (a) to live for the day, (b) to do as much as we could, (c) not to waste energy on stuff we couldn't do anything about. Above all, stay busy.

Caron didn't want to know that the cancer was outside her control, so she stayed busy with my mother's Plan A: do everything you can. I used her Plan B and kept busy. I had to let go of the negative energy too so I followed my father's instruction to live for the day. It didn't get me over the worry, and it doesn't get me over the pain and utter sorrow of losing Caron, but it does allow me to function on those days that I'd rather die. Work is therapy: staying busy is preferable to the black hole that sometimes threatens to swallow me up. Once again, Caron was leading from the front so it was impossible to be negative around her, about any of it.

And how was Russ during all of this? He was phenomenal. On that drive to Sevenoaks he imagined he'd never be able to cope. Well, he did. I think they were both exceptionally brave in their approach. They were a team, a fighting force, with Caron out front on the battlefield and Russ feeding the lines of support from behind. It was a test for both of them and they were in it together. But not everyone joins forces: trauma often forces people into lonely corners that they cannot get out of. No one knows how they will react in such circumstances until they are put into that situation. Caron and Russ had no warning, no trial run. It was thrust upon them, the golden couple whose worries in life up to that point had been negligible. So, Russ simply stepped up to the plate and said, 'I'll do anything you need me to do.' He doesn't think that was brave or honourable: it was what his heart dictated. He had a wife and two young sons for whom he would do anything to enable them to stay together. You can't be told you have cancer and be the same the day after as you were before. Caron had always been a little feisty, and at home she must have become even feistier. Russ says he's seen sharp businessmen take on the subject of their own mortality and watched them fall to pieces. Well, Caron didn't fall to pieces. She walked into battle. Just cutting out the chocolate and cappuccinos would have been enough to create a maelstrom in her life, but giving up those pleasures was just the tip of the iceberg. She had two little boys to bring up, no mean feat when you are facing your own mortality and trying not to get too tired or too hormonal.

Caron did everything she could think of to stave off the cancer and keep it away. She soared to ever more impressive levels in her ability to cope. My admiration of her, always high, was now stratospheric. She knew by then that the body develops cancer cells most of the time, but immune systems are in place to destroy them. Her rationale was, 'Keep the immune system healthy and it will look after the rest.' But cancer is cunning too, though ultimately self-destructive: if you're young and healthy, virile and active, cancer can grow and travel fast. Russ believes that even then it was taking hold and moving, unseen and unfelt, through her body. He thinks it must have been fast-moving from the beginning or it would have been stopped in its tracks when Caron had the radiotherapy and mastectomy. He says that oncologists he has spoken to say that perhaps she didn't have much of a chance right from those very early days. Were there rogue cells just waiting to ignite? Can it smoulder for years and years, then catch fire, spread and grow again? I don't know. We thought she was better, but maybe the embers were just waiting to ignite.

By September 1997 she'd had the lumpectomy, she had radiotherapy and she had changed her diet and lifestyle dramatically. She had worked a little, had rested and spent a lot of time on holiday in Cornwall with Russ and the boys. In fact she'd done everything by the book and had every reason to be optimistic. She and the rest of us were just beginning to put the horrors of the previous year behind us. Caron certainly looked wonderful and we had been knee-deep in wedding preparations for my marriage to Stephen. Needless to say we had shared many a plotting and planning lunch making endless decisions about the day and many more phone calls besides, but as the wedding day approached I sensed that something was wrong. Caron and I hadn't spoken for three days, which was completely out of character in normal times, but as she had been so closely involved in our wedding plans our daily conversations had doubled. I rang and asked her straight out what was wrong. 'Nothing, nothing . . .' she replied. But I could tell in her voice that wasn't the case. I said, 'Caron, this is me you're talking to . . .' And it all came out. She had found another lump. She hadn't wanted the discovery to spoil the celebrations, so she had been trying not to tell me. That was typical of Caron's generous spirit, that she didn't want to cast any shadow on our big day. Furthermore, she insisted on putting off having the lumpectomy and tests until after the wedding. I wanted to cancel our honeymoon in Italy, but Caron wouldn't hear of it. The biopsy was on Monday and we had an agonizing wait until Wednesday. Was the cancer back? Were all the changes she'd made to her life for nothing? Our honeymoon only really started when the call came through. Caron's voice said it all. The result was negative. The growth was benign. Caron was in the clear. We were all ecstatic, everything she had done since that first dreadful day of diagnosis had worked. Stephen and I went to Pisa to celebrate. By the end of the evening, it wasn't only the tower that was leaning!

Caron looked beautiful on our wedding day, as radiant as ever, happy, content and healthy. It is, as she said, a bastard disease. How could you possibly know what horrors were taking place beneath the skin, but once the results came in, we had been given back our chance at the happy ever after. It was a wonderful day and I was lucky enough to marry a wonderful man. As he says, dealing with a woman whose daughter is well is completely different from dealing with a woman whose daughter isn't well. She changes slightly all the time: he doesn't know who he's going to wake up to each morning and it's been like that since we were married, but no more so than since Caron died. I salute him for standing by me, for taking the swipes, for wiping away the endless tears, for losing his wife to grief without knowing whether he was ever going to get her back. I salute him for many other things, the trips to Australia, for being an adult male in my sons' lives, for making step-parenting look easy, which it isn't. I salute him for loving my grandsons as he does his own. There certainly is no end to the debt of gratitude that I owe him. Despite the shadow cast by Caron's looming second lumpectomy, the day we married was a wonderful day and Stevie has been a wonderful husband ever since.

11. A Terrible Secret

For five years I have been dealing with breast cancer – not all the time – but off and on and keeping it a secret. I didn't want many people to know because I was ashamed of having it – ashamed that something like that could happen to me. Not even many of my close friends knew initially – I remember hiding in the loo from probably my best male friend, because I couldn't face letting him know.

I tell myself, I don't want the intrusion – people seeing me as the usual 'cancer victim'. What I didn't realize then is that the only person who can make you feel like a victim is yourself.

There is so much fear connected to that world – statistics, brutal treatments, stacks of figures of those who make it and those who don't. That waking in the middle of the night, endlessly checking yourself, swaying between realism and denial.

It was like that one tiny lump had completely changed my life. And it has – though not in the way I ultimately thought – been a messenger from God to turn myself back to myself. I returned to love of myself, my family and God. Having had a serious illness has been one of the greatest teachers.

Caron decided on the very day she was told that she had cancer that no one was to know. She reiterated it on the drive home when they knew she had low-grade cancer and the doctor was going for cure. No one. Absolutely no one. What she did was completely close ranks on anybody having any information about what was going on. Gradually a few people were told, but most weren't. She did a million and one things with them and they never saw it.

Russ and I have read a lot of what she's written on the subject in her diaries, and he and Caron talked for thousands of hours about why she didn't want to tell anyone. He thinks, knows, that in the beginning she felt that maybe she had done something wrong. The inevitable question: why me? A question that leads to so many others. Maybe she had done something to deserve this? Or had she not done something that she should have done? Was God punishing her? She didn't want people to know that she had it because she didn't want people to know that she was flawed.

She was beautiful, she was intelligent, she was witty, she was exceptional, she had so many positive things going for her: suddenly to have cancer tacked on to the end made no sense. It wasn't right; it didn't work. We had all put her on a pedestal: I imagine they are hard to climb down from.

Basically Caron was not going to have it. There was absolutely no way. It was like a flawed diamond. You can have a perfect jewel that has this tiny crack in it, and suddenly it's worth nothing. She felt in the beginning, and it was not the right way to feel, that perhaps she had done this to herself. I don't think a day went by in the following seven years when Russ didn't tell her that you don't get cancer because of something you did or did not do. As Paul says, 'Sometimes shit happens.' But she couldn't escape the notion that there was something in her life, something she'd done, some relationship, some experience that had predisposed her to it. She explored this over and over again with different people, gurus, healers, spiritual leaders, for almost the rest of her life.

I understand it in a different way from Russ. Caron didn't think the lump was suspicious. It was a shock to find out it was. But it was small, they had found it early, and they were going for complete cure. Soon it would be over and she would forget all about it. She didn't want to be defined by it. She didn't want to be Caron 'cancer' Keating. She didn't want any label on her forehead. She just wanted to be able to get on with living. She was going to be fine. And when she was well again she didn't want to be seen as Caron Keating, cancer victim. Not even one who'd survived. Especially not one who'd survived. For then she'd be linked to it for the rest of her life and she just wanted to put it all behind her. She felt that people write you off once you've been diagnosed with cancer, but that shouldn't be the case. Cancer is such a wild card that no one knows exactly what the outcome will be. She didn't want people's pity, she didn't want to be a statistic, and she was absolutely not going to be one of X number of people who died of breast cancer that year. As the years went on, the secret became a barrier of protection, another crutch: she still wasn't going to be Caron 'cancer' Keating.

People often ask me how I felt about that. I believe you should be able to fight any illness in whatever way you want. That is your prerogative. So, I would go along with anything Caron wanted. She was the one with cancer, not me. Overall, I think that feisty attitude stood her in good stead and gave her the ammunition to fight.

Some people thought she didn't tell people because she saw it as a failure. All the processes she went through attributed cancer to something that the patient had done. The practitioners couldn't just say, 'You got ill, it's awful bad luck. There doesn't have to be a root cause or a direct consequence of past behaviour or experience. It's what you do once you are ill that matters, how you deal with it.' Caron needed to discover what she'd failed at before she could fix it. She would question every aspect of her life, possibly blame but definitely question whether her marriage to Russ was as good as it could be. Could it be better? Am I repressing something inside me? Should I be on my own with my children? Would I then feel freer? Is whatever I'm suppressing making me sick? Am I too dependent? Is my close relationship with my mother making me sick? Am I seen as being in competition with my mother and is that healthy? Caron was adamant that she could never be accused of springboarding her way to success because of me. It went to the very core of who she was. Caron was her own person. She was an individual in her own right. We were in the same business, but in completely different areas of it. That one of Don's and my children would go into broadcasting was almost inevitable: we were a media family. There are family businesses all over the world. Of course that hadn't given her cancer. She was married to a man who loved her unstintingly: that hadn't given her cancer either. But we went through all this questioning. It wasn't just Russ and me, it was everything, as I've said. She even asked Michael whether he felt in competition with her. Who got more attention? She went over Don's and my divorce with him. It was endless and exhausting.

I think the trouble was that if you consult enough people, you don't necessarily believe any of them wholeheartedly. Caron flitted like a butterfly from one opinion to the next, taking bits from here, there and everywhere. She ended up doing a million different things, questioning a million different things, taking on a million different things, and in the end was no closer to the answer. What is it that I'm doing or not doing to deserve this?

There were other reasons for not telling, easier ones to understand. She didn't like the tone people often adopted when someone got ill – she couldn't stand the simpering, whimpering voice and the soft limp hand. The sad eyes when they asked, 'How are you?' It would piss her off. 'Damn it, if you want to know ask me properly!' She didn't want their fear either: she had enough of her own, without taking on other people's. She didn't want to become a soap opera.

Whatever her deep-seated, oscillating, private or public reasons for keeping such a terrible secret, it gave her the courage to walk into the *London Tonight* or *This Morning* studio as if nothing was wrong. She worked a lot during that time. If anything it was her heyday. Working on *This Morning*, she was at her happiest in the business. She started out covering for Judy Finnegan on Friday mornings with Ross Kelly, and when Judy was away, she filled in for her with Richard Madeley. She loved it because it was Richard's programme, not hers: she wasn't carrying the responsibility, he was. He was as feisty as she, opinionated, and Caron fitted perfectly into that mould. Among the serious issues, her direct and intuitive questioning, there was a lot of laughter. When I watch reruns, they are always laughing. Proper head-back, wide-mouthed, guttural laughter. Richard has said publicly that if he wasn't working with his wife, the person he'd most like to work with was Caron. She had a pipedream that she'd come back home from Australia and work again with him. When she couldn't walk very well, she said, 'That cuts out TV, then.' But we used to say, 'Any time you want to, Richard will have you back and you'll just have to sit in a chair.' Pipedreams and fairy-tales. We were telling each other those things to the end.

In a funny sort of way her refusal to tell people meant that she couldn't be anything but her old self. She was almost able to bluff it out and, in doing so, forget. It worked because later, when things were getting worse, Russ would see her sitting in the bathroom, her head in her hands, pulling her strength up from inside. Then she would raise her head and smile. Everyone benefited. Russ delighted in watching her find enjoyment, positivity and solace in her own fun.

And what about the rest of us? Those who knew. Michael was amazingly positive: she was young and strong, we'd all be strong and beat this. To the end he thought she would. As he said, what was the point of thinking otherwise? That was wasted energy, energy he could have used to help Caron. Paul came to the same conclusion via a different route. He simply wouldn't accept the alternative. Their grandmother's ethos is strong in my children.

When Caron told Cathy she had cancer her second line was,

'And I don't want anyone to know.' Not even Johnny: Caron's best friend, Cathy's husband. That was a big ask. I know it was hard for Cathy to carry that burden: your partner is the one you lean on at times like that. Caron asked the few other girlfriends who knew not to tell their husbands either. She didn't want them feeling sorry for Russ or her. Maybe it was a girly thing too: she never flaunted her breasts so it makes sense that she didn't want them discussed around her friends' dining-tables. I'm sure having a scalpel taken to her breast attacked the very essence of her femininity. Also, I think she was very proud and did not want to have to deal with the extra fuss – like the acting: although she loved the theatre, she feared the stage. She loved singing, but only in a group. Certain types of attention she adored, but telling people she had cancer would bring the sort of 'singled-out' attention she did not crave, the unwanted solo spotlight she preferred to avoid. The other up-side of keeping it secret was that it freed others around her to be normal. She didn't have to deal with people dealing with her. All her life she'd been dealing with people dealing with her family, and wanted it to stop.

She told Janet Ellis in the kitchen in Barnes. It was one of those weird things: we were talking about plans and she said she couldn't make a certain arrangement the following Friday. When Janet asked why, she got a most unexpected answer: 'Because I'll be in hospital. They've found a tiny, tiny lump.' It was almost casual so Janet thought, Maybe it's nothing, she looks fine, she's talking calmly. As Janet says, if it had been her she'd have been doing the full Italian widow . . .

Yasmin, her great television friend, was the other person she told. Not immediately. She never told anyone immediately. She would deal with something first, then tell. Yasmin was pregnant at Gabriel's christening, as was Fiona Foster, the current-affairs reporter. Caron was ecstatic about that. Her motherly side came out and she fussed over her friends. Yasmin's children's walls were painted by an artist Caron sent over; she still has books that Caron lent her and her Moses basket. Caron loved being a mum and couldn't wait for her friends to be mums too. When Yasmin's daughter was born and she would ring, complaining about sleeplessness, Caron would say, 'Darling, she's only ten days old. What do you expect?' She never mentioned the cancer. When Yasmin was tired and complained that she had to give Sophie a bath, Caron would say, 'So don't. Put her to bed with food in her hair and do it in the morning.' The only clue to what was going on in Caron's world was those little tips: she'd started re-evaluating what was important in life and dismissing the little things.

One day Yasmin went to have lunch with Caron. Her mother had just been diagnosed with cancer and they talked about it over the meal. Then Caron said, 'I don't want you to tell anyone this, I'm fine, but I've got it.'

'What?' asked Yasmin.

Apparently Caron went bright red.

'Got what?' asked a perplexed Yasmin.

'I've got cancer.'

Yasmin could not believe it.

'It's fine, I'm fine, it's a bastard disease, but you've just got to be positive about it,' said Caron. And that was all she said about herself and her predicament. She went on to give Yasmin a list of things to do for her mother. The first thing Yasmin did was go out and buy her mother a juicer.

From then on Caron would deal with something first, then tell her few chosen confidantes. Even then she'd diminish what was going on to not quite the status of a broken leg but something to be dealt with, rather than her whole life. That made it easier for her friends to cope with. She was doing them an enormous favour because it meant their friendship could stay on the same track – they could still have silly times, the girly dinners. It was a nuisance that she couldn't drink coffee any more, but the others did and Caron just had the herbal substitute. She was very good at managing it, whatever place she put it in her mind, she made it very acceptable for the rest of us.

Cathy says, and I understand this completely, that even though she had known about the cancer for seven years, the day Caron died she was as shocked as if Caron had been run over by a bus – Cathy, who had seen her on that little metal frame in Australia, Cathy, whose husband had seen for himself her condition in Switzerland, was blown away by the news of her death. Such was the strength of Caron's courage, her positivity, her desire to beat cancer.

Even Paul admits that he didn't believe she could die from the disease. His business partner's mother was given six months and, thank God, is still alive twenty years later. The same man had a sister who had successfully beaten the disease, so why not Caron? Keeping the secret was pivotal in that. She taught us to believe in the miracle, and if everyone had gone around simpering and whimpering, with despairing eyes and fateful prognoses, she wouldn't have made it as far as she did.

Of course, that meant an enormous number of people were kept in the dark. Russ and Caron, as I have said, were magnets; they made friends wherever they went, and I think a lot of people were hurt that they hadn't been told. Her colleague at *Blue Peter*, for instance, Mark Curry, knew at the end but not because Caron had told him. He, like many others, had considered himself a good friend and was confused when she fell off the radar. I think it probably got quite difficult for those who did know. It wasn't as if they were part of some charmed inner circle – it wasn't a bonus to carry that knowledge around with no one to share it – and they could understand why some were thinking, Why didn't she just tell me? It was complicated. Caron didn't really know herself, but she was adamant that the secret of her cancer would be kept.

As time went on people began to wonder why she was pulling out of work and questions were asked. First she pulled out of *Attraction*, a new show she was due to present for Channel Five. Then, a few months later, the same happened with a programme called *Apparitions* for Channel 4. There was a strange pattern to it: she'd have the treatment, improve, get stronger, find work, something would happen and she'd have to pull out for more treatment. We would all say the same thing, 'She had a rotten time after Gabriel was born, but she's fine now,' and to most of her friends that was the truth. Some thought she was rude because she'd withdrawn from them, and wondered why certain friends were backing her up when others considered her behaviour unacceptable. Then the press reported that Caron had had postnatal depression after her father had died, and although she was angry about the stories and resented the labelling, they gave her a get-out clause. For a while. But as time went on, and she didn't get back into regular work, it got worse again. How long did postnatal depression last, for God's sake? Gabriel was walking and talking.

When people asked her directly why she wasn't working, or why she was spending so much time in Cornwall before she and Russ had moved down there, she'd dance round the subject, determined to keep her secret. People were confused as to why she was so removed. Actually, the removal took place in several stages, but latterly, once she'd gone to Australia, it was difficult for people to get in touch with her.

Even when she moved down to Cornwall, the friends who knew thought she was just doing what she wanted to do. Not something she *had* to do. Of course, eventually the rumour mill cranked into action: people wondered whether she'd had a breakdown, whether she'd turned her back on life. Was there trouble at home? Had she and Russ moved to try to patch things up? It went on and on, and although she hated every false story it never crossed her mind to set the record straight. She didn't like doing the publicity she had to do when she was working, and she certainly wasn't going to give interviews now. Even her friends in Cornwall, the people she saw seven days a week, didn't know. When she did her final disappearing act to Australia they were more perplexed than ever, but I don't think Caron thought they were hurt by her actions. She was forging ahead on a quest to self-heal. Not everyone could come along for the ride.

Of course, gradually the secret got out. Yasmin told her husband one day when he caught her in tears after she'd spoken to Caron about her chemotherapy. Her mother had died by then and she was gripped with fear because her mother had said, 'Look after your friend, she isn't well.' Her mother had been a doctor, so whatever Caron was saying, Yasmin was beginning to wonder. Yasmin told Caron that Johnny knew, and she was fine about it. Russ was chastised because at some point he had to tell his business partner, Peter Powell, what was going on in order to be able to facilitate the move to Cornwall. Caron didn't talk to him for four days. Russ says she was horrified that Peter knew she was 'flawed'.

One weekend when they were living in Cornwall something came out in one of the tabloids. I think someone had taken a photo of her walking on the beach and she didn't look so well. They charged her with the crime of burnout. Yasmin and her husband were staying at the time: he works for a tabloid newspaper and told Caron not to say anything. So she didn't respond. She didn't scream, 'The reason why I'm not looking so good is because my body has spent the last six weeks being pumped full of chemotherapy, I've had my breast removed, my hair has fallen out and I'm wearing a wig'. No. She held on to her secret and her dignity.

Turns out she needn't have worried. I now gather that the editors of several newspapers knew almost from the beginning. A porter took a photo in those early days at the Royal Marsden.

Others were taken throughout the seven years which landed on editors' desks. Thankfully none was printed. I'm told one paper even got hold of copies of her medical records, which is a bit too much for me to take in and I know because Peter Powell was perpetually putting out fires while Caron and Russ were in Australia, that another had information about the radiation she was having on her spine in the final year of her life. If that is the case, then a newspaper in England would have known more details of Caron's condition than Caron knew herself. However, none of these stories ever broke. I am sure I have Peter to thank for that but I've also heard from friends in the press that there was a general agreement to leave Caron alone. They liked her, she had never been one to court the press and so she and her decision to fight her battle in private was respected. So, although her secret was out, it was still safe. I will always be grateful to the British press for leaving her in peace as they did. I don't honestly think she could have fought as long and as successfully as she did if they hadn't given her that privacy. If what I've heard is true about the photos and the medical records, then that agreement renews one's faith in mankind and the newspaper industry.

I wonder if there wasn't a more fundamental reason for Caron not to acknowledge publicly that she had cancer. I wonder if the secret she was really keeping was the one from herself. For all her bravado and positive thinking, underneath it all she was petrified of dying, petrified of leaving her family and the boys. When you're dealing with a terminal illness, you can do whatever you want to do, tell or not tell, it's up to each individual. Maybe Caron didn't want to acknowledge it because that made it true. I totally accept that many people who have cancer will research it to the enth degree. That is their right. What is it? How long do I have? What are my chances? It is a matter of personal preference, of choice, and should be respected. Some people want to put their life in order and live the rest accordingly; others exist only because the cancer is denied. At the end of the day, there is no right or wrong way.

Like most of us, Caron never liked hospitals. She never liked the official side of things. At the end she made me promise she'd never go into a hospice or hospital. If a doctor could come to see her at home, she was happier. She didn't like the Royal Marsden, although it is the most superb hospital: she said it had 'Death' written over the door. It reminded her of the people who had lost their hair, and were already having chemotherapy. Just as she didn't want to be a statistic, she didn't want to face up to the fact that maybe one day she would lose her hair. You only went to hospitals because you were ill and Caron didn't want to be reminded that she was ill so she didn't want to go. She felt and looked good: a visit to the hospital reminded her of the disease that was raging inside her. Perhaps that was why she could be lax about visiting the doctor, because she dreaded the bad news. She'd send in the advance party. She would say, 'Don't give me all of the bad news, don't tell me the worst scenario, don't tell me that if it doesn't improve I only have a number of weeks, months, years, I don't want to know. I only want to know what I *have* to do. Tell me what I have to do and I'll do it. If it's more injections I'll do it, if it's more exercise, I'll do it, if it's another pill, I'll take it. But don't give me all the dressing, don't unravel my mindset or the positivity I've built up. Don't force me to acknowledge this disease. I have not invited it in. It is an impostor and it cannot stay.' I admire that. I've told my family that if I am ever unlucky enough to find myself in that position, that's how I want it dealt with. I don't want to know whether I've got six or twelve months. Who knows, if you're in that position, whether you can resist the temptation to ask, 'How long do I have, what's the prognosis?' But I like the idea of 'Just tell me what I have to do.' It is a very individual thing. I must stress that Caron was never deprived of the orthodox treatment she needed: she had it. She just never knew the nuances of it. She never knew or wanted to know the full extent. So, she sent in the advance party, Russ and myself, and we would sieve out what it was she needed to know, and what was in her opinion superfluous. It's self-protection, I suppose. So yes, mostly she was keeping the secret from herself. That was what gave her the strength to live. But whatever brave face she could muster for the outside world, there was always a quiet voice that whispered away to her in the dark.

Thoughts are very powerful things – if we let them. Like emotions they come and go. We have hundreds and hundreds of thoughts a day – they come and go and often when we start to notice what's happening, we just let the mind run away. But in this we have choice. There is a split second before the thought takes form when we can decide whether or not to let it in and then if we do, we have a further choice as to whether or not we let it through. Do we entertain it, place it down, lay a table for it and let it grow and grow in stature and size and importance? Sadly we often do.

For me, this dealing with fear has been one of the really, really challenging aspects of being ill. With serious illness, it is undoubtedly easy to let your mind go wild and create havoc. Even when I was clear, my mind loved playing 'what if – ?' 'what's happening in your body?' and so the endless checking around begins and the forever focusing on one part of the body. I believe it is essential if you have a strong mind to be given to obsessive thoughts, to train and discipline it. It's too easy to let it run wild and out of control, leaving you in pain and despair . . .

That pain and despair was to set in again. Just over two years later. On 15 December 1999 Caron went to the doctors, when her endless checking finally resulted in what she feared most. On the eve of the new millennium all our hopes were dashed. The cancer was back and this time in a more aggressive form.

12. Darling, I'd Rather Be Shopping

We were so confounded and devastated by the news that we asked the specialist, Mr Charles Lowdell, to come to our house in London and explain in more detail. On the eve of the new millennium, he gave my daughter eighteen months to live. The cancer had changed and become much more aggressive. Michael and I just looked at each other in total disbelief. The oncologists will still say that they don't have all the answers, but they do give time lines. Maybe it was a wake-up call. Caron had been resistant to certain aspects of the treatment on offer, like not taking Tamoxifen: maybe this was their way of making us understand that action had to be taken. Right up until that second we had been going for cure. Tough, yes, but cure. Whatever their reasons for giving us that prognosis, we never told Caron what the doctor had said. We knew better than that.

I had planned for the entire family to go to Florida for the New Year Millennium Celebrations; now I wanted to cancel the trip. The doctor talked about immediate mastectomy, so I didn't think we had a choice. But Caron wouldn't hear of it. We would go on holiday as planned, the kids were so excited and she didn't want to disappoint them. She booked the mastectomy for the day after our return. At some point before we left she found the time and, more impressively, the inclination to go over to Yasmin's house with Christmas presents. One of her girlfriends said with a little envy in her voice, 'Wow, Caron has everything, doesn't she?' She was looking effortlessly fabulous as always, Russ was being the gent as always, the boys were screaming and playing. Everything? Yasmin looked at her friend and thought, You have no idea what this woman is going through, no idea at all . . .

Stephen took a book by Caroline Myss on holiday. We rented a house in Fort Pearce on the east coast of Florida. Caron devoured the book. The author believes that we bring illness on ourselves and suggests how we can heal ourselves. It became like a Bible to Caron.

I read two books by Carolyn Myss – an American medical institution: *Anatomy of the Spirit* and *Why People Don't Heal and How they Can*. I knew from those books that it was possible to heal, although I didn't have the knowledge to do it, and realized/decided that going down the medical route would buy me time. Myss's theory is that before the healing takes place, we need to heal those things that cause the disease in the first place. The first time it happened, I was confident it was my dad dying: all the grief had formed small lumps. I never thought it would happen again. When more cells changed it meant looking at the situation a little more deeply and with more clarity. Surgery and six sessions of chemotherapy were going to give me plenty of spare time to gather the information I needed to heal myself . . .

For those glorious two weeks Caron was able to rest when she wanted to, eat fresh food, get some sun and take long walks on the beach. There was an undercurrent during all the celebrations, of course, the ever-present sword of Damocles hung over us, but we carried on despite it and had a great time. Caron was in no pain at that stage; the only pain was in our hearts and heads and stomachs. She and I had a long time to talk about the implications of the mastectomy and how she was now determined to explore more fully the realm of self-healing. But she didn't know what the doctor had said. That was the terrible secret that Russ, Michael, Paul, Stephen and I had to bear. Eighteen months! The words screeched in my brain as I listened to Caron talk determinedly about how she was sure she was going to be fine. She had no idea just how aggressive it had become, no idea at all. But she was so convincing that even though I had been told eighteen months, I said to myself, 'Well, the doctor doesn't know my Caron, he doesn't know she can self-heal, he won't believe about the positive route and, yes, she'll have all the drugs and the mastectomy and the chemotherapy, but she'll be doing all of this other stuff too and she will survive.' I distinctly remember Sandy, Paul's partner, saying to me that she couldn't believe how stoic Caron was being. She was bowled over that Caron could come away on holiday knowing the doctor had wanted to operate immediately. We were all very proud of her. We were all terrified for her.

On 1 January 2000, as the sun came up, Caron and I were on the beach together. She looked into the sky and said, 'Look Mum, it's going to be all right.' The clouds had formed into a beautiful angel shape. Caron thought it was a sign from God, given to her on the first day of the new millennium, that it was going to be all right. Who was I not to believe her?

My mother had a mastectomy when I was in my early forties. It was an emergency operation and happened while I was in the Seychelles. Six months earlier she had gone to the doctor with eczema under her breast and been given some cream. After that they never asked, and she never said, whether it had cleared up. Which it hadn't. Then the nipple inverted. My mother got scared and went back to the doctor. He sent her to hospital immediately and she was operated on very quickly. She was seventy.

I landed at Heathrow and got a message to call Caron. When I heard the news, I flew straight to Northern Ireland. As I arrived at the Craigavon hospital in Portadown there was my ever-cheery mother, walking down the corridor carrying her drip around in a Marks & Spencer's plastic bag. Even though she recovered really well, and everyone thought that was that, I was, and remain to this day, angry about the wasted six months,

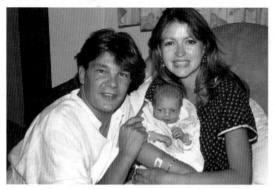

The magical first photograph of Caron with beautiful baby Charlie

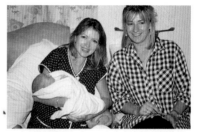

A family exhausted. Caron showing off her brand-new baby Charlie to her great friend Cathy Comerford, who later became his godmother

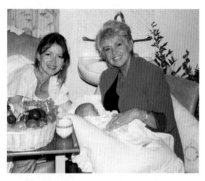

Newborn Charlie. I will always be grateful to Caron for asking me to be present at Charlie and Gabriel's births. What a privilege!

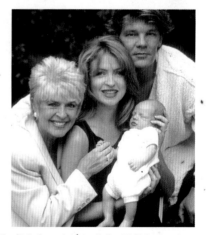

Charlie's first photo call for *Hello!* magazine, taken in the back garden in Barnes

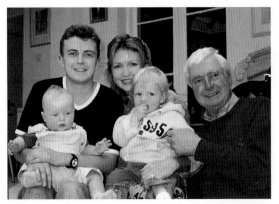

Proud grandfather Don, visiting his
first two grandsons, Jake and Charlie,
at Paul's house

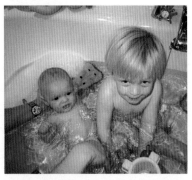

Nothing like fun at bathtime. Gabriel is
not so sure

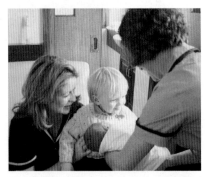

Charlie's joy – being presented with his baby
brother Gabriel. Charlie still looks after and
watches out for his little brother

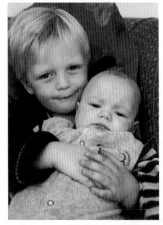

Charlie – a gorgeous caring boy, cuddling his baby brother Gabriel

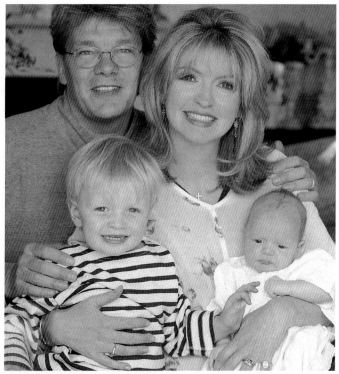

Gabriel *(right)* looking slightly bored with his first photo-shoot

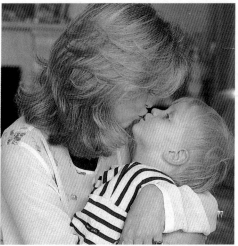

Beautiful boy.
Charlie aged two

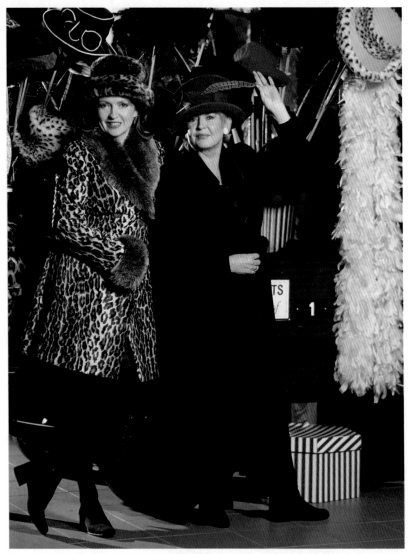

Consummate shoppers

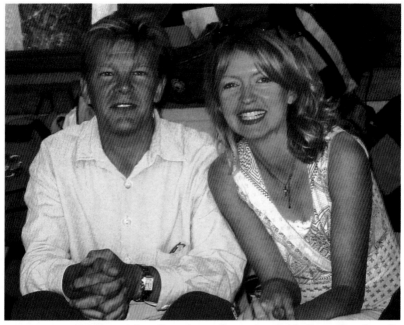

A great couple – Caron in a really good period in Byron Bay, Australia

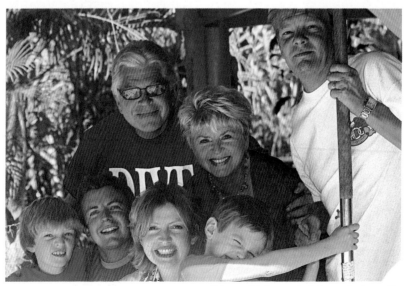

Taken at Taylors - their home in Australia.
The family all gather round for Caron's birthday. She adored special occasions

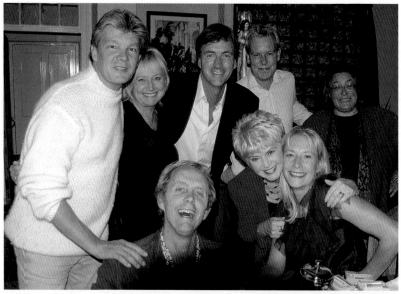

The Stalwart Cornwall Gang. *From left to right:* Russ, Judy Finnegan, Richard Madeley, Andrew 'Bill' Williams, Judith and Jono Taylor, Glo and Claire Williams

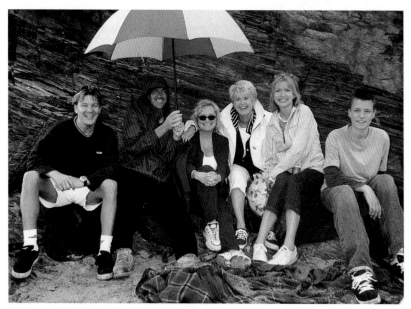

A very wet but happy day on a Cornish beach, with our dear friends Richard and Judy and their son Jack

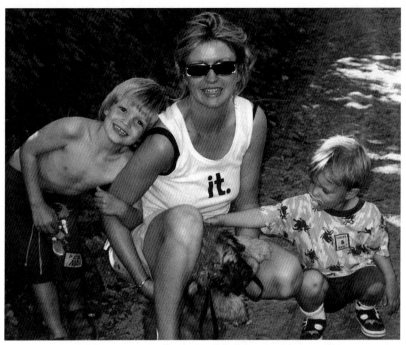

Happy days in Cornwall. Charlie (*left of Caron*) with one of his posey grins.
Gabriel (*right of Caron*) more interested in Candy, their wheaten terrier

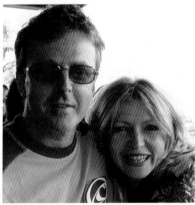

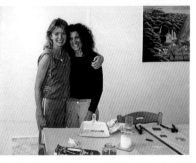

Caron's art studio, which she shared with
her friend Jen, a professional painter who,
for a while, was like a sister to her

A memorable and poignant trip for Paul
in Byron Bay. Photograph taken at the
Seven Mile Café, which Caron loved
because it offered really healthy food

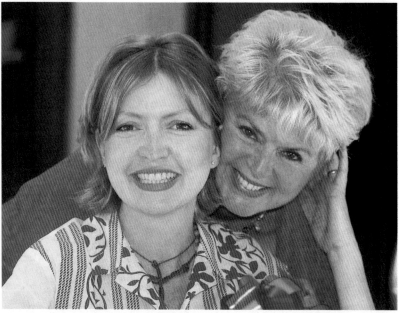

Caron's last birthday, 5 October 2003. She was in the middle of radiotherapy. Always that broad smile and shining eyes

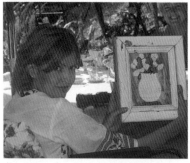

One of my last birthday presents to Caron, a painting she had been eyeing for weeks

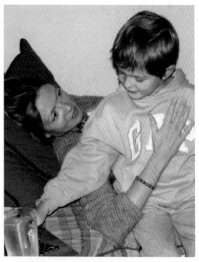

At their home in Australia. Precious time spent with Gabriel, aged six

that the doctor and my mother were so slack about following up the initial examination. In those days, no one questioned the doctor, and certainly not my mum. I was aware that she was unlikely to be able to come over to England any more to visit. On my birthday that year, four months later, we went to the local hotel for a drink. The bar was full of people, then the crowd cleared and there, in the corner, was my mum. Caron had gone to Ireland and travelled back with her. It was the best surprise present I could ever have had. Two years later she was getting on the bus one day and her arm snapped. It was classified as an involuntary break. The cancer had seeped into her bones.

So, of course, when Caron was advised to have a mastectomy, I was under no illusion about the possible implications. I knew it was huge. I was older, wiser and I treated this news with a new eye. Having said that, Caron was much younger than my mum had been. I thought Caron had youth on her side. I could not get my head round the fact that my beautiful girl, in her thirties, was going to have a mastectomy. I knew she'd have reconstruction, I knew it was for her own safety, I knew it was essential, but I just couldn't handle it. This new information was monumental.

On the eve of the operation we went to cook dinner for Caron in Barnes. I couldn't do much to make it better, but at least I could do that. We all went, her brothers, Sandy and Stephen. We were sitting around the table, false jollity, false conversation, false bravado. We knew what would happen the next day but none of us knew how to deal with it. I think we were talking about politics when she blew up. She stood up and shouted, 'Will you all shut up? Just f*****g shut up! Don't you know what's happening to me tomorrow? Why are you talking about everything in the bloody world, but you can't talk about what is happening to me tomorrow?' I was so upset and disturbed: I'd seen my baby girl in turmoil and couldn't do anything about it. I couldn't bring her any peace or comfort. I rang my friend Roberta in Northern Ireland, clutching my own breast in tears, crying into the phone. I could feel it being cut off. I could visualize it. But I still could not believe it.

As with all my children when they are sick – though, thankfully, apart from Caron, that is rare – I have always believed that you should be there at the hospital beforehand, there during the premeds, then go with them as far as the theatre. More importantly, you're there when they wake up. So that was what Russ and I did on the day of Caron's mastectomy. It was an agonizing wait. Despite the hours and hours that passed with nothing else to think about, we could not absorb what was happening to Caron somewhere else in the building. It was such a long operation because she had decided to have the reconstruction done at the same time. Some doctors say that, if you can bear it, it is better to have the mastectomy first and the reconstruction later. I'm told that removing the breast is relatively simple. It's the reconstruction that is complicated. But, understandably, Caron wanted it all done and dusted. She didn't want it hanging over her: she wanted to get on with living her life. Also she had 100 per cent faith in her surgeon, and he did a great job. She ended up with a great-shaped boob. She always intended to have the nipple remade – she was talking about that until the very end, but it was never a priority. I don't think it actually bothered her that much. At the time she'd been more concerned about the effect of the anaesthetic on her body and made sure she took everything that Jan de Vries recommended to counterbalance its effects and keep her immune system as strong as possible.

As always, Russ wanted to please Caron and made everything as bearable as possible. She was fortunate enough to have private treatment. He arranged for her to have a corner room, in the Lister Hospital in London, that was as light, bright and unhospital-like as a hospital room could be. Everything we could think of that might help her recover was brought into the room. She was heavily into doing mosaics then, and made a beautiful mask while she was in there, which she gave me the following Christmas. I wept buckets when she gave it to me because it represented all the agony of that time. Every little tile, every little piece of mirror had been put there so painstakingly. It sits in my bedroom. It still makes me cry.

We made it as much fun as we could. The tag team brought on a few more members so that we could take it in turns. Janet arrived with fairy-lights for Caron's room. She was so impressed by the reconstruction that she thought, Move up, girl, I'm getting in. I used to park on the other side of Chelsea Bridge, then walk across, all the while staring up at her bedroom window wishing myself nearer and nearer. In retrospect, all of the time we spent in isolation, in the wards while she had injections, the hospital rooms where she was recovering, turned out to be capsules of very special, treasured times. The worst for me was the new depth of despair to which I plummeted on the night before the operation. Afterwards, when Caron was sitting up in bed, recovering better and faster than expected, it was easier. Mentally you say to yourself, 'Well, they had to cut away the bad stuff, but the reconstruction is brilliant.' So once again, you turn the negative into a positive. Suddenly we were relieved that the bad stuff had gone. I said to Caron, 'Try to think of it as cosmetic. Think of all the people who have this done by choice.' Suddenly it was mundane, pedestrian: the fear had gone. Temporarily, at least. The cloud of doom, the fearful taboo, had lifted so much that even the little boys came to visit.

I think that God, or a greater force, gives you the strength to cope with each stage of the disease as it comes. In the beginning the lumpectomy, that tiny grade-one twelve-millimetre tumour signalled the end of the world to me. Eighteen months down the line we were faced with numerous grade-three invasive carcinomas, widespread invasion into the lymph nodes, surrounding fat and some of the breast ducts. The breast comes off, yet we found the strength to rationalize it. Once it's a *fait accompli*, it's amazing how you can turn it round and move on. Consciously or otherwise, and I suspect it is otherwise, you continue to do a head job for the other person, and you have to do one on yourself. And this is how it continued. It wasn't like a road accident which happens in one blow: this was step by step until the end. And each stage is worse than the stage before, yet somehow you learn to deal with it better.

We were advised to let Caron recover from surgery before starting chemotherapy. She and Russ had always gone to Fowey in Cornwall for holidays, and now they started going there every waking minute that Charlie, then aged six, was off school. Each time she came back, she found the city more oppressive, the pollution more aggressive and the pace of life too fast. So they said, let's reverse this. Hans Moolenburg in Amsterdam had told Caron early on that people who make a change in their lives have a better chance of life.

During the February half-term, Caron and Russ had been walking on the beach in Fowey where they rented a small white fisherman's cottage at Readymoney Cove on the seafront. Caron looked up at the row of houses on the cliff above them and said to Russ, 'I wonder what our lives would be like if we lived there?' On the way back to London, with the two kids asleep in the back of the car, she said, 'Let's move.' Russ turned to Caron to see if she was serious, then drove on in silence. He had seen the look in her eyes. She was like a rabbit caught in headlights. Russ knew what his wife needed. She needed the change that people had been talking to her about. She needed the privacy. She needed to get out of London, away from the pollution and overwhelming pace.

Maybe Russ is right. Maybe it was like driving with a chip in the windscreen. As the hairline crack begins to spread, you know there is only a certain amount of driving you can do before the screen breaks apart. It cannot last for ever and no amount of sticky tape will save it. His theory, unconsciously put into action, was: the slower you drive, the less pressure you're going to put on it. That was why he took his wife's words seriously, that was why he went into the office the next day and as good as resigned from day to day business. Peter accepted that his partner had to do what he had to do and made room for the change. Caron and Russ took their foot off the accelerator and got more mileage out of a windscreen that had been designated as flawed long before they were ready to lose it.

Caron's knight in shining armour moved rapidly. He called some estate agents in the area to discover what, if anything, was for sale. Nothing was. But one agent said that one of the residents had been thinking about selling, though they hadn't actually put the house on the market. That was Menlo, one of the houses they'd been looking up at during their chat on the beach. The agent gave Russ his estimate of the value of the house and said he'd set up a meeting. Sometime that week Russ returned to Fowey, flew in, saw the house and told Caron the owner was willing to sell. The property, although in good condition, had not been modernized. But it was in a wonderful location and had great potential. The price had mysteriously gone up by 30 per cent, but Russ didn't care. By May of that year Menlo was theirs. Russ had given his wife the change she needed to turn this journey around and get them back on their original path. Renovations soon began. So did chemotherapy.

Chemotherapy had been recommended because of the change in the grade of Caron's cancer and the behaviour of the tumour. The scan had revealed some small hard lymph nodes on the left side, which they had not removed, and, maybe a sign of things to come, a small nodule in the right breast. Thankfully, they all resolved rapidly with chemotherapy. Caron was faced with six intense sessions of high-potency chemotherapy, each session separated by a twenty-day gap to let her body recover as best it could. Chemotherapy works because it is so aggressive;

it kills cancer cells but if it is too strong it can damage the heart. At that stage the doctors were treating Caron with as strong a dose as they could; anything less would not have worked. For secrecy's sake, Russ would drive them up to the back of the hospital where they'd meet a nurse and sometimes Michael or Cathy Comerford if Russ had to get back to look after the boys. Upstairs, Caron would put on this strange headgear: a big metal helmet that keeps the head cool, to minimize hair loss, while the chemotherapy is being administered.

Whoever was with her would settle her in and get the television lined up, or would chat away. Michael was brilliant at it. He could gossip with his sister while they flicked through magazines, laughing about what people were wearing, discussing any scandal that was going on, anything really, rather than talk about what was happening. When it was over Michael would drive her to me in Sevenoaks. That was where the sickness kicked in – when all that stuff was inside her. Sometimes Michael would fall out of 'clown mode' and simply stare at the tube in Caron's arm and wonder, as she did, Is it this stuff that's killing you? Yasmin says that Caron could not have been more grateful for her younger brother's support during those six weeks. He was an absolute trouper. Chemotherapy isn't supposed to be fun, but somehow the two of them cast their maverick Irish spell over the room, and found a way to laugh. Michael, of course, believes that the hard job was caring for Caron in the days that followed, when she was really sick. The truth is, it was all hard, but Michael says that sitting with his beloved sister and talking nonsense was the least difficult part of it all.

Cathy would call up and ask, 'How's the chemotherapy going?' To which Caron would reply, more often than not, 'Darling, I'd rather be shopping.' As ever, she was making it easier on us all.

So Caron went home to recuperate, she wasn't throwing up but she couldn't eat for a while, she started to lose a little weight.

How ill she felt depended on the amount she'd been given and how it was administered. They did a great job, because she wasn't as wiped out as I'd expected her to be. She stayed in bed for the first day and didn't eat, but on the second she might manage a baked potato and beans. The day after that she'd eat a little more and would get up and come downstairs. Basically we did what we could to cosset her until she got her strength back. Which she did. We used to say, 'Regard it as a little holiday away from the daily grind.' She'd do jigsaws, draw, read, sleep and watch TV. By the time her friends saw her she looked pretty good. All the way through she just wanted to get on with it. I do not recall her ever sitting around and moping.

What she did find painful after the chemo were the ulcers: her mouth was full of them. It was very uncomfortable. I remember Johnny and Cathy coming down to Kent: they had a great morning, a real laugh, the usual Sevenoaks thing, all of us sitting around drinking tea, gassing away as if nothing in the world could bother us. All the while Caron's mouth was covered with sores.

Eventually she told the others. She left a message for Yasmin that she was at my house. That was the only sign Yasmin needed to tell that something was wrong. Caron always retreated there: it was where she felt safe.

'Are you all right?' asked Yasmin.

'I'm okay now,' she'd say. As before, Caron needed time to get her head round what was happening. Again, I'm glad she didn't tell a lot of people because then she didn't have a lot of people to update.

'They found some more lumps,' she'd say.

'In the same breast?' asked Yasmin. Because her mother had explained the disease more fully to her, she was probably more clued up than any of us.

Caron talked to her about the chemo: 'It's not too bad actually. Michael makes it a real laugh – he makes it like a day out. Then I go to Mum's house for a couple of days and eat baked potatoes and baked beans and lie around, watch *This Morning*, then go home. Just a few more and it's over.' And, as far as she was concerned, it was done. Physically, she coped amazingly with the extreme potency of the chemotherapy. Mentally, she drew a line under it.

Stephen said to me before Caron had the mastectomy, 'One of the best things we can give her is a really good wig made of real hair.' He made a template of her head with cling film, then painstakingly took samples of all her hair colours and shades. Then he went to the best wig-maker he knew, saying it was for a client, and 'Nancy' was born. In a way we were trying to be one step ahead of the game. We were hellbent that, if the day came that her hair started to fall out, the wig would be there as back-up. Thanks to Stephen, she never had a day when she thought, I can't go out because of my hair. When you feel helpless and hopeless, this kind of practicality is all you can do to feel you're making a real contribution. You can love, hug, comfort, stroke, kiss, run errands, look after the boys, cook and you still feel hopeless, but the wig was a coup. Stephen's coup. It must have been incredibly hard for him all that time: although Caron wasn't his daughter, he loved her like the daughter he never had. He was watching me watching her. So he was really pleased to be able to do something practical that made such a fundamental difference to the quality of her life at that time.

If you looked at her head from above I swear you couldn't tell that it wasn't scalp. Nancy was their neighbour at their first house who had helped to look after Charlie when he was a baby. Caron adored both Nancys, the real one and the wig. Because it was so tailored, it was very comfortable and she could forget she was wearing it. That, and that she knew it wouldn't fail her, gave her a great deal of confidence. Losing hair is traumatic: it tends to come out in lumps. She never lost it completely, but it was patchy and thin. I only saw it once. All her life she'd had a glorious mane: I had spent so many years plaiting it, brushing it and tying it with ribbons, and now it was gone. At times she looked twenty years older. Her desire for privacy protected us all from the horror of her hair loss. She never complained. I never heard her cry, 'Mum, my hair's falling out in clumps,' although by the third dose of chemo, it was. I don't think I could have dealt with it as she did.

If she wasn't wearing Nancy, she wore a scarf. You soon develop respect for someone who is going through what Caron was, and we were all careful to knock on her door before going in, and didn't turn up unannounced. Likewise, I never asked to see her reconstruction or later, when she had had a very radical poultice treatment, which scarred her badly. You have to honour the sufferer's self-respect.

Her friends never saw her without Nancy either. If Cathy dropped in after the school run, she'd be wearing Nancy. People would say, 'Have you had your hair done? It's never looked so good.' Those who knew would hide a smile and have a good old laugh about it afterwards. Nancy mark two became her great friend. She would set the alarm early and put it on so that when the boys came into her and Russ's room they wouldn't be shocked. But one day they overslept, the boys scrambled all over them as usual and didn't even notice the change in Caron's hair. The boys just saw their lovely mum. Your children, I have learnt, teach you more about life than you could ever teach them. And I don't mean just when they're young.

Before she moved permanently to Cornwall in the summer of 2000, Caron had a big lunch for the Soho House Mafia and the Barnes ladies. Some knew why she was leaving, most didn't. It seemed an odd choice to those who didn't, since she was doing so well at *This Morning* and was apparently on great form. It seemed to her friends that every time Caron went back to work and got into the groove, something happened to stop her. The move to Cornwall made them wonder if there was something they weren't being told. Cornwall seemed a drastic change, but that was exactly what Caron wanted.

It was a hot day and Caron was quite thin – she'd lost a fair amount of weight when she couldn't eat after the chemotherapy. Two of Yasmin's friends came who didn't know any of it, not that she'd had three operations, lost a breast, had radiotherapy, was halfway through chemotherapy, or that she was wearing a wig. Once again, comments were made about Caron's appearance but more in envy. She was thin and some of the women perhaps were a little envious and even wished they could be more like her. You have to be so careful what you wish for. Caron's weight loss came at a terrible price. Anyway, Janet Ellis was giving Caron some stick about moving to the country, saying she'd never survive in the back of beyond without Joseph or Harvey Nichols. Caron took a lot of stick – she could dish it out, but she could take it, and everyone was laughing about it, even the ones who knew. Caron had underplayed it all so much that they almost didn't take it seriously. That is not a criticism: it's how Caron wanted it. It was a really hot day, they sat outside in the sunshine, chatting, laughing and drinking. It wasn't until later that Yasmin, Cathy and Janet thought how hot it must have been for her to sit there in a wig. In fact, during that lunch they forgot themselves for swathes of time. It didn't even seem strange not telling people, as by then it felt that there was nothing to tell. Even I, who'd lost my mother to breast cancer, was taken in. I don't think any of us fully understood at the time what it meant. Maybe I remained naïve to the end and hadn't learnt as much from my mother's death as I'd thought.

13. Sea Air

The summer following the purchase of Menlo was a fantastic one. Which seems impossible, considering that Caron was undergoing chemotherapy throughout it. Russ and she bought the house in May and immediately got their teeth into their new project: renovating Menlo. This was no dab-of-paint job but a large-scale project to turn the property into a young, modern family house, and probably just what they needed. It was something else to focus on. It was wonderful for Caron to do something so positive towards changing their lifestyle. They moved back into the fisherman's cottage on the seafront that had housed them for so many happy holidays over the previous ten years, and from which they could look up daily and watch the process of building take place before their very eyes. They visited Menlo daily, with their lovely architect, Chris Jones, had a cup of tea with the builders, and Caron got creative, designing a completely new built-on kitchen and semicircular dining area. They were determined to get the most out of the property's location overlooking the sea.

They spent hours walking around the building site, high above Readymoney Cove, planning and imagining. The Cornish light distracted them from the shadow of chemotherapy. Everything became easier to handle. Caron had something wonderful to look forward to. She was making the change she thought would improve her chances of beating cancer. She was active on all fronts. It was an incredibly positive time.

During that summer they got the boys into the local school in Fowey, and in September they moved into their wonderful new clifftop, sea-view, glass-fronted, heavenly house. Yes, it was a lovely summer, the best since the cancer had been diagnosed. There was something innocent and free about it, and the boys loved it. Russ bought a wooden clinker-built boat called *Driftwood* and quickly taught himself to sail. They created wonderful *Swallows and Amazons* adventures for the children to enjoy, taking picnics to little coves, playing cricket and rounders on Alldays Field high up on the headland and looking down the estuary where the boats sail into Fowey harbour. I know who enjoyed those adventures most of all: Caron and Russ.

I, on the other hand, was selfishly thinking – six hours away! This is not where Irish mothers want their children to be. No more popping over for coffee on the way in from Kent or reading the children stories at bedtime. No more meeting up in the studio after work. No more easy shopping trips or long lunches without a six-hour journey first. And what about her friends, whom she loved so much, relied on so heavily, saw so regularly? If I had known then that another twenty-four hours would be added to that distance, I would have settled for six. As I came gradually to understand their move to Australia, I eventually understood their departure from London.

Caron was a family person at heart: she wanted her children to know their extended family, and liked small places where everyone knew your name. Life in Cornwall emulated her childhood in Northern Ireland. Fowey gave her that sense of belonging, which was why she loved it so much, so quickly. The local community welcomed the family and she soon felt very much at home. London is big and very impersonal: it was difficult to find the quirky one in the room when the room was so overcrowded. I should have known that Cornwall, or a place like it, would call to her. If Don had been alive, it might have been Ireland – I think they even looked at a couple of places there. I have a vivid picture of Caron in my mind riding her bicycle, along the esplanade, with a basket on the front with all the shopping, in Fowey. She could bike down to the local fish shop, buy something fresh from Graham and Sue, have a chat at the deli across the street with Sally and Jane and bike home for Russ to cook what she had bought. Russ, never one to do things by halves, not only took to the sea but enrolled himself on the Rick Stein fish course so that he could make the most of the local produce. Stephen and Michael joined him, and that short week changed our lives.

There is no doubt about it: Fowey gave Caron the new start she craved. Not only was she leaving the pressures of the city behind her, she was gaining a new zest for life. There is a beauty and spirituality in Cornwall that reaches into your soul. It gives you space, freedom, colour and clarity. All of the things Caron felt she'd lost. It gave her the time to do things she'd previously only talked about doing, or felt she'd never done enough of. She could paint more and go for walks; she could throw herself into the community, which she did with aplomb. At the Fowey parade during regatta week, she'd be the one in the pink wig dressed up as Barbie, standing on a float, embarrassing her children. More importantly, Cornwall gave her back her children.

The previous two years had been a struggle, coming to terms with Don's death and her shocking diagnosis. Cornwall gave her the space to nurture the boys. She liked getting to know the mothers at the school, beyond a cursory chat while the car is double-parked and the wardens are circling. Even before they had moved into their new home, they joined a local protest to stop a mobile phone mast being built near the school. We all joined in and there was massive publicity. In the end Russ went into the headquarters of the telecommunications company and negotiated with the top man to have the mast relocated. That sort of thing would have appealed to Caron: it made her feel she was doing something worthwhile for her community and in turn they warmly welcomed the family. Overall, she was comfortable living down there. They were extremely happy and, I had to admit it, the sea air was good for Caron. Cornwall was a good move.

When Russ and Caron relocated, their friends Wendy and Graham Bills moved with them. Russ and Graham bought another set of buildings, called Wild Thyme Farm, in which they set up Bluefin Productions. Attached to it was an organic field, which Caron loved, where they planned to grow vegetables and fruit. They even had a pottery room in one of the outbuildings. While the boys were at school, Caron and Wendy could do pottery, Russ and Graham worked on new business projects and all was well with the world. They had a dream, a Utopian vision, which, for a little while, they lived.

Then Caron found a new path to follow. On his way back to Fowey after a business trip to London, Russ stopped at a garage to fill up the car. Casually, he picked up a pile of magazines for Caron, *Vogue*, *OK*, *Hello!*, *Architectural Design*, and an innocuous-looking New Age publication that he thought would interest her. Caron was still making regular journeys to Matthew Manning, the healer, and the homeopathic reflexologist. She had even visited Jack Temple, who told her the black stockings she wore were carcinogenic. She was still searching for a miracle. Russ took those magazines home, and Caron, as with all reading material, devoured the lot.

When more cells changed it meant looking at the situation a little more deeply and with more clarity. I had time to do it – surgery and six sessions of chemo gave me plenty of spare time to gather information and have healing sessions. The move from London and the renovation of the house in Cornwall was something else to focus on, though I still wasn't sure that I had actually cleaned out the vast problem.

My search at that stage ended one day in Cornwall when Russ brought me a copy of a spiritual magazine and in it was a leaflet for a book called *The Journey*, written by an American guru called Brandon Bays. It told her story of how she had managed to heal herself of a baseball-sized tumour in her stomach without drugs or surgery but by using a process she had developed of gaining access to the cellular memory. Something inside clicked and I immediately wrote off for her book and tape. They were waiting for me when I got home some days later and I simply devoured them.

Here was a woman who'd had a baseball-sized tumour in her stomach and had managed to shrink it without surgery or drugs in just six weeks . . .

That was all Caron needed to read.

The book and cassette were waiting for me when I got back to London. Blonde, blue-eyed and smiling at me from the cover – an all-American gal glowing with health. I devoured her story in a day and decided to see her. She lived twenty minutes away and gave private sessions – I dialled the number at the back of the book.

'Sorry, Brandon's away at the moment and she doesn't give private sessions unless you've been to a workshop first,' said a brisk-sounding woman on the phone.

'I can't go to a workshop.' I tried to explain without really telling her why – although the main reason was a horror of 'opening up and sharing' with a load of strangers. Catharting in public was really not my thing.

'Then, sorry, but I can't really help you.' Brrrrrrr.

Undeterred I refused to give up. In her book Brandon had been desperate to see a reflexologist and hadn't been able to – determined, she kept going until she eventually got through to him. I decided to adopt her approach and use it on her.

Next day, the LSH [long-suffering husband] offered to ring for me and we contented ourselves with the thought that if it was meant to be we'd get an appointment. Much more of a natural diplomat, he charmed and cajoled his way through the conversation – and, probably more significantly, actually told them what was going on. This time she said she'd ask and get back to us.

Five minutes later a guy rang back asking for Russ. It turned out to be a childhood friend who had moved to London with him when they were seventeen and doing the guys-in-the-big-city thing. He was Brandon's right-hand man and had e-mailed her and got me an appointment.

I've come to the conclusion that we never really know what is going on, why situations present themselves like they do and how sometimes the direst of circumstances produce the biggest of gifts.

Just before the appointment I was due for another infusion of chemotherapy – but, much to the horror of the doctors, I'd been fasting and my body wasn't ready for the next session, which meant that by the time I was due to see Brandon, I was actually feeling pretty good.

I arrived early – this only ever occurs in my life when I'm frightened or deeply impressed with whom I'm going to meet. An Irish sense of time and dislike of waiting have meant a lifetime of apologizing for my tardiness. Anyway, there I was with no idea of what to expect or indeed how exactly she was going to help me.

A smiling girl met me at the door and offered herbal tea – and then there was Brandon herself, just as glowing, smiley and radiant as the picture on the cover.

This was a woman used to dealing with nervous wrecks on her doorstep and she talked to me gently in her reassuring voice before leading me into a vast light-filled room, overlooking a beautiful garden. It was calm, tastefully furnished with white, and Buddhas were dotted around.

It was like stepping into another world. This woman, whom I had never met before, treated me with so much care and seemed genuinely concerned about what was going on in my life. Having wrapped me in shawls and put cushions under my bare feet she began her *Journey* process and took me to a place so profound and different from anything I'd experienced that I couldn't speak about it for three days afterwards.

My lasting memory was experiencing my spirit as being so huge that I just kept wondering how I would ever get back into my body again.

Afterwards she asked me to stay for lunch, which was organic, vegetarian accompanied by freshly squeezed juices, all stuff I loved. It was served in a bright airy conservatory at a big table surrounded by more radiant, friendly people. Before we started everyone held hands and Brandon said a blessing for the food. Wow, I thought, people really live like this? It was like peering through a window into a parallel world, one that I quite fancied inhabiting.

As I write this I realize that is exactly what has happened. Not only do I still know Brandon – she has become a really good friend – just last night we had dinner with her in Byron Bay, where I now live. And, yes, before we ate everyone held hands and blessed the food and the company.

I don't quite know how I came to be living here – all I do know is that somewhere along the way I put out a really strong prayer and something or someone much more powerful and knowing than me heard and spun it into action.

Be careful what you pray for – you might just get it.

Russ said that sitting in Brandon's house the first time they went there was like being shown into Heaven's waiting room. It was the first time they had experienced a full-on spiritual house. Against an all-white background there were Buddhas and the colourful Indian elephant god, Ganesh. All the windows were open and white linen curtains billowed in the breeze. Joss sticks burned smoothly in the corners. Imagine what it was like to go from muddy boots, bikes, battle games, fighting and all the boisterousness of life with two small boys to such total calm. The depth of the tranquillity they felt was limitless and they were taken aback by the whole experience. For Caron it was a blessed relief and the perfect antidote to the clinical side of cancer she had been going through.

From then on, Caron and Russ travelled up to Slough every now and then to see Brandon and her husband Kevin. That was when Caron really started to work in tandem with the orthodox treatments, accepting that the chemo was necessary but happy to augment it with the inner strength that complementary therapy gave her. And it *was* giving her inner strength: you could see it in her eyes. Yasmin remembers seeing Caron stand in front of her on the deck at Menlo, in a big jacket, walking-boots and her stylish Maharishi trousers (a different pair for every day of the week, naturally). She closed her eyes, breathed in, and looked so strong it was as though she was drawing strength from some invisible force. Yasmin wanted to clap: she was bowled over by Caron because in that instant Caron was trying so hard to face everything that was happening to her without self-pity. Her inquisitive mind was taking on board everything that Brandon had to offer. She was trying to stop the wall of fear, which was threatening to imprison her, building up.

It must have been hard. The two practices, orthodox and complementary, don't always run parallel. Many orthodox doctors don't like self-healing teachings: they mistrust it and its promises. Equally, self-healing requires purity of mind, body and soul, which is difficult to achieve when you are required to take medication that Caron regarded as poisonous. So although she brought these two opposing sides together, I doubt it was an easy fit.

At times I am simply overwhelmed by the enormity of it – oscillating between the two worlds I seem to straddle. The world of medicine, with its talk of cells, genes, treatment, time spans, and my flourishing spiritual landscape where the illness isn't the issue but, rather, what has brought it about . . .

It is a little like childbirth. Mothers are told that natural childbirth is best for the baby and less likely to lead to intervention and complications. In other words, no pain relief. Statistically that is correct. But natural childbirth used to kill many women. Thanks to orthodox medicine, that is no longer the case. It is a fine line and can often lead to confusion because, no matter how hard you try, you may be one of those women who, a hundred years ago, wouldn't have survived childbirth, in which case intervention is better. I think the same applies to the juxtaposition between self-healing and orthodox treatment.

In the autumn, life settled down in Cornwall. Russ and

Caron had great friends down there and, once again, their home became a magnet. Jono and Judith Taylor regularly popped over for tea. Judith is a governor of the school that the boys attended and Jono is a retired barrister in his mid-forties. Both are very bright, ex-Cambridge, and appealed to Caron's inquisitive mind and her love of deep conversation. Sarah Matthews was another great mate, who was always the bearer of home-made chocolates and goodies for the boys. Then there were Nick and Navan. Also London business people who had moved to Cornwall for a life change and Clare and Andrew Williams from Lanhydrock, who have subsequently opened a health and well-being centre in Fowey. They had built up a group of friends on their previous visits and, of course, there was no shortage of visits from their old crew. Johnny, Cathy and their kids were regulars, as were Janet Ellis and her husband John. Even Yasmin started going on holiday there. Although Caron didn't tell anyone what she was going through, most of them probably knew something was up, but didn't let on to Caron and Russ or to each other.

Even Stephen and I bought a house down there, although we had no intention of doing so.

Not long after they'd moved into their own house my daughter looked at me with that twinkle in her eye and said, 'I'm going to show you a little house. It has fabulous views . . .' Wouldn't it be wonderful if we were neighbours? she said. Her sly suggestion seemed like a good idea. It meant that if she needed me I could be there without having to be on top of them. The views may have been idyllic but like Caron and Russ's house it needed a lot of work. The builders lived there for two months, and as they moved out on 18 December 2000, we moved in. I loved our times there together. They proved to be halcyon days. Caron would often pop her head through the kitchen sash window and say, 'Any chance of a cup of tea?' and we'd settle in for a nice long chat. Other days she'd say, 'Come on, I haven't had my walk today,' and off we'd go, trudging up the hill to the fields above the cliffs. There was a particularly favourite spot, Alldays Field, where she and Russ would go to watch the boats coming into and out of the estuary: most of the boys' birthday picnics took place there, and it was a place where Caron could walk off her fear. There was lots of emphasis on exercise, keeping everything moving, and general health. We all learnt to cook to Caron's tastes and values: organic food replaced non-organic in my kitchen, and, of course, there was the ever-present green tea. I think it did her no end of good because right up to the end she looked incredible. Her eyes remained white, never went that sickly yellow, her skin stayed clear and a good colour. When her hair grew back it had a healthy shine. I swear, if it wasn't for the change in her posture and the pain, you'd never have known how ill she was. But, like her positivity, her healthy regime lulled us all into a false sense of security – which at least let us enjoy her without always fearing the worst.

Of course, that meant that when the bad news came, which it always did eventually, we were shocked all over again. She did everything by the book, I thought, so why didn't she deserve to succeed? She'd put so much energy and dedication into it. It was so unfair.

At the end of this most testing of years, I wanted to organize something that was exclusively for fun. I didn't want that period to end with only thoughts of cancer and treatment. It was to be a punctuation in time. A full stop to those difficult times and the beginning to a new era. I organized a surprise trip to Paris, with Russ, as ever, aiding and abetting. A driver took me to her house early one morning, I crept into her room and said, 'This is nothing but good news. Pack a bag, we're going on a trip . . .' Caron was baffled when the car passed the exit for the airport and headed into London. But she began to piece things together as we arrived at Waterloo. We chatted for the entire duration of the Eurostar journey and arrived in the centre of Paris ready to do what Caron did best – shop. We had the most glorious day out and in the evening, happy and weighed down with bags, we headed off to the George V Hotel off the Champs-Élysées for a reviving glass of champagne. It was closed. Caron couldn't understand why I was so worried: there were many bars in Paris we could go to. Then, from the shadows of the adjacent building, we heard a familiar voice and all was revealed. 'Hey girls, you looking for a night out?' Stephen and Russ stepped out into the cobbled street. The surprise was complete. Off we went to Sacre Coeur in Montmartre to celebrate.

Eventually Caron's hair grew back, and like all her periods of recovery, she looked well and healthy and happy. For a while she had a lovely bubbly short haircut that I adored. I often stare at pictures of her from that time. How is it that she could look so great when the reason for her hairstyle was so ominous? Understandably, the reassessment of her life became more intense after the mastectomy. Her diet was put under even more scrutiny. Her research into prevention and cure became more widespread. The days of sneaking the odd cappuccino were over. Everything was a little more serious now. She gave up red meat. Then she gave up chicken and fish, though when the cancer spread to her bones she relaxed that ban because by then she needed whatever strength she could get. At the end, she also allowed herself to indulge the chocoholic that had lain dormant since her trip to Amsterdam, and she nibbled on Green and Black's 70 per cent cocoa chocolate. You've got to live, right? Jan de Vries kept an eye on her general vitamin use, adding things like Spirulina to cleanse the liver, linseed and IP6. Research on IP6 said that the husk around whole wheat was particularly anti-carcinogenic because it assisted in the renewal of the good cells, the ones chemotherapy had depleted. She was eating scoops of IP6 every day. She would eat porridge in the morning. Everything was now organic. In Cornwall she found a farmer who'd deliver whatever was in season every week. She started using vegetarian cookbooks, cooking lentils and growing herbs. By the time she went to Australia, she was seeing a lot of dieticians and was always tinkering with her diet, adding things and taking away others, but her dedication to the cause was constant. Coffee enemas became a daily routine. And she gave up drinking.

It is true that Caron liked her food, but she had always been a fussy, picky eater. I have a lasting memory of Caron eating her peas, two at a time. What she loved about food was company, going out for dinner with friends and the chat. She missed her carefree girly dinners with red wine and poncing fags, but she stuck to her new regime. The food could change; the company she kept.

All this was done under the umbrella of her oncologist, Charles Lowdell. She did tests regularly. She started taking the Tamoxifen that she had chosen not to take earlier. There was more reassessing to do, however. Diet was not enough to satisfy Caron that she was doing all she could to keep the cancer at bay.

Towards the end of 2000, Brandon told Caron that she and her husband were going to Australia to do a series of workshops. Why didn't she, Russ and the boys come out for four weeks in the new year? It would do her good to get away from the harsh Cornish winter, and Brandon thought she would benefit from some intense self-healing. Frankly, the sunshine alone was a pull. Russ recognized the look in his wife's eye. It was the same look he'd seen in the car driving back from Cornwall after their chat about reversing their life. She wanted to go. She *really* wanted to go. Russ was not so keen. Their new life was good, he and Caron were a strong team, the boys were in a routine and had made friends. It would be another upheaval in less than a year. Four weeks was a long time: it would mean Charlie and Gabriel missing school, falling behind, being different from everyone else. Something kids don't relish until much, much later in life.

But when Caron had decided she wanted to go, that, as usual, was that. She made it happen. Christmas was nearly upon them and finding a house to rent in Byron Bay was no mean feat. There were houses either at the very bottom end of the market or at the very top. No guessing which end they went for. By now Russ had sold the shares in his Internet business and had a bit of money to burn, and burn it they did. Wategos House overlooked Wategos Beach, in the most easterly part of Australia where traditionally Aboriginal women would go to give birth. It was a large six-bedroomed house and overlooked the ocean. Caron loved it. It was wide, open-planned and enveloped by Australia's roaring nature.

They spent Christmas Day in Cornwall, and Caron, by now a fully paid-up vegetarian, proudly cooked her first full turkey dinner for the rest of us in her new home. Then the whole family flew first class to Australia for the first time. It was a monumental decision with far, far-reaching consequences: that Christmas was the only one we all had together in Cornwall. But at the time Caron was simply investigating the positive sides of the mind, body and spirit world and finding out what more, if anything, it could offer her. If there was nothing, it was a great excuse to have some sun. The answer was, she soon discovered, it offered her everything. But Byron Bay turned out to be the shopping mall of the world when it came to alternative therapies and, as we all knew, Caron was a proficient consumer.

14. Instant Calm, Sudden Chaos

Because of their connection with Brandon, they were soon meeting a lot of people in that area. Russ, with Bluefin Productions, had been toying with the idea of making a video, with Caron fronting it, about relaxation, meditation and the art of letting go. There seemed no better place to do that than Byron Bay, where every area of complementary therapy was represented. There was sound healing and music therapy, Roger the wonderful *tai-chi* expert, Brandon, who did the 'journey', of course, and many others. Everyone was game on. Russ rang Universal and pitched them the idea. They liked it. The video would be made, *Instant Calm*, with Caron Keating. Even a British yoga expert who was popular at the time came over to cover the yoga section. The idea was to show each of the practices, then teach the viewer a ten-minute relaxation technique that was an amalgamation of them all. This is Caron's introduction to that video:

I'd always felt I had led this very charmed life, I have a family that I absolutely adore, lots of friends, jobs that I love doing and yet throughout my life I've had this sense that there was something more. I didn't know what it was or how to get to it, but from time to time I had whisperings of it so I knew of its presence. Then about four years ago a couple of things happened that just made my life, as I knew it, totally disintegrate. Whatever I did to try and get it back again wouldn't work. So I decided to go on a quest to find myself again. This search took me all over Britain, abroad, and I met all kinds of inspiring teachers and each of them gave me another piece of the puzzle. But in the end what I discovered was that what I had been looking for had been inside me all along and I'd

just forgotten it was there. And it's inside all of you, and all you have
to do to get in touch with it is really listen to yourself. Listen to your
heart . . .

News of the video spread like bushfire, and every practitioner
of every kind of complementary therapy flocked to Wategos.
They poured in. While Caron kept her illness private, she
listened acutely to the theories behind the lotions and potions,
the methods, the pills, the practices. If she liked the idea of any of
them, she would take the person aside and explain her situation.
Having said that, generally people did not know that Caron had
a terminal disease: they weren't coming up the garden path to
cure her, they were coming to get on to a video destined for
the European market. Some were fantastic – they truly believed
in what they did and came with a lot of love. Others were
extremely questionable. The problem was that Caron treated
them all with the same attitude. Maybe this person can heal me.
Maybe *this* person can heal me. Although Caron had survived
chemotherapy, and even though it had shrunk the tumours in
her neck and other breast, no one could tell her whether she
was out of danger. It was too soon to say. Cancer has a habit of
rearing its ugly head again, and Caron didn't know if or when that
was going to happen. So, from that day on, she was looking to
these people to provide her with a miracle. It may sound barmy,
but all who came calling did so with a history of alledgedly having
performed miracle cures.

Caron was immediately enamoured with the scope of complementary treatment and healing available at Byron Bay. But
maybe even she wasn't prepared for one particular day.

It's not every day that someone claiming to be Jesus walks up your front
path, having driven twelve hours non-stop from Sydney. However,
by the end of that event-filled day in February, I had learnt that just about
anything is possible.

From my early Sunday-school experience, I knew that he had some of the right attributes: long hair, beard, piercing eyes, a gentle manner. The stigmata had faded, but perhaps they would over two thousand years. He had a rather tubbier body than the traditional lean Christian version on the cross – oh, and I don't recall Jesus being quite such a chain smoker. But my six-year-old son seemed to like him – always a good sign – and apparently the Pope had also liked him and picked him out of a 10,000-strong crowd at the Vatican to bless, possibly a more reliable sign. One more thing: he was Australian.

This small detail didn't faze me – at that moment, he seemed a lot less worrying than some of the people who were already in the house. It seemed that everyone that night was masquerading as someone else. A ringleted yoga teacher from London confided that he was actually the Archangel Michael, came to tell us that we were all angels but hadn't realized it. There was a wizard clad in black – supposedly the Prince of Darkness – here to scare us all back to God, with his white-bedecked shaman goddess, me, Russ SCLSH [slightly confused long-suffering husband] and our two small sons, whom I'd completely forgotten to feed. Thankfully Russ hadn't.

It seemed entirely plausible that Jesus might have also rocked up to join our merry band so we welcomed him in.

The wizard, a well-known author and teacher in the mind, body, spirit field, had somehow ended up coming to stay with us and for the first twenty-four hours had seemed a slightly unusual but harmless guest. Towards the afternoon of the second day things suddenly took an interesting twist when he decided that there were things he had to help me with. 'Come outside. I have to talk to you,' he suddenly announced. Once seated at the table, he started: 'You have to open your heart up. Now, do you want to go fast or slow?' I wasn't sure I wanted to go at all. At that moment I was torn between intrigue and telling him to F off and mind his own business. It is pure arrogance that allows one person to assume the role of telling another where they're going wrong in their life.

Paying to go along to a workshop and have the error of my ways pointed out was one thing, but having them highlighted by a virtual stranger who'd kind of invited himself to stay in our holiday house was an entirely different matter. Maybe he thought he was doing me a favour. This 'holiday' was turning out to be something quite different.

'Put your hand on my heart and tell me whether you trust me or not.' Gingerly I placed my hand on the black T-shirt over his heart, closed my eyes and asked for a sign. I don't know what I was expecting – thunderclaps or disembodied voices saying 'Retreat, retreat!' There was nothing. No sign. No inner messages – nothing.

While I waited for my heart to burst open or whatever was going to happen, the shaman goddess insisted that I, too, dressed in white. The only white clothes I had were silk and brand new, having been bought just days before to wear in a video we were making. This suddenly seemed like a much better use.

She kept dragging me into the bathroom and making me look at myself in the mirror. 'What do you see?' she demanded.

I didn't quite know where it was all leading. 'Me?' I answered sheepishly.

'But look at how powerful you are.'

Apart from looking quite dazed, I couldn't see any difference, but I didn't want to tell her that. 'Oh, yeah,' I mumbled.

Anyway, part of me wanted to believe that maybe it was true and I had changed into this all-powerful goddess-like creature whom she claimed to be seeing.

When we returned to the garden there was a heap of bodies on the ground. Oh, my God, they're having an orgy in my garden! was my first thought. My Northern Irish upbringing hadn't prepared me for moments like that.

On close inspection it turned out that everyone was having an innocent out-of-body moment, lying on the grass, looking up at the stars and generally feeling in love with the world. I joined them, covering my new outfit with grass stains but having too interesting a time to care.

Eventually the charm of rolling around on the lawn, gazing up at the moon and stars and supposedly feeling our hearts erupt grew thin . . . The LSH (long-suffering husband) had retired to bed, the wizard and his moll had vanished, leaving me to chew the fat with Jesus and Angel Michael until six in the morning. It was a strangely comforting night – I was just another lost and lonely seeker looking for happiness, fulfilment, a cure and an ability to love myself – whatever it is people leave home and go searching for.

The next morning my bearded friend started talking about miracles. Apparently he'd performed his first the night before and I was the lucky recipient. This came as a bit of a surprise: I'd always assumed that miracles came complete with lightning or at least a bit of a show – picking up one's sick bed, regaining sight, that kind of thing. In the midst of all my heart activity I hadn't actually noticed anything different and certainly not a miracle.

A year later I discovered there wasn't anything different – it hadn't come true, there was no miracle. The cancer was back. But I didn't know that then. At the time, it was just one more bizarre thing that had happened . . .

No, there was no miracle. Caron was wrong about those people. But when you are battling something like cancer, you are prepared to try anything. Until that point Russ and Caron had worked together as a unit to fight the cancer. He was running with her, in whichever direction she wanted to go. But the candy store that was Byron Bay was too much for Russ, too much for both of them. Caron was trying everything, her hand in every jar, darting from one 'teacher' to another. Russ was trying to keep it all together. Their four-week trip became six, and during that time Russ was producing a video, working hard. He was also paying bills in the UK and in Australia, overseeing Charlie and Gabriel's home tutoring. He tried to keep up with Caron and remain vibrant about whatever she was trying out next, without letting her go too far or get too lost. He'd managed that until the fateful night that Jesus walked up the garden path. He says that was the writing on the wall. He became conscious that staying as positive and open-minded as Caron would get tricky.

Free your spirit, open your heart, self-heal – Caron was intoxicated by it all. Even after her doubts about that night, she booked a week-long course with the same wizard in Italy for the following May. Russ was trying to protect her, but she saw it as him holding her back and probably resented him for it. After all, she was the one with cancer. Russ says that was the moment at which he stopped being only a partner and started being a parent too. Their relationship changed. The only thing to stop her diving headlong into the 'freedom' they were offering was Russ and the boys. So, the seeds of doubt had been planted and the questioning, which – apart from the few weeks when she'd distanced herself from me – had been mostly inwardly oriented, was about to change again.

In March 2001, they finally came home and settled back into Cornish life. Once they were home, things seemed to sort themselves out. As Russ says, once you'd taken Caron away from the candy shop, she stopped wanting more. It was almost as if all that extraordinary stuff hadn't happened. In fact, she told her friends about Jesus and the angel, the wizard and his witch. She laughed when Cathy or Johnny listened with disbelief on their faces. Yasmin loved hearing about the loonies and the nutters. When Caron was away from it, they lost their intoxicating power. She could reason with herself, see things more clearly. Her good mates, the ones she trusted, who had her best interests at heart, were telling her it all sounded bonkers and she came down to earth with a relatively small bump. Russ was happy to have his wife back. Her interest in the field didn't waver, mind you: she still went on a Caroline Myss self-healing trip to Stonehenge, but it was no longer insidious and all-encompassing. She didn't have to distance herself from those who loved her to do it. So, after a few weeks, Russ and Caron were back in a great place and she had got herself together. They both worked on editing the video, which gave them a chance to laugh about their trip to Byron Bay. It seemed that it was all behind them. They were still working with Brandon, and I'm sure she helped to mend a few doubts and niggles.

But on the horizon, looming over them, was the trip to see the wizard in Italy. By the time May came round, Caron no longer wanted to go, and Russ definitely didn't want her to go. She came within inches of forgoing the deposit and putting an end to the whole thing, but someone from his organization phoned and she changed her mind. Or her mind was changed for her.

Russ was not happy. He told her, 'We survived the last episode but it's going to be harder to come back from this.' Not only was she going against Russ's will, she was going against us all. But, as an alcoholic goes back to the booze, Caron went back for more. She regretted it almost as soon as she got there. It wasn't opening your heart, this was scary stuff. She wasn't allowed to contact anyone at home and was completely alone. The odd call she sneaked to Russ made him worry all the more. He learnt that someone else who was there that week had parents waiting at the airport to fly stand-by to get their daughter back. Scary stuff indeed. Caron didn't go into full details about it with Russ – she probably told Michael more, but Michael isn't telling. Russ doesn't mind that he doesn't know the details. He wouldn't have wanted to know anyway. He suspected that it would be too hard to understand and possibly damaging.

She came back, and for three weeks they struggled to return to what was deemed normal daily life. It was a difficult time. Even Caron didn't know why she'd gone. She hadn't enjoyed it, and was desperately grateful to be home safely. Russ met her at the airport: he'd never seen her so happy to be back, but they argued all the way home because she refused to draw a line under it and move on. If she hadn't liked it, if it wasn't helping her, why did she go on justifying it? They reached breaking-point. Russ simply couldn't understand why she was doing what she was. Once again, he was telling her off like a parent and, once again, it created an atmosphere between them. Over the following summer the same bunch of eclectic people started to

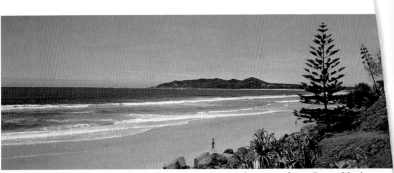

Belongil Beach, Byron Bay. One of many beaches in the area where Caron liked to walk and body surf

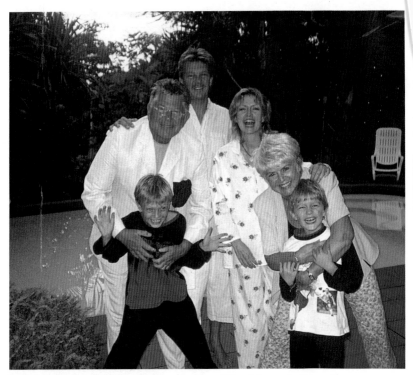

Just out of bed – poolside at Taylors, Caron and Russ's home in Byron Bay. Stephen (*left*) and I were on an early morning flight back to London

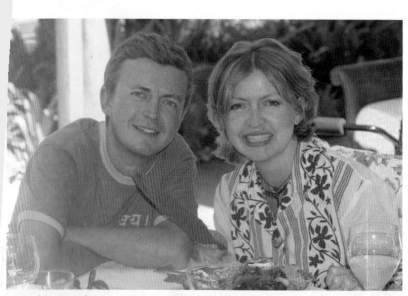

Michael in Australia. A surprise visit for Caron's birthday

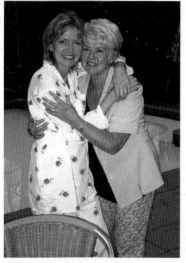

We never could say goodbye.
Another farewell on one of my many
trips to Australia

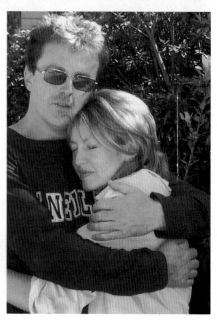

Paul's heart-wrenching farewell as he left
Byron Bay. One of my favourite shots –
seeing their love for each other.
It sits by my bedside

from all over. She made a wonderful speech, thanking Russ for everything he'd done for her and all that he'd put up with. Some in the room knew what she was talking about, but most thought it was simply an apology for excessive shopping, a tantrum or two, or her failings on the domestic-goddess front. But she needn't have apologized for any of those things: those were the things that Russ loved about her, always had. Once again, they had been through a lot, had changed as a result, but still loved each other deeply.

They also went to the Scilly Isles to celebrate Russ's birthday, this time with just the boys. Caron was as loving, giving and caring as she had ever been. Russ and the children relished it. When Caron wasn't thinking about herself and her illness, she had an amazing capacity to love. The terrible irony was that she was so worried about living that, after diagnosis, everything else came a poor second. For Russ it was hard to have that love diminished. But what could he do? What could any of us do? Stamp our feet and say, 'What about me?' We weren't the ones facing death. All we could do was keep our fingers crossed that Caron would be given the all-clear, and that we could put this dreadful anxious time behind us.

Whatever peaks and troughs Russ and Caron were going through, dreading those regular medical check-ups she had to have, Cornwall stands out strongly in my mind as a time of particular contentment. It is often the case that the closer one is to one's children, the more turbulent the relationship can be. Well, not in our case. After the boys were born she understood just how much I loved her, how unconditional that love was, and she was thrilled when Stephen and I bought the house in Fowey. She had always wanted us to be neighbours.

She and Yasmin used to talk about death when Yasmin went down to Cornwall. Perhaps because they'd both lost a parent, Caron found it an easier subject to broach with her. Caron told Yasmin that she believed we were all part of a bigger picture.

turn up in Fowey, some of whom Russ really didn't want in his home. The differences were exaggerated when the old friends and the new 'friends' collided.

As Janet says, 'We had a fantastic time in Cornwall despite the weird Australian people who would pitch up.' That summer, two of them were staying, walking around barefoot, opening the fridge and helping themselves to whatever they wanted. They didn't contribute a great deal, didn't offer to help, and always left a mess. It annoyed me: I thought Russ and Caron were being taken advantage of. They were always so generous: everyone was always asked to stay for dinner, wine always flowed, there was food aplenty. Many of those people seemed to have no focus in life, and some appeared to be drifters on the make. Janet found them intrusive but while they took and took, they talked about spiritual energy and freedom, openness and love. If you rejected what they said it was because *you* had the problems and *you* were really uptight. One said to Janet, 'Your body language tells me you don't get where I'm coming from.' It's all well and good to be a hippie but, my, they were happy to accept a lot of hospitality that was only 'free' because somebody else was paying.

Not all of them had the best intentions. Not all of them had the worst. Russ, Caron's friends, her brothers and I were in the tricky position of trying to bridge the gap between the two. We didn't know if they were amazing or not but, of course, like Caron, secretly we hoped that the genuine article would walk through the door, take away her fear and therefore our own.

As they had after Byron Bay, Russ and Caron managed to overcome the hurdle that was the Italian trip. There was never a point when their relationship wasn't strong, but certain elements of it had changed. However, by Russ's fortieth birthday, 12 July 2001, everything seemed smooth and their relationship was as strong as ever. She organized a huge party for him, taking over the Fowey Hotel and filling it with their friends

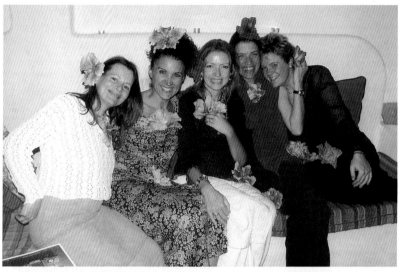

The girls from Caron's 'women's circle' who gave her endless love and support

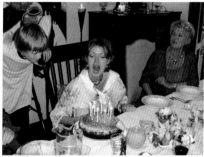

Charlie making sure his mum blew out all the candles

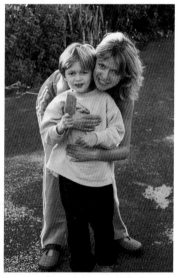

A chocolate-coated moment with Gabriel in Austrailia

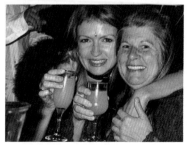

Denise, the pooh fairy. Enough said!

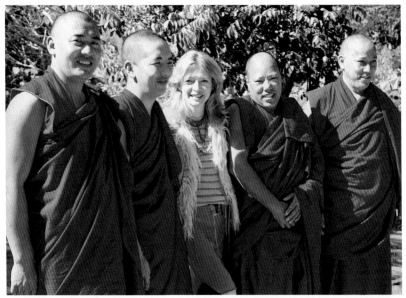

Caron wrote in 2003: 'A miracle happened when four Guyto monks came and chanted for me – to bless me and for healing. I feel so blessed and full of peace and happiness'

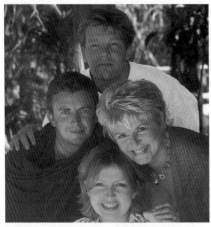

Caron's last birthday, on Michael's final day in Australia. Michael is wrapped in Caron's gift to him, a Guyto monk's robe. He said he wore it all the way home to London to keep Caron close

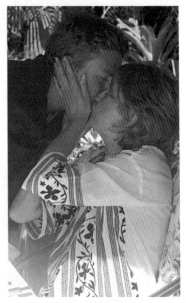

Caron's last birthday. Michael wearing the monk's robe, which he treasures

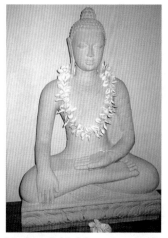

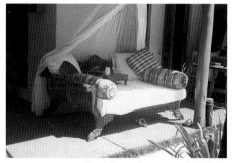

Caron's much-treasured daybed.
Respite in the afternoon for tea, chats
and catnaps

My fortieth birthday present to Caron.
5 October 2002

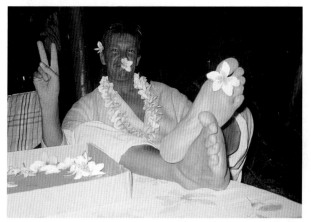

Those frangipanis get everywhere! Peace, man!

Two of the Guyto
healing monks with
Charlie and Russ. Taken
outside Caron's beloved
summerhouse in the
garden at Byron Bay

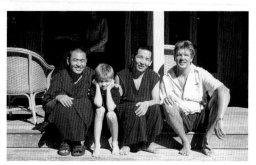

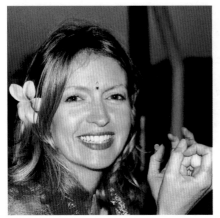

Thankfully not the same frangipani that Russ had between his toes

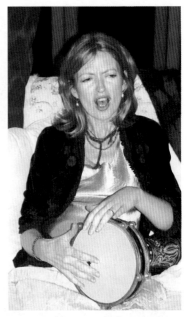

Always ready for a sing-song

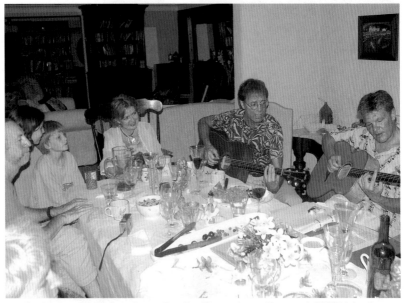

Family sing-song at Taylors, Byron Bay. Duelling guitars - Russ and Cliff Richard on one of his trips to Australia

Compared to dark winter days in Britain, no wonder this Byron Bay setting brought hope and light

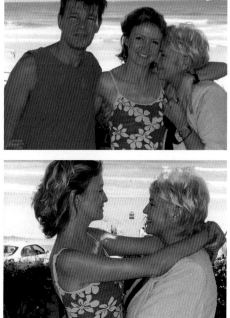

A tender mother-and-daughter moment. Just one of those emotional goodbyes

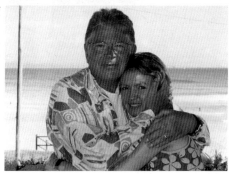

For Stephen, the first of many trips to Australia. Watergos Beach, where Caron loved to bodyboard

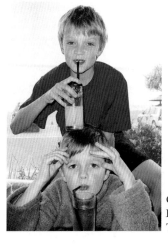

Charlie and Gabriel. A juice stop at Belongil Beach, near their home at Byron Bay. They often went there after school

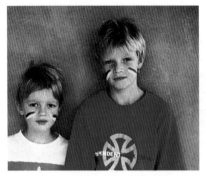

England v. Australia. Charlie and Gabriel off to the cricket in Brisbane. Best part for the boys? Getting home at 1 a.m.!

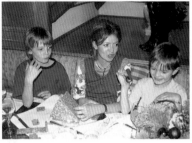

Making gingerbread houses. Caron's first visit to the Paracelsus Clinic in Switzerland, October 2003, with Charlie and Gabriel

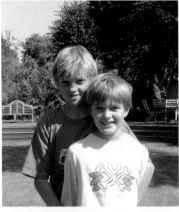

Brotherly love. Charlie and Gabriel

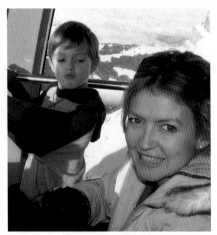

Caron defying the odds by taking Gabriel on a trip up Santis Mountain in the Swiss Alps, even though she had fluid on the lung

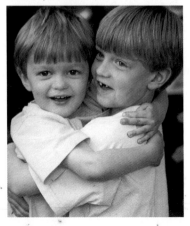

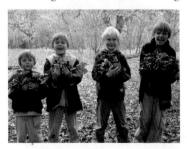

Cool cousins, April 2004

She had faith. This life wasn't all there was: more was to come. She also told Yasmin that she could never imagine being without me, that she couldn't comprehend losing me, and was very sensitive that Yasmin had lost her mother. Her criticism of me for having been too busy when she was young seemed to have passed. She had matured and, to her friends, appeared much more accepting of things.

There were many, many good days, when she was feeling strong and brave. Days of picnics, sailing, walks and rounders, days that she'd squeeze Yasmin into a wetsuit and get her surfing. I would wave them off from the safety of the beach and watch them run screaming into the freezing water. They caught a few waves, got tumbled about. Of course, the boys were great at it by then. I can still hear Caron whooping and screaming as if she hadn't a care in the world. It is one of Yasmin's best memories. Mine too. Even when she'd been for a scan and they'd found more hotspots, debris, they said, which they wanted to investigate further, she found the extra strength she needed to keep the fear at bay. She sat very quietly on a beach in Readymoney Cove, felt an enormous sense of well-being, and thought, Whatever happens, it'll be all right. Her friends think that when she said, 'Whatever happens', she meant her own death, but I don't know. Perhaps Caron didn't exactly know what she meant either.

But there were other days. Days when she went for solitary walks above the cove to a bluff where you can see across the estuary. People believe Jesus – the real one – came there on a trip to Europe and a little cross marks the spot. She would go up there to stand in the wind and scream and rage. It might be easy to criticize some of her actions, many of them appear misguided and irresponsible, but we weren't the ones standing on a clifftop screaming into the wind, prepared to do anything, anything at all, to keep the cancer away and stay alive however extreme that seemed to us.

Despite scaring herself in Italy, in October she signed herself

up for a three-week sound-healing course in Australia. She did
this despite the re-evaluation of whether what she was doing
was really benefiting her. When she told me, I just stared at her
in amazement. What was so strong that could make her put all
those bad memories of Italy aside and go back, leave Russ and
the boys, her family, our love? Sound healing may be very
pleasant, but do you have to go 12,000 miles away to do it? I
can understand that it can move people, but can't it move people
here too? Yes, it was a beautiful sound that, like chanting,
resonated deep in your core, but I didn't want her to go. There
was drumming involved too, which Caron loved because of the
sense of release it gave her, but even she had to admit that it
wasn't going to cure her. She boarded the plane anyway. Her
bravado, however, was only skin deep.

I went to a three-week workshop in Australia to do some sound healing
and was convinced I was going to die on the way over. The terror was
huge but I sat with it – sobbing in the loo at Heathrow and outside of the
terror was a calmness that stayed with me for the entire glorious trip. But
still the fear struggles on . . .

Despite her outward appearance of positivity, of faith in her
chosen quest, the fear never left her. In the year since the
mastectomy, the sword hung over her head. Others may have
forgotten that Caron had cancer, but she never did. Neither did
I. There was a constant gnawing in my mind, stomach and
heart, day and night. We all had it. Then the silent terror we
shared rose into the open again. On 3 December 2001 Dr
Charles Lowdell confirmed that the lump Caron had found in
her right breast was malignant. The cancer was back. None
of it – the screaming, the praying, the positive thinking, the
regression, the organic food, the sound healing, the drumming
– had changed the course of events and Caron was terrified. So
she ran. Straight back to Byron Bay. This time, alone.

15. Searching, Searching, Searching . . .

By December 2001 Caron knew she was in deep trouble. As a family we understood why she was searching, searching, searching. The fact that her grandmother had died of breast cancer couldn't enter the equation. If it were simply a matter of genealogy, then what was happening was outside her control. And that meant there was no way she was going to find a cure. Those demon cells continued their march through her body despite everything she had done to stop them. Her search, her questioning up to that point had augmented the orthodox treatment, lent her a crutch. The reflexology, the healing with Matthew Manning, the homeopathy with Jan de Vries, even the mad characters from Byron Bay, were a device she used to give her extra strength. But then everything changed again.

On 3 December 2001 I went for an ultrasound scan full of fear and trepidation. I used to dread those check-ups and felt as if the doctors were searching for some small cell change to seize an opportunity for administering all sorts of brutal treatments. I do know, of course, that they carry out a brilliant job and save many lives. I guess it's just that my belief system is that illness is not something that comes for no reason. I believe there are many factors, not least emotional and spiritual issues, which have registered deep within us. Strong emotions that we've shut down, stored in our bodies, got on with life and simply pretended they don't exist. But left to their own devices, these emotions can start to fester away in those dark, hidden places – with us totally unaware of their very existence. Or maybe, catching glimpses of them from time to time, we make an extra effort to bury them – smiling bitterly, ignoring what's going on until the day that something emerges physically and we can ignore it no longer.

For me, the most difficult part of having had cancer has been dealing with the fear. It steals up on me unawares in the middle of the most glorious times. I cuddle up to my children before bedtime and a dark thought will invade my mind. Sometimes it's hard to entertain the confusion/resentment in my mind as I sit on a beautiful beach looking at someone's perfect breasts, resenting the fact that they've never had to work on their mind or wonder what the hell is going on, or indeed had to live without a nipple. I play spurious games with myself – which would be worse, I wonder, to lose a breast or lose a leg?

Once in my self-pity mode, I glanced at a man playing joyfully with a child at the market in Byron Bay – confident and joyous. He looked as if he didn't have a worry in the world. It's all right for him, I thought unreasonably. Then I casually glanced down and saw a false leg protruding beneath his shorts. It was a strange reminder that we all have challenges to deal with. They may come in different packages but basically they're the same and no one really escapes. It comes down to how we choose to deal with them and I do believe we all have a chance.

In a way, we are so used to dealing with the future by referring to the past. It's the only knowledge we have and we drag it around with us, making it fit with totally different situations, allowing the past to keep reoccurring . . .

Janet saw her on the day of her check-up. Caron had been to the hospital, then went to Janet's lovely, cosy house in Hammersmith. She said, 'They've found something on the other breast.' Janet was completely shocked: she looked so well, had been fine when Janet had last visited her in Cornwall – it didn't seem possible. Caron appeared calm but we know from her writing that inside she was in turmoil. 'Don't worry,' she said. 'It happens every time I go. There's always something. It'll be fine . . . I get the results tomorrow.'

Janet said she'd call the next day, then didn't want to because she was worried that Caron would think it was the hospital. Finally she cracked and at about ten thirty p.m. she called Caron and got the news. She said, 'It's in the other breast and I'm leaving tomorrow.' Janet was confused. Leaving for where? Back to Fowey? No. Back to Byron Bay where Judas, Jesus and the Angel Michael were waiting for her with open arms. Oh, yes, she was desperate all right.

When I heard the numbing news that the cancer had spread to her other breast a new type of sickening knot grew inside me, yet I heard myself on the phone saying calmly, 'Don't worry, darling, you'll deal with this like you dealt with it before . . .'

But Caron had other plans:

In December 2001 I found out that the cancer had returned a third time. The small thickening in my breast that I had touched endlessly, prayed about and feared was not the harmless cyst I had been hoping for.

I am numb. Trying to shore myself up against the shifting, quicksand parameters of my world. As, yet again, it spins out with this ever-shifting landscape of illness.

I feel like someone who almost gets away with shoplifting, and just as they walk through the door a hand is clamped on their shoulder and they are dragged backwards into some nightmare. Except this is worse. A full nightmare, in Technicolor. Life can turn on a pinhead: a clear check-up and I walk out of there a free woman, able to get on with the life she knows; a small clump of dodgy cells and the landscape is shattered.

'It's like trying to gather warm Vaseline,' my girlfriend has observed, of my previous attempts to reshape my life into something vaguely resembling the old one. Perhaps that's the point – I'm not meant to. But I don't know that yet.

I grasp for something solid to hang on to. Small, insignificant details are given the weight of a Holy Grail and become safety ports in the storm. I try to cling to anything positive while a wall of grimness teeters above my panicked mind – threatening to sweep away all rationality the second I let it in.

'This happens to a lot of women my age now, doesn't it?' I ask the radiographer, desperate to make it an everyday occurrence, like going to Asda.

'No,' she replies. 'I hardly ever see it in people as young as you.'

'Liar!' I want to yell at her.

'Why didn't you get it checked sooner?'

She has no idea what it is like to have lived with this for three years, dreading every check-up, terrified of this precise moment. It's not as if some warning light has appeared on my breast flashing 'check-up required', like the petrol light in a car.

I hate her.

Numbness is somehow easier. I go through the motions, talk to the people, walk to the car.

'Couldn't it just sort itself out and disappear?' Russ asks my doctor hopefully.

'Not without a miracle,' he mutters.

A light goes on in my mind. Of course. A miracle. And I know just the place to find it.

'The only thing I know,' I say to my mother, 'is that the times when everything seems like it's falling apart, we're being looked after the most.' But my faith is not that solid yet. I can almost kid myself – though deep in the night I wonder. What have I done or not done? Why me? Why again? I've done everything I know how to do – or so I think: is there more? Am I to be stalked by this relentless hunter until I give up, give in, roll over, feet in the air in submission? Or will this ferocious guide gently leave me one day – take the pointed stick out of my back – satisfied that I am at last on my path and living the life I'm meant to live? I don't know – none of it makes sense . . .

Russ and Caron went to have supper with the Comerfords. Since Caron had done everything by the book and more, they were assuming she would be all right and had champagne at the ready. When Russ and Caron came through the door, it was immediately clear from their faces that it wasn't good news. Caron was incredibly calm, considering, and Johnny and Cathy tried to fill the air with optimism. But there was little to be optimistic about.

It is late that night when I reach the safety of my mother's house. Relieved to be away from the world of hospitals, ultrasounds and serious-faced specialists. My mother and I weep in the kitchen. Tears of frustration, sadness, fear of losing each other, and at the enormity of the love we have for each other. I feel safe in her embrace. I smell her smell. It is at once familiar and reassuring. A mix of her, her perfume, her lipstick.

Wherever she goes in the world she leaves a trail of lipstick stains. On people's cheeks, on teacups, on tissues. She says she can talk better with it on. Once when we were bored we counted how many lipsticks were in her handbag. There were fourteen.

Tonight, frightened as I am of being swept away, I cling to her. I need the strength and security even though I know I will have to face many moments alone in a place where none of my family can come with me. But not tonight.

Not now when the fragility of life seems all too apparent. Tonight I will bask in the familiar feel of family, of tea at the kitchen table, of my mother and my husband's love enveloping me, shielding me from a wildly unpredictable universe. I will rest until I am strong enough to face it all again . . .

Caron didn't give herself much time to rest because the next thing we knew she was asking Russ to book her on to the next available flight to Australia. They had been planning to repeat their winter holiday in Byron Bay, but not until after Christmas.

The following day was very strange. I was in turmoil. Trembling. Confused. But outside the mask went on. I went on comforting her and being positive while we walked round the nearby town of Westerham buying bits and pieces for Caron's imminent flight. The shops was full of joyous decorations, a scene that would normally make our spirits soar, yet we were facing this. All over again.

We went into a friend's shop and Charlie saw a soft, cuddly leopard, which he immediately took to. Caron bought it for him. I remember her crouching down at her small son's feet and saying, 'Every time you're feeling lonely, or you miss me, you hug your leopard and I'll be with you . . .' Unsurprisingly, Spotty sits in pride of place in his bedroom. I could not believe she was really going to leave us all, but she was adamant. Byron Bay was the only place she could bear to be.

We returned to Michael's house in Fulham and sat around the dining-room table, eating a Thai takeaway as the minutes ticked by. False jollity returned. I cannot fully express how surreal it was. We stood in the street with the little boys and watched Russ and Caron drive away, waving until they turned the corner. Then she was gone. I stared at the empty space at the bottom of the road, unable to register what my eyes were telling me.

Caron called from the airport in tears. I listened in tears. She was adamant, but she was confused. She was trying to be so brave, but she was terrified. It was like the Italian trip and the sound-healing exercise all over again. She was torn. But eventually the pull of the teachers and gurus, the self-healers and spiritual advisers won over our pleas to have the orthodox treatment first, then go. Caron flew back to Byron Bay.

What the serious-faced specialist had found was a tumour mass in her right breast measuring 4.3 centimetres with a gland in the left neck. A biopsy showed grade-two invasive ductal carcinoma. They were also concerned about the lymph nodes in her neck and an area of bone in the first left rib, which they noted with a 'high degree of suspicion'. Their overall conclusion was that this was a resurgence of the original breast cancer, rather than a new primary tumour. They recommended adding Zoladex to the Tamoxifen, and if the tumour turned out not to be hormonally sensitive, as before, then more chemotherapy. Caron's medical records note that she had not been taking the full dosage of Tamoxifen in recent months. She was resisting medication. I suspect the collision of the two worlds she straddled had created another grey area. She was in the middle of a tug of war and didn't know which way to go.

Once she was back there, the power Byron Bay had over her took hold again. There was no Janet to tease her that the healer fancied her, or Cathy to tell her that the reason she fainted when she first went to a healer's seminar was because it was forty degrees Celsius outside and she was in an airless room with a crowd of people, all packed in like cattle, rather than because she'd been 'moved'. She didn't even have Russ's ever-watchful eye, reminding her that not everyone was as genuine as they appeared to be. No doubt Caron had been predisposed to their promises prior to rediagnosis: it was in keeping with her spirituality, her curiosity about unexplained phenomena. But after 4 December, she needed them more than ever. She needed a miracle and, as she said, she knew exactly where to get one. If she hadn't been over in October, maybe Byron Bay would not have been the place to provide her with one. But she had. And, as far as she was concerned, it was. So in her panic Caron fled. She left Menlo, the boys, Russ, everything. Jono and Judith, their great friends in Fowey, said life had changed for them when Caron and Russ came to Fowey: a light went on. That light went out on the day she left.

It went out for Russ too. The bikes were wrapped and waiting, hidden in the garage to give to the boys. Christmas was all planned. The turkey had been ordered. The family was organized, the decorations were ready to go up. Not only that, she had started work again: *Rich and Famous* at peak time on Friday nights for ITV. She only managed a few editions – interviewing *Coronation Street*'s Curly Watts at home in Spain, Mike Reed and Bruce Forsyth. They had been well received and had competed highly in the television ratings. Again, the rumour mill started to grind. Where had she gone and why had she gone alone? No one accepts that you leave television by choice because it leaves you, so why had she pulled out of yet another show?

Yasmin remembers that they'd planned to meet up in Soho House for one of their infamous dinners. Instead of a girly catch-up, she was told that Caron had gone to Australia. She was stunned, but suspected she knew why. Most didn't. To most of her friends, it seemed as if she'd simply vanished. Despite her calm exterior, Caron had been poleaxed by the doctor's findings. The huge wall of fear she'd been trying to get past crashed in. With the fear came the question, again and again and again: what have I done to make this happen to me?

I think the hardest thing of Caron's entire battle was thinking the cancer was her fault. First, it was had she partied too hard? Then she thought it was the television studios, which had pumped her full of electricity and radio waves. She said over and over again to her friends, 'I have to find the reason for this. If I find the reason I can deal with it.' She was demented by it and she was out to find something in her life to blame.

We all went back under the microscope for further investigation. Sometimes it was hurtful, mostly it was just desperately sad, because there is nothing you can say to somebody who believes they can change the course of events if only they can find the cause. If you say, 'There is no reason for this', you're telling them they can't change that course. It was a terrible *Catch 22* position to be in.

And it got worse because she refused to have a second mastectomy. Her flight back to Australia was perhaps in part so that she didn't have to fight her corner on that front. Just as Byron Bay had lost its potency once Caron was back in Fowey, we lost our power when she left us. I know that during that time, and probably during her first visit and throughout the subsequent courses she attended, people had said to her, 'This is your life. You have to do what you want. You've been held back by your cancer, your mum, your husband. You're not your own person – they've been holding you back from your own will,' perhaps not directly, but indirectly through suggestion and hints. There is even a term for it: neuro-linguistic practice or NLP. It is used by cults as a way of making what is said more believable. Mediums use it. Fortune-tellers use it. Tarot readers use it. Advertising agencies use it. Therapists probably use it – not all, but some. It can be extremely positive, but it can, in the case of cults, drive families apart. Dangerous seeds are planted, watered, nurtured, and when a full thought grows, you are left thinking it is an original one, and that, no, you haven't directly been told to do anything, your mind is your own. But it isn't. When we all said, 'Don't go,' we were watering those seeds ourselves. It's all very clever.

The healing chimed with her. She loved the regression. She liked the process. Actually, I agree with a lot of the teachings: I believe you can do a great deal for yourself, that you can achieve incredible things with the right attitude. I believe in changing your diet and taking supplements. But a lot of it led to questioning that was painful and full of resentment. And I think during that time, while the panic subsided, Caron took herself to some dark, lonely places when she could have been enveloped in her family and her husband's love. She was searching for a reason that might have predisposed her to her condition, something deep in the mists of time that would explain everything. That, of course, included having a career in the public eye which is so competitive, a mother who wasn't like most 'other' mothers, and all the other issues in her life. Then again, who am I to judge? Maybe, just maybe, if she hadn't gone on that journey she wouldn't have survived as long as she did. Maybe it was the process of asking the questions that kept her alive: her investigative mind desired to find an answer, and that desire was stronger than the destructive power of cancer. What she found when she got there, that hope of life, outweighed the desolation she'd left behind.

Janet had said to her over and over again, the notion that a particular type of person or a life situation could bring cancer upon themselves was destructive and wrong and too much of a burden. She would reason with Caron that we are all going to die of something and, right now, it will probably be either cancer or heart disease. It's just damn bad luck if it's early, but it happens. Janet was incensed by the idea that people bring everything on themselves, yet it had seeped into the public consciousness and Caron believed it. Well, it's true that eating fried food all day, smoking cigarettes and working too hard can bring about heart disease and cancer, but a good many people defy this logic and live to a ripe old age. As Paul has said, he has worked with electrical equipment and microphones all his life. Did the radio waves just bounce off him? A lot of people live at the end of cul-de-sacs: do they all get cancer? No. Do you get cancer because you have fun in your twenties? No, no, no. But since the answers weren't forthcoming, the search became more intense.

Caron would look at Paul sometimes in wonder and say, 'How come you're so content with life? Why are you so happy?' He had found his niche: he was doing something he loved, which made him enough money to provide for his family. He was fulfilled. Caron had not found that fulfilment. Due to her illness, she was more analytical than ever. She was on a carpet-bombing exercise, and everything was in the firing line. Her career. Me. Russ. Even Don was pulled off his pedestal. Preconceptions of domestic life. Modern society. Everything.

Caron was hard on all of us at some point during her search for a cure, her quest for life, but the person she was hardest on was herself. She could never decide what she really wanted to do with her life, or get out of it. Should she have been a writer, a painter? Maybe she should have stayed with her childhood calling and become a doctor. Yet to many it might have appeared that she was blessed with a charmed life and what could possibly be missing? After all, few get to cherry-pick their way through a television career as effortlessly as Caron did.

After moving to Cornwall she took over from Judy Finnegan in *We Can Work It Out*, a consumer programme. She'd be collected by car, taken to Newquay airport, flown to Leeds for two days' filming, then brought home again. For this she was paid a substantial amount of money. But she complained: she didn't like the subject matter, it was too pedestrian. It made Paul quite impatient to hear her: 'Do you have any idea how long it would take most people to earn that sort of money?' he asked her. She didn't care. She pulled out of the job. Well, that's all well and good if someone else is picking up the bills. And, of course, someone was.

Caron had always experienced total devotion from Russ, so I suppose after a while she took it as read that he would continue to support her. After all, he had completely masterminded the move to Cornwall. He also masterminded the extension of their first trip to Byron Bay by making the video. They created the monster together. But in December 2001, the pandering came to an abrupt halt. Russ told Caron she couldn't and shouldn't go. She couldn't leave them just before Christmas. But Caron had that look in her eye: she was going, with or without his blessing. She said she 'had' to. Then she vanished. Just like that.

There were people she knew over there, of course, but she was on her own, scared, vulnerable and completely out of control. Russ was left to deal with their two boys at home.

Caron's escape to Australia had been so swift that she had nowhere to stay when she arrived. For the first few weeks she was on a put-you-up bed in a friend's sitting room. To leave the comfort of her family home, back-up and support without knowing exactly where she would lay her head took guts – even more, when you consider how desperate we all were for her to stay at home. It was a terrible, terrible time for each and every one of us, for slightly different reasons and in slightly different ways.

Was Cornwall, and now Australia, really the place she was likely to live longest? If Russ had said, 'No, I need to keep my job in London. We have all our friends and family around, we're going to need them now, more than ever,' what would Caron have done? Russ says she'd have gone anyway. He was caught between the devil and the deep blue sea. How could he keep his precious sons away from their mother, who was now battling a more aggressive form of cancer, for one minute longer than was necessary? He couldn't.

Yes, of course Cornwall and Australia turned out to be amazing in many respects. But have we convinced ourselves that it was the right thing for her and Russ to do because it was what they did? Have we convinced ourselves that the search took Caron in the right direction and prolonged her life? I don't know. Russ is convinced that had she stayed and had the second mastectomy her self-esteem, her general well-being would have left her: she was at such a low ebb, had nothing to hang on to, and therefore staying would have killed her. I'm not so sure. Of course, you can't possibly know what it's like until you are faced with it. But if I'm being totally honest, I would have preferred her to stay at home, have the second mastectomy, then go back to Australia for all the 'good' treatment she craved.

And did it really have to be Australia? Yes, it's lovely to walk on the beach and be in the sun, but why couldn't she and Russ have done that in the South of France, or Italy? Yes, it was nice to surround yourself with lots of spiritual people, but you're cutting yourself off from your age-old friends and family who love you and want to help, and can support you just as well, if not better. Yes, it's good to do all the alternative therapy but, please, have the second mastectomy first. Please follow up with the orthodox treatment. All of us who knew her plan thought, Stay here and get help, then go. Please, God, have the treatment first. Janet thinks Caron knew, even if she'd rather have had her fingernails pulled out than admit it, that further treatment wasn't going to work. It was the same with Janet's mother, who also stopped taking her pills. Your sixth sense takes over.

Maybe Janet is right: maybe the thing Caron wanted at that point, above all, was control. Some modicum of decision-making rather than giving herself up to further invasive treatment. Russ agrees. He thinks she was in such a delicate place at that precise moment, teetering on the edge of total meltdown, that whatever confidence she had left, whatever strength, would have been torn from her if she'd been forced back into hospital where they would have operated on her again. She'd faced it the first time with stoicism and bravery, and didn't have the strength to do it again. She said, 'If I have these operations I will die.' Perhaps, somewhere in her system, she knew it was too late for surgery. What would she gain? What would they chop off next? Also, she knew she couldn't have the full dose of chemotherapy she needed because she'd had such a high dose the first time. So she'd have had to have a reduced strength, which, of course, hadn't worked the first time and therefore was unlikely to work this time when the cancer was more aggressive. She looked death in the face and knew then that it couldn't be beaten. Staying meant more hospital visits and every visit brought more bad news.

Now she was going to try something else. And that meant going back to the searching. Back to Byron Bay. At the time I wanted to shake her into reason, but at the same time I was walking on eggshells, not wanting to shatter any of her hopes or dreams. So instead of shaking her I would say gently, 'Wouldn't it be better to have the other breast done now?' She'd say, 'No, I'm going to self-heal. I know now that I'm bringing this on myself and I have to go down this road.' It wasn't that she was giving up when she ran away. In fact, she was taking on even more. She needed that extra mythical layer of hope to continue her battle. She asked more questions, she separated herself further from us. She became more discerning as time went on, but at that moment she would have done anything. *Anything.* Her motivation, as always, was to stay alive for the boys. How could we question that? We couldn't. How could we not go along with it? We had to, Russ more than anyone had no choice but to bend to Caron's wishes. How could he keep the children away from their mother at Christmas? So, he made arrangements and reluctantly followed Caron to Australia.

16. Another World

Christmas that year was a nightmare, as bleak a time as there ever was during Caron's illness. As usual, Russ managed to sort everything out and a few days before Christmas he took the boys over to join their confused and beleaguered mother. By then Caron had found a very small house on the beach – there wasn't much available: not only was it last-minute, it was the busiest time of the year. Most of their friends had gone elsewhere for the holiday season and they found themselves alone and adrift. Apart from Caron's death, I honestly think it was the unhappiest period of Russ's entire life. Caron was questioning absolutely everything. The poor man was relegated to a bedroom at the back, which was dark and dank and stiflingly hot, Caron slept alone in the bedroom at the front. Yes, she was healing and needed time to meditate, but mostly because in the turmoil that followed this latest diagnosis, their relationship was under considerable strain. The children slept in bunks in a tiny room off the sitting room. They looked lost, all of them, no one more so than Caron. There was a forlorn tree and one string of lights, which reflected their mood. There is no doubt about it: Caron was a frightened woman and difficult to live with then. The children were confused while Russ was frustrated and disoriented and just wanted to go home. Once again, they were no longer fighting the same battle. Nor were we back at home in England, we wanted her home too, but she was adamant. Caron was staying.

Finally arrived in Byron – in the rain. It feels very good to be back here – there is something in the fabric of this place which I recognize and connect with right away. Of course, I miss my mum and the family, but this is where I want and have to be – at least for now . . .

Russ could not believe it had all so suddenly come to this. He was being pushed beyond his limits. Caron was at breaking point. There was no one to help and I don't think either of them could fathom out what was going on and so they found themselves sitting opposite one another at the small kitchen table with Caron saying, 'Well, if you have to go back to England, go. But I am not coming with you.' She was making it extremely easy for him to fold, wave his white flag and leave. From Swallows and Amazons to possible separation in the blink of an eye. Russ went and lay on his horrid single bed and thought and thought and thought. He couldn't leave Charlie and Gabriel. Caron was off trying every trick Byron Bay had to offer. Who would care for the boys? All their friends were somewhere else. He couldn't take them with him. Who knew how long Caron would stay? By morning he knew he had no choice. He had to stay with Caron in Byron Bay. Once again, she'd got her own way.

I too was beside myself. I spent Christmas in tears. The cancer had spread and Caron had gone. So, too, had the boys and Russ. We had all been looking forward to Christmas together in Cornwall, and suddenly they weren't there. But the bloody cancer was. I was broken-hearted. For the first time in my life, I had to teach myself to be without Caron. For her to go to Australia at all was the biggest blow I personally could have had and that was without any illness – a healthy Caron going there to live would have been bad enough. But to have her going when she was ill, knowing the cancer had spread, was of such magnitude that I have no words to describe it. It was unbearable. I was bereft. Having not been to Byron Bay myself, I could not understand her decision. Michael and Paul tried their best to pick up the pieces that I was in, but Caron's sudden departure was hard on them too. I have described it in the past as a mini-bereavement and it was. I mourned the fact that she was not living in Cornwall, and I hadn't liked it when they'd moved down there from Barnes. Australia was a blot on the horizon. I resented it. I simply couldn't get to grips with what it could give her that we couldn't. Turned out I had a lot to learn. Things my daughter would teach me.

Once that bleak Christmas was over, Stephen and I started plotting our own trip to Byron Bay. Long before the resurgence of the breast cancer, Caron had thought it a good idea if we went to see for ourselves what it offered her. We arrived in January just as they were moving into the huge house they had rented the year before on Wategos Beach. Instantly I could see why it appealed to Caron: it was a fantastic house in a wonderful location. But Australia was not my natural habitat. First, it was hot as hell – forty degrees Celsius – there was no air-conditioning. Secondly, I'm severely allergic to mosquito bites and, of course, ended up covered with them: they swelled and itched like crazy. Then I was bitten by a spider: one leg grew to three times the size of the other and required a visit to the local hospital. As much as Byron Bay was Caron's new-found panacea, it was not mine. Still, I was thrilled to see her and be with her. Except I wasn't with her very much: in fact, she was away for most of the first week.

Caron was doing something called body electronics. It was a six-week cleansing process undertaken by a group of eight people, led by Brandon and her husband Kevin, who were once again in Australia for their new year convention. They ate specific raw food and drank minerals until their bodies were cleansed and free of toxins. Then, over a three-day period, the group would touch the energy points on Caron's body, chanting mantras and using acupressure to heal her. It was a very old ritual that took up to four hours every time. These people went through considerable adversity for Caron, but she loved and appreciated it. The hands-on body work was done with love and good intent and, like all the Byron Bay treatments, had been known to cure people in the past of their particular malaise. Caron was in the mode of shifting growths; it was a very intense part of the self-healing process she was undergoing.

We landed in Brisbane at six thirty in the morning and after a two-hour drive were extremely excited to arrive in Byron Bay. We had our written instructions on how to find the house but we had to wait all day to see Caron. Finally she came in with a lovely bunch of roses and explained the process. Our re-education was about to go up a level. For all of those people to go on that radical diet and do hours of hands-on work with Caron was a very generous, beautiful thing to do. It gave Caron enormous strength and positivity. She felt special, treasured and loved. Caron needed to be loved. She was very sensitive and, let's be realistic, who doesn't need to feel loved? She was charged by the whole process. Excited. Serious-faced doctors weren't just handing over bad news, people were doing something positive, and doing it all for her. 'Can you imagine all these people giving up all this time for me?' she said. It made her feel privileged, cosseted in the mind-body-soul sense. It was a territory that none of us understood or knew about at the time. If I hadn't seen it with my own eyes I wouldn't have believed it. The shattered girl who had run away from England was body-boarding in the sea, relishing the warm air, with a wide smile on her face and a complete sense of freedom. I don't think she would have been doing that back in England. Charlie and Gabriel were beginning to relish the beaches at Byron as much as their mum. We spent a lot of time playing in the surf and climbing over the rocks, investigating whether the crabs were any bigger in Australia.

I talked to her oncologist before I went out to Australia, distressed and willing him to give me a good reason to encourage her to come home. But he said, 'Don't knock Australia. If being in the sunshine makes her feel good then go with it. As long as she also takes guidance from her new recommended oncologist, then anything that makes her feel good is fantastic for overcoming cancer.' I could see it now for myself and, despite the mosquito bites and excessive heat, started to look at Byron Bay through Caron's eyes. Gradually I stopped resisting, resenting Australia for taking Caron away and began to walk this new path with her. After all, it appeared to be doing her good and was only for another month or so. Or so I thought.

Caron was keen that I understood some of the treatments she was having, and I was intrigued to find out more and meet the practitioners she saw regularly. First I visited Serge, a healer, although not hands-on. Perhaps Caron was breaking me in gently and knew I wouldn't like too much hands-on activity while I was so green to the subject. He was very good and took time to explain the mind–body–spirit arena to me. He could pick up vibes from my body and tell me where my weaknesses were. He was also good at helping Caron to relax and meditate; after the maelstrom, she needed that more than ever.

I also had acupuncture with Neil. He had spent years studying in Japan, and used Japanese needles, which were thinner than the Chinese ones. He was fantastic, a mainstay in Caron's life until she left Australia.

That was probably as far as I wanted to go in trying it out for myself. Caron was always mad for me to have colonic irrigation, but she was doing it in a hut in the middle of the rainforest, and frankly if I was going to have something stuck up my bottom, I wanted it done in a more clinical environment. I liked the woman, Denise, who did it, and I agreed with the principle of cleansing, but I couldn't get my head round the hut and the hose. Denise the pooh fairy, as we all came to call her, was also pivotal in Caron's life, but more of that later.

We stayed until the end of January, when Stephen and I had to return to England for work commitments. It had been a truly enlightening trip. I suppose I felt a little more settled, having seen Caron *in situ* and got more of a handle on the place. I could picture her pottering around their beautiful house. I could see that in Byron Bay she was beginning to learn how to say, 'I have cancer,' without the fear that someone was going to go running to the press. No one knew who or what she was and she liked that. She was just Caron, a lovely being, an independent soul. It gave her a freedom that she relished. There were some characters I didn't take to, but Caron didn't seem as possessed by them as she had been; most were as vulnerable as she was. A pattern emerged with all the new practices: Caron would soak them up, then spit them out. Soon she realized that most people had gone to Byron Bay looking for answers for themselves or to make a living. So, yes, I suppose that on the whole I was comforted by what I'd seen – but the journey back to the airport and saying goodbye to her was extreme agony none the less: I couldn't help wondering how many more times we'd have together and what the next few months held in store.

At Easter Russ and Caron were still at Wategos Beach when Johnny and Cathy flew in from England. They saw Cathy's brother in Sydney, then set off to Byron Bay, which they'd thought was a little way up the coast. Distances are not what they seem in Australia, and it turned out to be a ten-hour drive on a single-lane road. Johnny did most of the driving and was almost hallucinating by the time they pulled up at Wategos Beach. He unpeeled himself from the car and stretched out a dozen knots and aches. The man was knackered.

It became immediately apparent to them both that Caron was not in a good place. Their welcome was not as they'd imagined. Caron was agitated and on edge, and although she was pleased to see her friends she said that a sound-healing therapy session was taking place in the rainforest and admitted that she really wanted to attend. It was rather like me turning up to discover she was on the body electronics course. A thirty-hour flight, an excruciating drive, and now Caron wanted to get straight off in the car for an hour's drive. She obviously felt bad about leaving just as they'd arrived because she asked them to go with her. Cathy gave her husband a look that said, 'No way.' So she turned to Johnny. They'd had many such experiences over the years – Caron was always making Johnny try new things – and although he really didn't want to get back into the car, he could see that it meant a lot to her. One thing he was certain of: it would be an interesting ride. As he says, when Caron had an enthusiasm you were just carried along with it. A hard-to-refuse combination of charisma and force. He could tell that things were out of kilter and decided it was better for all concerned to indulge her. So back into the car they got, and they headed out into the night.

Russ had ordered a Thai takeaway and there were a couple of bottles of wine in the fridge so he and Cathy settled down and put the world to rights, which was probably exactly what he needed to do. Russ was frustrated by Caron. He couldn't believe she was proposing to go when the Comerfords had made such a huge effort to come and see her. He was right. But so was Johnny. In this instance it was better to indulge her because if she hadn't gone she wouldn't have been able to relax and have fun.

As Johnny says, it was a most amazing evening. They chatted all the way there and back, and in doing so reached an understanding of where she was going with all of this and what she was trying to achieve. He saw for himself how it was helping her on a spiritual level – giving her strength to carry on the fight. Strength that had deserted her on 4 December. She was completely on form on the way back, the old Caron. It showed Johnny how committed she had become to the process of self-healing. She was put out when the Comerfords arrived because, although she was desperate to see them, she believed she had to do these things. The only way she could cope with her life was keeping to the routine, keeping her faith in everything she tried.

So, once she'd attended that course, she relaxed and they had a wonderful few days.

The course itself was more of the pure sound healing that Caron had done before. Johnny enjoyed it, although it was very hippie. Who else could he have found himself with, meditating in a 'temple' built to Aboriginal design in the middle of the rainforest, open to the elements, chanting and making sounds that vibrated through his body or humming quietly to the cacophony of tree frogs and crickets? It could only have been Caron.

So their holiday began in earnest. Caron took them to the Byron Bay market, an experience in itself. There is a market culture in Byron Bay that is really the essence of the place. There, you can get any kind of crystal, herbal remedy, reading and massage. Dangly things hang everywhere, incense burns prodigiously, there are bells and chanting bowls, drums and pipes. You name it, you can get it – art, craft, sculpture, jewellery – along with all the colourful people. As Cathy says, you could have got the crowd from Central Casting: they all looked exactly the same – the plaits, the jewellery, no one in shoes or bras, wafting cotton, all drinking funny tea. Like many of the practitioners, most of the other people had gone there to discover something about themselves. They had their own language about the journey they were on. Cathy found it very funny and, as she always had, continued to take the mickey. She thinks that's why she and Caron stayed such good friends. She was always the more cynical of the two and, like Caron, never minced her words. She wasn't about to change now, cancer or no cancer, hippies or no hippies. That was one of the great things about Caron: you could always be honest with her. She'd always listen to a point of view. She didn't necessarily believe Cathy, just thought she had got it wrong, but she never tried to convert her or decided she wasn't spiritual enough. Accepting to the end, our Caron. As long as you accepted her.

They got to meet Brandon too. Cathy says she was like a mermaid with long blonde hair. They went out to dinner and Cathy said she wanted the squid. Brandon immediately piped up and said, 'Darling, you can't eat squid. No one eats squid. If you want to be pure and clean, squid is the worst food to eat.' Any guesses what Cathy ate that evening? Oh, yes. Squid. As she says, 'I think they had me down as a bottom-feeder from that point on.' It didn't stop them having a great time.

One night Johnny and Caron stayed up talking late. It is one of the rare times that I know she talked directly about dying. It was a personal conversation, which started with a discussion about faith and progressed from there. He hasn't told me the details, and I wouldn't expect him to because it was a very private moment, but he has said that when the boys are older, if they ever want to know the content of that conversation, he will tell them. What he has told me was that for the first time Caron revealed the true depth of her fear. In the past they'd always talked about 'getting through this', 'recovering', 'having the strength to recover'. But this was different. Russ was right: she had looked death in the face and realized she might not beat it. She was wrung out and upset because, although she suspected the worst, she desperately wanted to live. Sometimes I would complain about getting old, and she would say to me, 'Don't knock it. I dream of being that old woman sitting in the chair watching her grandchildren . . .' Johnny says that listening to Caron talk so uncharacteristically negatively was dreadful. When they returned eighteen months later, for Christmas 2003, Caron was physically in a much worse condition but she was calmer. She was a different person. She didn't talk about dying but was much more accepting of the situation and living for the day, each day, one by one and whatever it might bring.

Of course I missed Caron desperately. I resented Australia because it took her away from me, and I fought with myself over the possibility of going there permanently. But the reality was that we couldn't just up sticks and go, as she and Russ had. Although I feared from that first visit that the three months would be extended again, I didn't know they were going to stay permanently. I didn't know whether it was going to be another month or whether they'd simply stay until winter. It just drifted on indefinitely, and all the while we were hoping and praying that she would come home.

When they went to Fowey, I had had no intention of buying a house there, but I did so that I could be near her if she needed me. I couldn't go on doing that. First, I didn't know that Byron Bay would hold her affections for as long as it did. Sometimes I felt her decision to run off like that was purely on a whim and Russ was just giving in. For me to buy a house in Australia to be up the road from her in case she needed me was an immense undertaking: what if she'd decided to come back or go somewhere else? We couldn't just go on buying houses and moving around the world. Caron wrote many times in her diaries how she needed solitary time to meditate and heal. She needed the space. Anyway, I have a husband who has a business in London: he left it behind for the second time so that we could go to Australia for Easter. During those two years Stephen was away from work for months at a time. I will always be thankful for his support then. In the back of my head, too, I was also aware that for Caron to have me there sometimes brought complications she didn't need.

The anonymity and freedom that Byron Bay gave her was lost temporarily during the busy periods. English tourists would recognize us, and the mutterings she longed to escape would begin again. Conversely, she wanted the infrastructure she was used to, and that was her family. It was difficult to know what to do. So back on the plane we went, and arrived for our Easter holiday.

'Holiday' is a misleading word. We never thought of those trips as holidays. We went there to be with Caron, Russ and the boys. I could never wait to see them again, but also to cook and care for them. Most of the time we tried to take the load off Russ, who was single-handedly running the household. In that respect, we were there as much for the whole family as for Caron. We went to be practical, to nurture and provide back-up for the boys, whom I was always desperate to see. I loved the chance to be back in the simple routine of packing their lunches and driving them to school. You could almost believe that life was back to normal. But, of course, it wasn't.

As for Caron, we saw her as much as she wanted to or could see us, depending on her health. Like our first trip, there was a lot of time when she was away on courses and she was always having treatments of one kind or another. By now she was into doing a daily yoga session, acupuncture, oxygen treatment, *Reiki*, to add to the body electronics, sound healing, reflexology and colonic irrigation. She was busy healing, so we got busy in the house, with the boys, and were always on stand-by to drive her to whatever treatment it was that day. I liked it: it made me feel as if I was doing *something* to help. The tag team took over again.

On reflection, there is nothing to dislike about Australia and I have wonderful vivid memories of it. My gripe with the place was purely personal: it was holding my sick daughter hostage, and I wanted her home so that I could take care of her all the time. But the more I got to know the place, the more I could see that Russ and Caron were building themselves yet another charmed life. Easy, slow-paced, spiritual and balanced. But the moment when Caron announced their decision to stay on was gut-curdling. I remember it as if it were yesterday.

Charlie was furious. Russ and Caron had been extending their trip week by week and the boys believed they would be heading home sooner or later, as they had the first time. Their friends were at home. Their home was in Cornwall. So was their school. I wanted her back so that she could have more orthodox treatment, as well as everything she was experimenting with in Byron Bay. But Caron was adamant: they were staying. Charlie shouted at his parents, 'You promised we'd go home. You promised we'd only be here for a short time and I want to go back!' I remember Caron saying, in a very calm, quiet voice, 'When you're old enough you can decide where you want to live but in the meantime while you're with us and under age you have to accept our judgement that we're doing this for the right reasons.' He was so upset that he ran upstairs and locked himself in his bedroom. Nothing could placate him. It was not an easy thing to do, but Caron had a multitude of reasons, the depths of which Charlie or Gabriel could not possibly have understood.

Part of it was that she couldn't even face going back to the airport. She didn't want someone taking a photo and saying, 'This is how Caron used to look. Look at her now.' Some people knew it was cancer, but in Caron's mind it was still a secret. England meant the risk of being under the spotlight again, and the spotlight was the last thing she wanted in her life. She was learning just 'to be', and the spotlight is diametrically opposed to that. Every time it came to a feasible point of going back, she'd say, 'Please, let's not go back yet,' and so it crept on and on until they made that final decision: they were staying. And I suffered that same sense of bereavement and powerlessness all over again. The tangled feelings that consume you when you have a child who is suffering from a disease you can't fix returned. It is the most hair-tearing, frustrating, heartbreaking, deepest hurt that you can ever go through because you are helpless. You can't take it away, and now I couldn't even be with her while she was going through it.

At one point Caron started a girls' weekly get-together, which I enjoyed going to when I was there. I believe it goes on even in her absence. Everyone held hands at the beginning, then Caron would welcome them, they would listen to a mantra, and the forum would open. It was a spiritual, peaceful form of group discussion, therapy almost. It was wholesome, good and pure. We would decide on a topic, either a world event if something big had happened or something personal. Caron might say, 'I am finding my cancer very hard to deal with at the moment. Let's think of all the other things we find hard to deal with . . .' I remember that I once said, 'I find it very hard to deal with the fact that you are twelve thousand miles away.' It was the first time I'd been able to explain on an open platform without judgement how I felt. I said, 'What I find really hard to deal with is that my precious girl, whom I've loved intensely since the second she was born, has made a decision, which, although I understand it, I hate. Caron has come here to heal, but it is a decision outside my control. My instinct is to be with her all the time, but now I can't because of a decision she has made. It just isn't possible for me to pick up and move to the other side of the world.' I felt a huge release to be able to share how I felt and it was good for her to understand it in the company of her friends, who not only empathized but backed me up with compassion.

It was great to be honest, and that was what Caron loved about Byron Bay. Let's get it out in the open. She found it very refreshing. She found the anonymity refreshing. She had no television history and she learned that it was enough just 'to be'. You don't have to be anybody, anything; you don't have to drive yourself if you don't want to. A great thing to learn, hard, but by the end she had learnt it. We left Australia, having stayed over a month, and flew home. Once again, the journey to the airport was excruciatingly painful. Caron and I were both torn. She didn't want me to go, but knew I couldn't stay. I didn't want to leave her there, but knew she couldn't come with me. No one was better off. Cancer was dictating our lives.

During one of Russ's business trips home alone, Caron did something that enraged him. A practitioner in the Blue Moun-

tains professed to be able to draw out cancer with personally
formulated poultices. Russ had been dubious from the outset. I
hadn't heart of poultices being used for cancer, but I explained
to him the old practice of putting a bread poultice on an abscess
or boil and letting the bread suck out the poison. Was Russ's
disapproval the reason she chose to go while he was away? Or
had an appointment just appeared, like a calling, enabling her
to go? I don't know, but whichever it was, she and her friend
Melinda flew to the mountains west of Sydney to visit this
man. It was September. Her right breast had been swelling and
hardening to the size of a grapefruit since she ran away from the
doctors in England and their recommendations to remove it.
She must have known that all the work she was doing was
failing on some level. Her painful, puckered, swollen breast was
testament to her particularly powerful cancer. This man applied
a thick, black tar-like substance to her breast and the suspect
lump on her neck, then covered the area with white muslin
patches. He sent her home with jars of the stuff. Russ was
furious when he discovered what she had done, and we were all
concerned: it reeked of the desperate behaviour we'd witnessed a
year before. But just when you give up any hope of a miracle,
strange things happen: it was drastic action to take, but the
poultice appeared to be working. Her breast slowly reduced in
size. By the end of the treatment, the muslin was thick with a
green, pus-like substance. Was this stuff actually sucking out the
cancer? It seemed impossible. And yet the swelling was going
down.

As Caron's fortieth birthday approached, I realized I could
not miss such a landmark occasion. We were scheduled to go
to Australia for Christmas, but I was going to be there somehow
on 5 October too. We decided to surprise her so told her that I
couldn't get out of work – I was doing *Open House* daily for
Channel Five at the time. With only Russ in cahoots, we
planned our trip. They had left Wategos by then because it had

become too expensive. A lot of money was going out and little was coming in. Instead they were in a rented house which I had seen briefly on my previous visit, and knew vaguely where it was. As we drove through the gate, the nanny, a wonderful girl called Deesha, was leaving. She gave us a most perplexed look – back already? My heart was pounding with excitement as we crept into the house.

Caron was in the kitchen with her back to the door, talking on the phone. 'Any chance of a cup of tea around here?' I asked.

Caron swung round. 'Ahhhh! My mum's just walked into the kitchen!' she screamed, then promptly dropped the phone. We flew into each other's arms and, within seconds, Charlie and Gabriel had noisily joined the mêlée. Then Stephen's strong arms wrapped us all up into one tight, happy, loud bundle. I've no idea what the person stranded at the other end of the phone thought.

I had brought out a caseful of presents for her landmark fortieth birthday. We started opening them that afternoon and the gifts kept coming all week until Caron's big day. The one she loved most was an album I had put together of her life from birth. All the people who had meant so much to her were proudly displayed. For days afterwards I saw her showing it to her new friends, pictures of the old ones, Nana and Grando, her brothers and nephews, her schoolfriends, the gangs from Bristol, Barnes, Cornwall and television.

Caron had arranged to celebrate her birthday at the house they intended to buy, Taylors. It was a most beautiful guest-house, away from the beach, set back against the rainforest. The whole family went there for the weekend and we had the party on the Saturday night. It was a breathtakingly wonderful evening. Russ, as always, had made everything perfect. He had had dozens of sets of angel wings made up, all decorated with sequins, feathers, rhinestones and beads, and left them at the foot of the steps leading up to the house for the guests to choose the pair that suited them. By the end there were forty angels in the garden, which was awash with fairy-lights, twinkling from the eaves of the house and the trees, around the summer-house and the pool. Russ had woven his magic again. There was even a fire-breathing act that turned out to be Deesha, the nanny. I have never seen two little boys look more stunned – I don't suppose she had much trouble with them after that night. Only in Byron Bay would the nanny end up breathing fire and dancing like Darcey Bussell. Caron wore a fabulous black lace trouser suit and my overwhelming memory is of watching her rock and roll to jive music as if she didn't have a care in the world. It was probably the last time I saw her dance. I often look at the photos of her on that evening and wonder at her beauty. But one small detail stands out: she is wearing a choker round her neck attached to a fabulous silk flower. It covered the poultice on her neck, which was still working its dark magic.

My impression of that visit is that everyone had settled into their new life. Charlie had started playing cricket, roller hockey, football, you name it; he was a busy boy. Gabriel, as always, had adjusted to the change with ease and had made new friends. Caron and Russ had spent a great deal of time choosing a new school for them and had finally decided they should go to the Rudolf Steiner school. It was set in lush countryside five minutes from their new home. Each classroom was a round wooden hut. Parents had to sign a release form for their children to climb trees at lunchtime. It was bliss. There was nothing for a child not to enjoy. And that was why they chose it: so that the boys could have structure but as much fun as possible. At home they were in and out of the pool all the time, playing cricket in the garden, spying on the grown-ups. Caron was away a lot too – the courses and exploration rarely ceased; I think she loved the environment of them. Charlie used to say, 'Not another course, Mummy,' when she went off for the weekend, or several evenings in a row. Sometimes, as I've said, she went away for a week at a time. I know that she returned to the Blue Mountains, for example, that December to repeat the poultice treatment on her right breast. But, as with all these treatments, what could anyone really say? She was giving it everything she had, trying every kind of healing on offer to stay alive for the boys. She was doing it for them and could justify her absences to herself in that way. All she would ever say was, 'I don't want my children to grow up without their mum,' and off she went. That was as close as we got to referring to death during those years of searching in Australia.

Although their mummy was sick and spent a lot of time resting or away, I think when they cast their minds back to Byron Bay their overall memory will be one of joy. There was always music in the house – at night Russ and his pals would play the guitar. They wanted the boys to be happy and live a full life without the spectre of disease hanging over their heads. The following year got harder but, by and large, they succeeded in their mission, an accomplishment I know Caron was proud of, and I'm sure Russ always will be.

All the time I was in England, pretending that Caron and her family were in Australia by choice, she was the person I thought of when I awoke, she was the last person I thought of at night and a million times during the day. She was the one I thought about in the early hours of the morning as I paced the corridors until it was time to call. One of the first things I did when Caron moved was have a cheap telephone line to Australia put in. On days when something was worrying her I would call several times. I would call Russ to see whether she had made an appointment to see the doctor. I would be back on the phone to get the result. Barely a day went by when we didn't talk. She rarely called me to say she'd had a bad day, but I could tell from her voice when she was feeling worse: it was softer, quieter, fearful, perhaps. The reality of her symptoms would come out

in little bits. She did the same with the close friends who knew
of her illness when they chatted on the phone. It wasn't that she
was covering things up: it was more that she needed to get her
head round things before she told anyone she was feeling worse,
not better.

And so the year came to its close. It was high summer again
in Australia, Christmas and New Year. This time Michael went
out to visit Caron for his 'holiday', terrified of what he would
find when he got there. In fact, he was pleasantly surprised.

17. Living on Borrowed Time

I am in Byron Bay, Australia, home to New Age hippies, surfers, back-packers, gorgeous beaches and one of the best and most stimulating communities I've ever lived in.

I am healing and have come here to do it in a town that has the highest concentration of spiritual healers per capita in the Western world. There are over seventy yoga teachers alone, Kudalini, and belly dancing, people to sing your chakras back into balance, psychic life readings, tantric-sex workshops, colonics, colour therapy, flower essences, reflexology, sand therapy . . . Incredible things happen here. Incredible things happen every-where. Maybe they just seem more intense here. I have tried everything from colonics, sound therapy, body electronics, acupuncture, crystal heal-ing, fasting, poultices, orthodox medication and a whole lot of prayer and I'm still not certain that I'm completely clear of cancer. In fact, some of the drugs I've been taking had so robbed my bones of calcium that my body has been in a very depleted state. Help, though, is flooding in thick and fast . . .

Russ and Caron were renting their great friend Melinda's house over that Christmas period while they waited to move into Taylors. Michael arrived to find Caron in brilliant form. She was upright, her skin and hair were glowing, she was active, positive, a picture of good health. She took him straight into town to her favourite café, where he got his first taste of life in Byron Bay. A dandelion soy latte and an everything-free cake, which he was astounded to discover was absolutely delicious. Hey, this is pretty good, he thought, and any resentment he'd been feeling started to slide away.

It was Christmas Eve, Michael happened to have a couple of

friends in the area, which was just another excuse to have a party. Caron's friend Paul came over with a box of booze and they had thirty or so people over to the house, made apple martinis, played music, danced round the Christmas tree and had a great time. Okay, so she kicked everyone out at midnight because she was getting tired, but, as Michael reasoned at the time, wouldn't any mum of two boisterous kids?

On that activity-filled trip they swam in the sea, went boogie-boarding, walked and talked for hours. The Hari Krishnas were in town and, of course, Michael, too, sampled the Byron Bay market. Multiply the crystals-and-incense experience that Johnny and Cathy had by ten: it was Christmas. A busy time of year. There were people with tambourines, the prayer flags were out, people wafted around in swathes of tie-dye and the smell of cooking veggie-burgers hung in the air. Michael loved it. He found he could talk to those of Caron's friends who knew she was ill and, like me, found it a relief to have things out in the open. Melinda had sussed out that Caron was sick before Caron told her, and explained that in Byron Bay Caron was finding her path in life, her heart and her passions, so that she could communicate more clearly to her family and friends who she was and what she wanted out of life. At first he probably didn't quite understand, but over time, the place seeps into you, and slowly he developed a better picture of what was going on in Caron's mind.

The truth is when you are facing death you ask yourself all the big questions that we normally brush aside. Have I lived? Can I dream? Am I free? And maybe the hardest question of all: who am I? As surreal as it looked to us, the uninitiated, standing on the sidelines, Caron was calling reality into her life. It was a slow process but she was doing it. As Melinda said, she moved through all the major issues she felt she had, got through some and not others, but, as we witnessed, she gave it her all. What was the main thing she didn't get through? Fear, I think. She was terribly afraid of dying, and who wouldn't be? I have been told that people who heal themselves from cancer develop the ability to be really present for the 'now' – this is Byron Bay speak – but that Caron was too scared. I don't know what to think about that: I believe that that puts a terrible pressure on the patient, who suddenly becomes a victim of themselves.

There were other things she couldn't get past: she wanted me there all the time, however unrealistic she knew that to be, but then oscillated back to wanting more space. She missed her father too. She would tell Melinda all about her long chats with Don at the kitchen table in Northern Ireland. Caron was scared. But she was doing everything that those who had supposedly cured themselves had done. My daughter came to the end of that first year full of hope because she had done everything there was to do and, as Michael found, she looked wonderful, active and happy. Could it be that the miracle had happened?

Throughout all this time the biggest lesson has been learning to trust and NOT PANIC. To learn, in the midst of everyone telling you how fabulous their treatment is, to listen to myself. To really check it's what my body wants. This is so difficult when all you really want is someone to come and take the cancer away from you. It is really tempting to cling on to anyone who claims they can. The truth is though, it is different for everyone. There is no one way. For some people Western medicine is absolutely the answer; for others nutrition, herbs, visualization and cleansing will do it. A wonderful healer friend says that it doesn't really matter what you do, it's the change that you make inside that heals . . .

Michael met Brandon for the first time too. He, Russ and Caron, Charlie and Gabriel were invited over to her house for New Year's Eve, but Russ stayed in the back room with the boys and didn't really join in with what Brandon had planned. Of course, Michael went expecting a party but, no, this was Byron Bay. Brandon was sitting in a huge chair wrapped in orange while everyone else sat in a circle round her. He was handed a notebook and pen, not the drink he'd been anticipating, and a plate of vegetarian food. It was his first experience of 'vision questing'.

'Think about all the beautiful things that have been special to you,' said Brandon.

Michael started to write.

'Think about what makes you happy.' And so it continued. Michael liked it. He pictured himself cycling through Battersea Park on a crisp spring day.

Then she asked a question that forced him to grab the moment and do something with it: 'Turn to the person next to you and say something that you really mean from your heart,' said Brandon.

Michael turned to Caron, rather as I had in the women's discussion forum, and said, 'I forgive you.'

Caron was startled. She stared at her baby brother. 'You forgive me?' she asked, perplexed.

'Yes,' he continued. 'I forgive you for leaving us and coming here. Now I'm here I understand why you've done it. I've been pissed off and angry because my big sister has not only left us but taken the boys as well. Paul doesn't see you, Mum doesn't see you, she is devastated that you've gone, and it's us who have to try and piece her back together again. Something we can't do, because she's incomplete without you. It has been a terrible year for us back at home but, yes, I forgive you . . .'

Cancer, as I've said, is a lonely business for both the sufferer and the family watching from the sidelines. It is a selfish business too. We were selfish because we were without Caron. Caron was entirely wrapped up in herself, completely involved in moving out her 'blocks' and the 'debris of life' that we all, according to complementary medicine, carry around with us. It was the debris that Caron believed caused disease. So she hadn't considered Michael's angle, or ours. Of course it was all about her, which it had to be, but it was an interesting junction they came to at that meeting. A lot more things came up, whose edges Michael and she might only have skirted round. The vision questing opened a portal to further revelations. So, while Michael missed his midnight new year glass of bubbly, he got a deeper connection with his sister. And when you are living on borrowed time thousands of miles away, as Caron was, those moments are the most precious, the most vivid, and the ones that make her death almost bearable. By midnight Brandon hadn't finished her summation, so while the fireworks were going off all along the beach, she was still inside, talking. It didn't matter. What is time anyway? Finally they went outside and were given sparklers to write their dreams in the sky. I don't need to say what Michael's was, or any other wish he made from that point on until 13 April 2004.

Michael also met Denise the pooh fairy, the queen of the colonics. She would only 'do you', as it were, if you had a good aura and she liked you. She was a great person for Caron to talk to, older than her but not as old as me. She was a very spiritual woman, and some would say she had great healing powers although she didn't trade on them. She was keeping Caron's body clean, moving that debris on. Most people who detox and cleanse say that keeping the colon clear is good for the system. I think Denise was very good for my daughter, not only physically but mentally too. She was kind and reassuring, and I think she made Caron feel safe.

The first time Caron took Michael up to the hills behind Byron Bay where she lived, he was bowled over. Her place is like a grotto. The blue ironwork over the gate spells 'Angel Grove'. There are fairies everywhere, and in the middle of this enchanted forest there is a hexagonal gazebo with purple glass where she does her colonics. It wasn't the sort of procedure you see on *You Are What You Eat*, it was more like a hosepipe and a swill barrel on the other side of the room. Denise would talk away in her broad Aussie accent while she did it, believing as she did it that all those old emotional anxieties we cling to were being dislodged and flushed away. On one famous occasion she said to Caron, 'Oh, darling, there goes your father . . .' We all thought she was amazing because she could put a smile on Caron's face. She made her laugh, even when the pain got bad. Caron swore by her. Sometimes she wanted to visit Denise more than once a week, which Denise didn't recommend, but towards the end, when Caron's tummy was swollen and she got into difficulty, Denise was always on hand to calm her. She would sing to her and stroke her head, which soothed her. Afterwards she gave Caron specially concocted drinks to replenish her system with good things that were high in antioxidants, enzymes and vitamins. All that goodness flowing into her gave her confidence in her body's ability to continue the fight and she always felt wonderful afterwards.

Like me, Michael didn't partake. Instead he sat outside with Denise's friend Mary while she told him how UFOs were floating over Byron Bay, drawn by the special energy that emanated from the place. These things were not suggested: they were delivered as a matter of fact. Aliens were walking around Byron Bay among the tambourine-rattling tie-dye hippies, but Michael couldn't see them because he wasn't tuned in to them. Mary, however, could see them perfectly. They had another cup of green tea and the conversation continued. Like the dandelion soy latte, and the vision questing, it was all very Byron Bay. Michael could see why his sister loved it so.

The other person who was of enormous help to Caron was Neil, her acupuncturist. He, with Denise, was undoubtedly at the top of the list of those who, at the end of the day, actually made a difference. Caron went to him every week, and when she was really in pain she had extra sessions with him when he would also burn the dried Asian herb moxa to help draw out the pain down her legs. He was very down-to-earth, not as airy-fairy as some in Byron Bay. He was practical – in fact, he was the one who finally said to Caron, 'Stop going here, there and everywhere. Stop going from me to the shaman to the Bible-study group. Decide on the three things that really help your body and stick to them.' She was chasing therapies, as I've said, driven by fear. But it was difficult for her to stop because what if the one miracle that would work for her was the one she missed? I think all her friends out there would agree that she put enormous pressure on herself and spent too much valuable time getting into the car and going to this or that therapist when she could have been having fun at home with the boys, or indulging in painting. But they don't think it damaged her and, anyway, who were they to criticize? Judgement of others is not in the Byron Bay mandate – although, weirdly, it is. Bottom line is, no one can know how it feels to be dealing with the possibility of dying, except the person themselves, and so, like us, her friends in Byron Bay stepped aside, and let Caron continue on her own unique path of self-healing.

Like all of them, Neil had great stories about people who'd had cancer, people he'd helped, but unlike some of the practitioners, there was no false hope with Neil, which I particularly liked about him. He was one of the few people I saw regularly. Apparently we all tend to have one weak meridian and mine was my kidney. All the flights to Australia were taking their toll and I had begun to notice that my legs were puffing up and getting sore to the touch. He had it cleared up within two weeks. I felt that Caron was in safe hands with Neil but, none the less, her brothers, husband and I would urge her continually to see the cancer specialists in Sydney she continued to shy away from.

What an extraordinary time. I'm having conversations with God on an almost daily basis – am I imagining it or going mad? – no, it's happening.

I've had fear coming up about Monday's check-up. Although I know in my heart that all is well, it's as if I've been clinging on to the fear – afraid to let myself believe I am completely healed.

What this brings up in me is a sense of powerlessness which is what happened every time. I was told there was something wrong – all my power left me. Right now I feel strong, I have reached a part in the road where I have chosen to leave the old paralysis behind – the one where I was ill and worrying continuously about it coming back. I have chosen the left fork where I am completely healed and whole. There is no worry about future illness because I don't choose that route. It is reclaiming one's power and believing and strengthening. I feel like I'm finally saying goodbye to the cancer. I have made that move and just have to bring it through physically – on a spiritual level it's already done.

I have already gone through next Monday and it's all clean. I feel really odd – stuff is leaving me, this is letting go of 5 years of being consumed by fear and uncertainty and this is the dawning of a whole new era.

I am finally about to do what I came here for. How exciting. Nothing will stop me and I choose not to be ill again, to cause any sort of delay. I think that that's what the fear was – that somehow something was going to happen – but it won't without me wanting it on some level and I choose that plan from God and my higher self – that contract we drew up so many years ago. My positive contract is finally happening and I needed to go through this time to finally shift the last bit of fear.

I am so grateful for all of this.

My prayer is to let go. To live and love, truth, joy, health and service. To fulfil my soul's destiny on all levels and now there is nothing to be afraid of. Not now, not next Monday, not ever.

There have been strong days – it's as if I must get clear and stand powerful in my own light, not looking for healing from anyone or anything else, outside the divine love and healing of God. Know thyself and what you believe in. To look for it from someone else is to give your power away – you don't need to.

I love you and am always with you and remember Goddess – your illness has been removed from every cell in your body – never again will you be ill – you are the miracle.

From out of the darkness a small voice whispers to me,
Of freedom, love and places unseen
In my dreams it calls me home
How skilfully I ignored it

But when the whisper became a roar – I listened
In my delight, a river burst through, shimmering and golden
On which words and sounds eddy and swirl
It flows from my heart, so you may hear my song.
Now sing me yours.

The Bible-study group, to which Neil had referred, was an American-originated 'church' called the 'Course of Miracles'. Caron got embroiled in it during that first year. She would go on two-day courses, or three-hour-long midweek sessions, or sometimes she just went there to hang out. It was headed by a controversial figure who preached to the congregation about the scriptures. I believe he had been banned from preaching in the States, and although Russ was aware of the controversy surrounding him, he was not concerned. Caron got a great deal out of the sessions: she came to know and understand the Bible, and reunited herself with God. Although, as the spiritual being she was, I don't think she had ever really lost that connection. As with many high-profile preachers, there was an element in this one of 'We are all equal but I'm a little bit more equal than the rest of you,' but overall he was not a dangerous influence. The Bible-study group was a positive thing in Caron's life during the first year but in the second, when she took a turn physically for the worse, she tended to dip in and out of it on a sporadic basis, as and when she needed to.

It would be fair to say that in that first year she flitted between treatments, but her healthy-eating regime was constant. It was very regulated, very definite and very strict. She had a dietician who kept her on a controlled diet but it wasn't excessive:

nothing much had changed from the Cornwall days but it was more strictly adhered to. It was easier too: alternatives of every variety were on offer in Byron Bay. There was a juice bar on practically every street corner, while no alcohol, no coffee, no meat, no dairy, no sugar was mainstream there. Burgers and shakes were anathema. So, diet-wise, Caron was at home and fastidious about it. She didn't have to take her rice to a restaurant: they served all the lesser-known varieties and certainly no white rice. They served 'allowed' cheese from goats and sheep, and there was an abundance of fresh fish so she didn't feel as though she was denying herself. Every afternoon she'd make herself a beetroot, apple and carrot juice, and in the morning it was often fresh pineapple juice. She bought a machine and trays of wheatgrass so that any of us could juice it for her. There was a lot of goodness going in, and, as Michael and I now had to concur, what was there not to like about Caron and Russ's life in Byron Bay? Except, of course, that it was in Byron Bay. Sometimes Caron would admit she longed for a glass of wine, and I would say, 'Have a sip of champagne,' but her reply was always the same: 'It's easier not to.'

At the time of Michael's visit the poultice treatment that Caron had administered to her right breast, armpit and neck was complete. She had never been one of those girls who paraded around the pool topless in the summer, and had always been private about her body. Michael, like me, would never have presumed to see what the poultice had done. But on this trip she showed him. There was no doubt about it, the size of her breast had reduced, and in February 2003 when she finally went to see the oncologist in Sydney, after a nine-month absence, he noted that although there was some 'nodularity' there was no tenderness in the breast, the swelling was down, and there was no longer any mention of suspicious activity in her neck. However, the poultice had left its own deformity. At first sores had developed, which, over time, had scarred, leaving the skin puckered and raw. It was not a pleasant sight. Michael had to hide his shock and, as always, focus on the positive: the swelling had gone down, the lump in Caron's neck had disappeared. He ignored the pockmarked, sagging skin. There was cause for tentative celebration. What he and Caron did not know at the time, however, was that she still had a two-centimetre growth in the right axillary lymph node. And there was more to come. Much more.

On the penultimate day of Michael's trip, the two of them were on the beach planning to walk up to a tea-tree lake nearby. Tea-tree oil is a natural antiseptic, one of nature's wonders, good for the hair and skin, you can float in the brown, pungent water of the lake and let the tea-tree sap work its restorative magic. Caron loved it. She and Michael were on their own in the ocean, frolicking around. Michael remembers holding Caron's hand in the Pacific Ocean, facing the horizon, the vastness of it all, with the glorious healing sun beating down on them, and thinking what a special moment it was. Almost as if anything was possible and yet literally a second later everything would change. Suddenly she said she had felt something go in her back. She looked at Michael, a little scared. 'I want to get out,' she said plainly. So they did. They started towards the lake, but Caron stopped and said she wanted to go home. She went from dancing in the waves to lying crippled in bed the next morning. He remembers thinking, What's happened here? Something has shifted again. And yet when Michael first arrived, he and Caron often walked two or three kilometres over the cliffs. He just couldn't take on board what had happened.

Most of the bad news has blurred together now, time does that, but every single setback was, as Russ has said, like a baseball bat to the stomach. As Michael said his goodbyes, Caron was unable to get out of bed. His eyes didn't dry until he reached Brisbane airport ninety minutes later, as he wondered whether he would ever see Caron again. That was probably the first time he was faced with the prospect of Caron actually dying. Until then he, along with the rest of us, had been living the myth. I think the only person who really knew what lay ahead was Russ. And Caron, of course – not of course: perhaps.

Michael left Caron behind and came home. Another Christmas and New Year had gone by, but a new era was beginning. Caron and Russ moved into their first proper Aussie home, Taylors. It was a ranch-style house that opened on to a wonderful pool area right on the edge of the rainforest. The garden was five acres, there were lush palms, frangipani trees and birds of paradise everywhere. At the bottom of one path, there was a blissful summerhouse, which Caron considered hers. It was where she went to read, meditate and do her coffee enemas every morning. It was her private sanctuary, which she filled with little bits of art, rugs and the typical Caron trinkets and objects. It was a place to gather her thoughts and harness her strength. The boys knew instinctively not to go in there. Between treatments she was enthused with cementing their new family home. She started a collection of rose-printed china to which I added every time I went out. She was forever painting furniture, lining drawers, getting the family's roots firmly into the ground and tapping into her vivid awareness of interior decoration. The move was great: it provided excitement and furthered the adventure. It was a happy house, despite the threat of illness. I must reiterate it wasn't all suffering and down moments, but the shift in pain she had experienced that day on the beach with Michael wouldn't go away, and the next few weeks were hard. Something had obviously happened that she and Russ had to face up to, whether they liked it or not. Unknown to either of them, the cancer had travelled to her bones. Pain was to become a factor in Caron's life. Not the mental anguish she had carried with her since diagnosis back in 1997, but real, debilitating physical pain. But she was not alone.

After a year in Australia she had some really good friends who rallied round them both in times of need. Caron was incredible, really: during all this time of uncertainty she was rarely down, never depressed – in fact, quite the opposite. She exuded a phenomenal warm energy, which was what had attracted those wonderful people to her. Some real gems. Caron had less time now for those on the fringes who, at the beginning, had been grabbing their generosity and feeding off their desperation. Now she had prioritized: her last year was a time of solidarity with Russ and finding more strength from him.

As her friend Melinda says she knew nothing about Caron being famous: her previous life was only of consequence because she was examining it so closely. Other than that, her time in front of the camera was irrelevant. Melinda recalls meeting a woman who was fun and full of laughter. They clicked immediately because they both thought outside the box and were always ready to jump into the car and go on a journey of discovery together – often to do things that others thought they shouldn't, but to hell with it! It was the twinkle in the eye that Caron had always possessed, the 'it's time for the *craic*' twinkle, which always meant fun to her friends. Though Caron wrote of Melinda that she was 'a woman with the energy of five people', Melinda feels it was she who was keeping up with Caron. Even when Caron was really sick, she'd say, 'Come on, let's go to Belongil Fields.' It was a site for alternative concerts, fairs and festivals, and off they'd go.

One of Melinda's fondest memories of that first year is of a warm, moonlit night, when the women's group had gathered. After their discussion they went outside to dance and, moved by the glorious moonlight, decided to walk out to the point by the lighthouse. Charlie was invited to go with them, and together they traipsed down to the ocean like the wild things they were. The waves were silver, the sky was inky blue-black, peppered with a million stars, and they sang at the top of their lungs a song that came to mean a great deal to Caron: 'There Is

So Much Magnificence In The Ocean' by Mitten and Premal. It was a moment without fear. A moment so much in the now that it remains with Melinda and, I hope, Charlie. It was a moment of oneness with the universe, a powerful moment that encapsulated the essence of whom Caron had enabled herself to become. She personified the celebration of life, even though, or because, she knew she was sick: life had to be celebrated. That was why we chose that song for her funeral, hard as it was, and it was hard – damn near impossible – but even in the darkest moments life must be celebrated. If Caron left a legacy then perhaps that is it: celebrate life, celebrate love, celebrate yourself.

18. Divine Intervention

Caron's back pain grew progressively worse. It came in fits and starts and began to radiate down her left leg. Although acupuncture helped, she realized eventually that she had to go back to Sydney to find out what was really going on. She had been resisting Russ's urges to go since Michael had left because she didn't want any more MRIs or X-rays than were absolutely necessary. She didn't like them because they pumped more radiation, 'badness', into her body. Stephen and I went back again in the new year of 2003 and, after a spate of ongoing severe back pain, she asked me if I would go to Sydney with her. She hadn't seen her oncologist for nine months, preferring instead to concentrate on her mission to self-heal. Because of her pain the car journey to the airport was difficult. The walk to and from the aircraft was slow and arduous. It was frightening to see her like that. We checked into a hotel in Sydney and I remember looking across the harbour thinking, Same view, very, very different situation. My heart was racing about what this visit would reveal.

Previously Professor Martin Tattershall was responsive to Caron's needs – he had once had to give her some bad news, but then said, 'Go home, enjoy your children, surf. You're doing everything you can.' I think Caron trusted him as much as she trusted anyone in the field of oncology. However, on 20 February that changed. He ordered some X-rays of her chest, spine and pelvic area, and tested her reflexes. His maverick bravado attitude, which we were used to, failed him. While before he'd remained ebullient, without pussy-footing around, this time he looked up from the X-rays on the computer screen and said to Caron, 'I don't know how this happened but the cancer has spread to your bones.'

I was almost afraid to look at her. My stomach was heaving and my head was spinning. Bone cancer! How could that be after everything she'd been doing? I was reeling. Until now we had been dealing with breast cancer. But this was huge. I can only imagine what took place inside Caron's head, but mine was going a million miles an hour trying to second-guess what it meant as I tried to keep a calm expression on my face and remain in control. What I really wanted to do was throw myself against the wall, or the doctor, and scream and shout. He said, 'But, look, we're going to treat it with bisphosphonates and they're really good these days. It's a monthly injection, which is terrific.' Things were looking up. Then he took it all away. 'Sometimes they can give a patient six, eight, maybe even ten more years.'

Now I looked at her. For the first time since Caron's ordeal had began, she had heard a prognosis. From the horse's mouth. It did not concur with what she had forced herself to believe. She looked stunned. She had always been, and still was, going for cure. Or, at least, full-time management. It was one of those terrible moments, like the day when Russ had rung me in Sevenoaks and told me it was 'bad news'. Caron was led into a day ward to have the treatment there and then. They put a needle into her arm and left us. It takes about two hours and other people in the room were having it too. We didn't know what to say to each other – it was terrible.

After a while I made an excuse to get a cup of coffee, and went and stood outside the doctor's office. I knew two women had gone in after us and I just waited in the corridor. A few people asked me if I was all right. I reapplied my lipstick, searched my bag for a miracle, and eventually the two women came out.

Just as the doctor started to close the door, I stepped into the frame. I said I had to talk to him in absolute confidence. I know I can be steely when I need to be, and he let me in. I gave it to him straight. With his sudden gloomy outlook he had effectively signed my daughter's death warrant. 'You have absolutely demolished her confidence,' I told him. 'She has been positive from the very beginning and you have annihilated that in one tiny bombshell of a sentence. I cannot bear to see all her hard work go to waste. You have to do something.' I explained to him in detail how she had got by, that I wasn't being the over-protective mother, that this had been her survival strategy and how *she* had wanted it to be. She had always said, 'Just tell me what I have to do.' Nothing else. Some leading specialists might be too arrogant and proud to back down or apologize, but not Professor Tattershall. At once he replied, 'I'm sorry. Leave it to me. I'll rebuild her confidence, I promise.'

I left, still feeling shaky and unsure of how he was going to do that. I fetched Caron some lunch and returned to the treat-ment room. A little while later Professor Tattershall bounced into the room with a bundle of X-rays clutched to his chest and knelt in front of her. 'Right,' he said. 'I've now had a good look at the actual X-rays rather than on the computer, and they're not nearly as bad as I thought. This is where you've had radio-therapy, which has responded really well . . .' and on he went. He showed her all the good bits in her spine – 'See how clean that bit is, how strong that bit is . . .' Of course, the average person can't read an X-ray so Caron didn't know what she was looking at but, as is often the case, people see what they see. He was smiling, ebullient again, oozing with confidence. Afterwards he said, 'Now, there are a couple of suspect areas in the lumbar spine and that's what we're going to concentrate on. What's being put into your arm right now will deal with that.'

I watched, fascinated, the transformation that took place before my eyes. Suddenly Caron straightened up, a victorious smile returned to her face, the fear went out of her eyes. It was wonderful to see and I was filled with gratitude for Professor Tattershall. But, of course, I knew the truth, so deep down I remained terrified. The prognosis rang loud and long in my ears as I continued to smile at my rejuvenated child. I don't think she ever suspected I had had a word with him. Of course, you could hear questions rummaging around in her mind, but she took his re-evaluation at face value, and her positive outlook returned.

I must make it clear that she was not being deprived of anything: the treatment was the same, whether it was for six suspect areas or two. All we were depriving her of was negativity. Everyone is different, and others may not agree with Caron's methods. Or with mine, for that matter, doorstepping the doctor and telling him how to do his job. And maybe a small part of me would agree, but at that moment I would have done anything to protect her. People have a right to know, if they want to, but why not live whatever time you have left in a positive fashion, stronger for it? After all, miracles do happen: drugs change, new ones come on to the market. Isn't that the joy of medicine in the twenty-first century? Look at the HIV virus: people with it live long, full lives now, when they would have been written off twenty years ago. So, you can never afford to give up. Buddhist monks say you should never take away anyone's hope of life. You pray and stay positive because, until the very end, there is still a chance of life. While there is life in your body, there is hope. Who in this world has the right to take away your hope, and therefore your chance of life? No one. And after all, miracles do happen.

We returned to Taylor's where Caron would digest this new information. She was shaken. Not because of what Professor Tattershall had said and then unsaid, but because the cancer had not left her body as she had hoped and prayed it would. She realized that the doctors were not going for cure: they were going for management. And if that was the case we would back it up in whatever way we could. I rang Jan de Vries from Australia to get advice about bone-strengthening treatment and Caron quickly found other new treatments to help ease the pain and disappointment.

She started a water treatment with a wonderful woman called Mukti, which took place in a pool in Mukti's garden. The water was exactly body temperature, so you didn't know where your body ended and the water began. When Caron's back was bad, the sensation of floating was incredibly soothing for her. Mukti held her in the water so lightly that she felt as if only her own buoyancy was keeping her up, and she had total confidence in it. Then Mukti would swish Caron around in certain movements, sometimes dunking her under, sometimes letting her float. My fear of water kept me on dry land, but Stephen tried it and loved it. When Paul eventually made it to Australia, he did it too and it had the most surprisingly profound effect on him. Caron, though, loved it most: it helped her leave behind the pain and worry and return to a more carefree time of mobility:

Later in life, when I became immobilized for several months, I started water therapy, and after a few sessions the therapist remarked, 'You're always walking, walking, walking. It's what your body wants to do.' And so I was, eyes closed, floating in a spa pool in Australia, my mind and heart back in the North of Ireland, dodging the bull, sighting foxes and coming across great swaths of primroses. Banks of them would appear in the spring and they were always what I picked for my mum on Mother's Day. I still get them for her, but they're not the same as those wild Irish bursts of pale yellow, freshly picked on one of my long walks and lovingly given . . .

She also found Satya, who came to the house to massage her in a way that was tailored to her needs. Satya knew she must not touch Caron's back and instead concentrated on her limbs and other areas. Sometimes when Caron was in pain, she'd come in the evening and work on her until she drifted off to sleep. Caron also had a private GP because, of course, she wasn't eligible for treatment on the Australian national health system. The GP's name was Albert Salmona: he was very attentive and would come to the house to give her booster vitamin C shots, administer the monthly infusion of the nerve treatment Pamidronate, which Professor Tattershall had started that day in February, and the injections of biphosphonates. On top of this Caron was taking what is now being lauded as a new wonder drug, one milligram of Arimidex daily on top of the Zoladex she was already having. She loved being able to have all that treatment at home and not having to go the hospital route.

Meanwhile, Russ continued to foot the hefty bill for the treatments and to shoulder the responsibilities. Not to mention forking out for all the complementary therapies. Mukti, Mukti's boyfriend, who also became one of Caron's therapists, Satya, Neil, Denise – friends or not, everyone was on the payroll. We thought she drove herself mad doing too many treatments and I would say to her, 'Why don't you just do one a day?' Sometimes she was doing two or three. But she loved it and now, more than ever, she needed to feel that she was doing something to help herself, and Russ was not prepared to take that away from her. Often she'd do acupuncture in the morning, after which you should go home, relax and do nothing. But Caron would go on to have a colonic in the afternoon or reflexology. Her day, and ours when we visited, was planned around buying and preparing the right food, resting and those treatments. It was a full-time job, and she went at it with complete commitment. But the back pain would not ease. In fact, it was getting worse, and Caron was getting scared all over again.

A couple of other things happened around that time, which added to her fear. Matthew Manning, the healer Caron had seen so often in England, lost his wife to cancer. Caron was stunned and confused. How could a healer have been unable to heal his wife? She had also believed that Brandon had cured herself of cancer. The book describes how a tumour the size of a baseball had manifested itself in Brandon's stomach; she had shrunk it, then made it disappear through diet and self-healing. But Caron had understood that tumour to have been malignant. When she discovered that the presence of cancerous cells had neither been proved nor disproved, Caron was shaken. The two women remained firm friends, and Brandon was at Caron's funeral, but Caron's belief systems were rocked for a while. Then Linda McCartney a woman who appeared to be on the same path that Caron had chosen, Caron's shining example, died. Caron was devastated. I am sure Professor Tattershall's first, unchecked words kept returning to her mind. She had been planning to return home that April, but the back pain was too temperamental and she couldn't face the flight. It wasn't going to be the joyous return she'd imagined, where she could miraculously pick up where she'd left off. Her friends knew it wasn't a good sign that she had decided not to come. It was one of the few times that her voice belied her words. Uncertainty had crept back in.

Caron was now living constantly with pain. She had sleepless nights. She used hot-water bottles to ease her back. She had a special reclining chair to watch TV. She took more pain medication. Normally she lived in her Ugg boots, but she got fed up with them because they were too hot. I started to notice little things. In the garden, by the school gates, Caron would lean against a tree. The other mothers didn't. I bought her some shoes that gave her feet better support, but they didn't seem to bring her the relief she wanted. Her diet changed a bit then, and she started eating some chicken. I think she realized she was going to need some extra strength, but her strength continued to deteriorate. She was worried about the strength in her legs: her reflexes seemed to be getting weaker while the pain got stronger. Sometimes she used a walking cane for extra support. I will never forget the boys' first day back at school after the Easter holidays: all the parents were at the school gate and there

was Caron with her stick. She heard Gabriel telling everyone
that his mum had a bad back and that she didn't always use one.
Which was true, but she felt terrible that her sons were so aware
of the one thing she had tried to protect them from for so many
years. If you had said to me that my beautiful girl would be
using a walking-stick at forty, I'd have been broken-hearted,
never mind the thought of what it meant and the real reason.
The cancer was on its inexorable march through her body. The
unimaginable was happening.

The boys noticed other things. They would say, 'When you
have this treatment will you be able to ride your bicycle again?'
to which Caron would bravely respond, 'I may not be able to
ride my bike or skate, but I can read with you, draw with you
and paint with you.' She did all of those things. She used what
she could do to compensate as her mobility got worse. Of course
I found that very sad: she should have been riding her bike,
prancing about in the waves – just walking, damn it, as she used
to. Sometimes she would say that her left leg was cold, or felt
weak, or that she didn't have the same sensation in it as she had
in the other. Sometimes she would say, 'I can't feel my feet.'
Sometimes she would just look at me and say, 'It's scary.' And,
my God, it was. It was scary for all of us who were watching.

It was at about that time that she and Russ started talking
about death, although always in an indirect way. They were
organic conversations that just happened. Were they conscious
or unconscious? We will never know. They were playing with
both sides of the coin: remaining positive while accepting the
inevitable. It was a trick of the mind. Sleight of hand. Caron
would put a hypothetical question to Russ: would you prefer
to be buried or cremated? Russ would reply, then turn the
question round and, in doing so, have an answer stored away
for another, unimaginable, time.

Another sleight of hand that Caron played began around that
time too. She started a process with Russ that was akin to passing

over a baton in a relay race. She'd remind him that Gabriel didn't like a certain type of food or preferred one thing to another. She asked Russ to read to them if she was too tired. Russ is not a big reader, and he usually resisted, but he knew what she was doing. She was reminding him to read to the boys after she was gone, because she loved reading and it was such an integral part of her. None of this was dramatic and it didn't happen overnight, but they were little pointers to her husband about the boys. At the time Russ thought it was subconscious but, looking back, he thinks now that it probably wasn't. She just dropped them in bit by bit, over time, which implies to him that she had a fairly good insight into what was going on. Although she never admitted it, even to him. Like the conversations about death, it always remained in the abstract. She never said, 'I'm dying . . .' She never even made a will. But inside there was turmoil. And, just as it reached overwhelming proportions, Caron's prayers were answered.

Not having been in touch with my body for trying to work out what it needed was like being told to find a small village in India without a map. For the sort of mind I have I'd need the body of Arnold Schwartzenegger to keep up. My own voice and guidance seems very quiet sometimes, lost as it is in the whirl of my brain trying to work out what to do. And then something happened, which made me realize that I didn't need to worry, that all I had to do was ask for the help, and trust that it would come. Pray, and know that the prayer is simultaneously answered.

My girlfriend Mel was organizing some Tibetan monks to come to Byron to chant. On the night that the performance was happening I wasn't feeling very well, my back was aching, it was wet and cold, and I decided to stay at home with the boys. For once I listened to myself, and Russ went down to help and ended up being the most fabulous doorman.

At the end of the night he was telling Mel – the woman who organizes the monks – that I would have loved to hear them, but couldn't make it. 'Does she really want to hear them?' asked Mel, in her no-nonsense Belfast accent. 'Well if she can't come to us, we'll go to her.' The head monk, Sonham Dorje, is a healer, she explained. 'We'll go and see her tomorrow.'

And that was how on a wet Tuesday night in June I ended up with four Gyuto Tibetan monks resplendent in their crimson robes, cross-legged in our sitting room. Here we are, drinking tea and eating chocolate Tim Tams. It's quite a normal scene, really, except these are Tibetan monks, for heaven's sake.

There are moments in your life when you look at what is taking place around you and know that it has had nothing to do with you. That some higher power is weaving miracles around you. That a fervently made prayer has been answered.

It is said in India that to see a Gyuto monk is a blessing – but to hear one is transformational. When they have finished their tea the monks offer to chant for me. They are such joyful beings and exude an air of peace. It is a deep, resonant, vibration, which reverberates throughout your body.

I have no idea what they're saying, what any of it means, all I do know is that these men, who come from a completely other existence on the other side of the world, are there chanting and praying for me out of pure love. There is no other motivation. It is what they do. And it doesn't matter that we met ten minutes ago. They want only the best for me. This is love. Purely and simply . . .

Of everything Caron discovered in Australia, the monks were the most incredible. As she said, it was as if they were sent by God to help her in her darkest hour. Pain is physically debilitating, of course, but it is mentally debilitating too. It is depressing. It is a huge contributing factor in suicide, because living with daily pain is near impossible. I have no doubt that Caron was a tormented soul in the early hours of the morning when sleep could not give her the respite she so badly needed. And I am sure that Russ saw what it was doing to her. It comes as no surprise, then, that he orchestrated the visit from the monks and, having seen what an immediate and wonderful effect it had on his wife, was soon planning a return trip.

On one occasion they were all in the garden, when the Rinpoche, a senior leader, asked Caron if she would like to have some time with him alone. They went into the bedroom together. There, he told her through an interpreter that although he had dedicated his life to worship and had been a spiritual man his entire life, he, too, had been plagued with illnesses since childhood. 'You have not been singled out,' he said, and as if by magic, the guilt, the shame, the need to search left her. It was a monumental turning-point. Suddenly, everything fell into place. *She had not been singled out.* Neither had he – nor the Pope, for that matter. She hadn't done this to herself.

Grief breaks our hearts wide open and in the midst of our despair there is often a sense of exhilaration somehow bursting through the veil of life. Droplets of blistering clarity illuminate before you. Like you've been given the map that you have searched for your whole life. Suddenly bits of the picture make sense and you see straight through to the truth in a way that would otherwise have taken years . . .

I realise today the relief of the Rinpoche saying, 'You have not been singled out – you have not brought this on yourself.'

I have felt so different. In the past I always felt as if there was something wrong with me which I could not let anyone else see. Could not let anyone else in on, so that I could know how to be 'OK/fine'. God, how I hate that now. It's been so fantastic since my chat with the Rinpoche. Get a new mindset – he is right. Yes I have difficulties at the moment, so has he, with his health. He is not a bad person – he is next to the Dalai Lama.

Look at all the love around you, he said – you are a good person. We cannot ever know the natural reasons why things happen – it is a fruitless task to seek.

Accept these difficulties are a part of life at the moment – be grateful for the help from all your family and friends.

Her faith had returned. And, with it, hope.

19. A Happier Girl

When I came home I would tell the family what was going on. In fact, throughout the whole thing I was the mouthpiece. From that time on, it was sometimes difficult to talk to Caron because when she was in pain she didn't want to yack on the phone. Also, her days were our nights so it was difficult to get quality chat. I didn't mind pacing the corridor until it was time to call, but I didn't expect Paul or Michael to do so. Since I was passing on the messages, they didn't have to. Sometimes I'm sure they couldn't face it. Even Michael admits that he would purposely space his calls: it was too difficult to remain the buoyant brother if he spoke to her too often, especially after her back got bad. He needed time to gather stories and gossip, so that what he had started in the Lister Hospital during chemotherapy could continue. Also, she didn't want small talk – to repeat what she had already told me. I think Paul had found the distance and the situation hardest to overcome. But there was always the hope that Russ and Caron would suddenly announce they were coming home.

Paul met Russ in London every six months or so for a catch-up, and heard from him about the highs and lows. Sometimes Russ would say, 'You've really got to come,' then a week later she'd be better and the panic had subsided. But once he said to Paul, 'You really need to go.' It wasn't because Caron was in a particularly bad way but because too much was being left unsaid between them, and Russ knew that Caron was living beyond her borrowed time. But Paul in a way was in denial about going to see her. Why was Caron so different from all the other people with breast cancer who had to go to work, maintain

normality, stay with their family? Why was she allowed to run
away to Australia, live in a beautiful house and be allowed to go
off on any whim, anywhere, irrespective of what others thought
or felt? Paul knew how devastated we all were when she left;
he also knew we were all doing everything we could to support
her. Many of the treatments and therapy sessions she did threw
up more questions about our past and our relationship. There
continued to be ups and downs; the questioning never stopped,
I think that probably bothered him, because he knew how
desperate I was to make her happy. My relationship with Russ
had got a bit strained too: I wanted him to stop paying the bills,
end the adventure and bring her home. Now that we knew the
cancer had moved to Caron's bones, we all felt that Byron Bay
was no longer offering any benefits. We didn't know why Caron
was staying, why she was continuing to try to self-heal when it
clearly wasn't working. We wanted her to come home and have
more closely supervised treatment. I was battling about how
much time I should or could stay in Australia, knowing what I
knew. Caron's move had affected Paul, Michael and me con-
siderably. She was in the middle of the illness and we had every
sympathy with her situation, but this was also happening to all
of us. Hurting all of us.

June 2003

Hi Darlin',
Here I am back in Bangalow keeping a table for us! Not long now
(hurray).

I've just had a physio session. She thinks I'm doing really well and
that you and Stevie would be welcome to join the yoga class – though
I think you're probably a *bit* more flexible – still, you never know!

It is cold (I may need the thermal long-johns) but sunny – the boys
are at home with Sam and Rosie having a sausage cook-in outside,
with marshmallows for after – completely blissed out. Charlie got

new boots and is out traipsing round at 7 a.m. Gabe thinks if he could get a pair he'd be twins with Charlie and Sam but they're too big – he's very sad!

Enclosed are a few of the monk pictures and I thought you might like a couple of the 'butter lamps' from the ceremony. We put tea lights in them and I lit 100 every day to increase my lifespan. The summerhouse seems very empty without them all, though I think they're dropping by in few weeks.

We said goodbye to the Merc last night, my gorgeous fortieth birthday present which isn't practical any more. We went for a final drive into Byron Bay to buy an ice-cream. The boys say they're going to search for the car when they're older and buy her back!

Russ's office is nearly done and we're busy planning a potential radio show! – 'The Hookey Spookey Show', full of Byron's more colourful characters.

Apart from that, all else is normal. I'm gaining more strength all the time, tho' still having to 'take it easy'; which I don't always remember. It's great to be able to drive again – my freedom back.

Really looking forward to seeing you both – and Paul.

All our love and kisses,

Caron, Russ, Charlie and Gabriel xx

Paul hid his anxieties and denial. Mentally it was safer to assume that, like his partner's sister, Caron would beat it. Now other people were saying to him, not just us, 'Your sister is really ill.' He didn't want to hear it. He didn't want to have to fly to Australia. He would say, 'No, she's been here before. She has this habit of getting back on her feet. She will come home.' But finally Russ persuaded him to go. And thank God he did. It was only a ten-day trip, but in many ways brother and sister lived a lifetime together during those eye-opening days.

It was July, and Paul was at Heathrow, checking in, when

the ground stewardess informed him his visa wasn't in his pass-
port. He hadn't even considered that he might need one. His
first thought was, Great, I don't have to go. He admits that if
he could have got out of it he would have. He was afraid of
what he was going to see. Recently his and Caron's sporadic
conversations had been difficult and strained. But the stewardess
smiled brightly and told him to go to the visa desk: he could get
one there and then.

Reluctantly, he boarded the plane dreading what he would
find when he arrived. He had heard the stories about Caron
being bedridden for days, about Caron walking on sticks, getting
a frame. He'd seen photos of when she wasn't looking well so
when he walked into her kitchen he was terrified, nervous
and edgy.

Caron looked at him and smiled. She said, 'You look exactly
the same as when I saw you two years ago.' Paul couldn't believe
it: the same applied to her! She looked fantastic. She wasn't any
different. It turned out that his visit corresponded with one of
those extraordinary times when Caron appeared once again to
defy logic and medicine. Not only was she up and about, she
was driving. She had organized a range of therapies for Paul to
try and, taking himself by surprise, he found he enjoyed them.
He had read an article on the plane that said, 'If you've never
been to Byron Bay you might find a connection with people
you don't experience elsewhere, and you'll probably notice that
people look you in the eye all the time and really talk to you.'
On his very first day Paul realized that people were indeed
looking him full in the eye, and it made him really self-conscious.
But he soon relaxed and entered into the spirit of the place.

He noticed how much Caron and Russ had changed. They
were relaxed. Calm. Peaceful. Happy. Paul and Caron spent
many hours together, chatting, and he was overcome by what
an incredibly good place she was in. The Caron he remembers
from that visit was the Caron who walked the dogs on the

beach, laughed and cooked pancakes for the boys. He never even saw the frame. Or the cane.

He did things he would never have done at home: he had his cards read, his crystal energy rebalanced. He went over there thinking he was going to drink some beer and chill out on the beach with Russ, but it had turned into an enlightening experience. He found himself drawn to a lot of the therapies – even Denise the pooh fairy. I was stunned to hear that he'd gone to the purple gazebo in the forest, but he found it a really good experience. I think Denise grasped that it wasn't going to go as far as letting go of his dad, but with Paul being so anti that sort of thing normally, it seemed remarkable to me that he could make the connection between physical and spiritual cleansing. But that's Byron Bay for you. As Paul says, it's easy to dial into it. There was the pooh fairy, singing to Paul and rebalancing his chakras while she stuck a tube up his bottom, and all before breakfast. He thought happily, If only people could see me now.

And then, most surprising of all, Paul did water therapy – this for a man who'd nearly drowned when he was a boy and eyed a deep bath with suspicion. But Caron thought it would be good for him to deal with the issue of water and swimming, so off they went. He had never met Mukti before, of course, and was completely thrown when she changed into her swimsuit in front of him. Like Caron, Paul is a bit of a prude. He didn't know where to look, started mumbling in a Hugh Grant, very British sort of way and proceeded to pull up his shorts under his towel. Then she went for a pee outside, in full view, and he nearly ran.

But when he got into the pool, things changed. She cradled him and moved him around in the water in smooth movements. He found himself in the foetal position, being swayed around by a woman he'd never met before and not wanting the treatment to end. She started to manipulate him, press on his chest and slowly change his heartbeat. He started to take up the rhythm of her palm: at first his heart was racing, but hers was slow and steady, and eventually his matched it. She whispered into his ear, seductive but reassuring. His feet started splashing vigorously in the water. Part of the therapy is about releasing withheld tension and anxiety, trauma. His feet had kept running and she said, 'Where are you going? Where are you running to?' She asked Paul the same question and he couldn't answer, but he knows that when he's stressed he dreams about running. Now when work gets too much, or he is upset by something, he puts on his trainers and runs. It gives him the release he needs to remain on an even keel. After an hour and a half of the therapy he was exhausted.

But he went back for more and in the end did three sessions. After the final treatment Mukti took a man who couldn't swim and was terrified of water right under. She moved him round quite quickly, up and down like a dolphin, and by the end he was under the water for twenty seconds at a time. Before that there was no way he could have done it. Eyes open, nose clamped, listening to wonderful whale music, suspended – like a fish or a foetus, he wasn't sure. He loved it. Can you imagine how Caron must have felt? Byron had worked its magic on the most discerning of souls: he was buoyant. Caron loved helping others, and the buoyancy would have rubbed off on her. She also loved to witness others' scepticism subside. No one was more sceptical than Paul. But what a conversion!

He did a lot in those ten days that he would never have done before. It was life-changing, a completely positive experience. Only a couple of things happened to remind him of why he was there. Although Caron looked really well in comparison to how she'd seemed in the pictures he'd seen, Paul became conscious when they went to the beach that people were looking at her. By then her back was more arched than it should have been. She'd occasionally take his arm for balance and he'd remember that now Caron was different from other people.

One evening she asked to borrow a book he had bought for the long plane journey home. She said, 'Don't worry, I'll give it back to you.' She did. The next morning. She'd read it from cover to cover. It wasn't until then that he realized how much pain she was in. She was unable to sleep because of it, so lay awake, reading the hours away. But she never went on about it, so it was easy to forget. She referred to death but Paul, now more than ever, wouldn't allow himself to go there. Although he had gone expecting to help her, she had helped him. She had shared Byron Bay with him, and passed on that inner knowledge to him, that feeling of connection. There was not one wasted moment: they did not stop for ten days.

I wouldn't describe Paul as New Age as a result, but he is much more connected to good and negative energy. People who are bitter, who cannot communicate and are full of negative energy often live less. He tries to avoid such people. If you are positive and your cup is half full, life *is* better. I'm not saying these things are carcinogenic but people can make themselves ill through worry. Like Michael, Paul will pack up and go home now: he won't stay at the office until ten, he'll go home and hug his kids. They are both more acutely aware of their well-being and health.

Paul has just left – he was here for a week and it was so good to see him. You do forget how much fun you can have with people – particularly with family – regaling all the stories down the years, etc.

I feel we've been too serious at times and we just need to laugh and have a good time. I'm sorry Paul has gone home – special days, special times to treasure.

Like the rest of us, back in London Paul hadn't been able to understand what Caron was doing, but after he'd been to Australia, it all made sense. He appreciated why it was so important for her to be there, understood why it worked for her, and with understanding came forgiveness. He no longer felt angry about what it was doing to the rest of us. Byron Bay was where she needed to be, and that was that. He believes that if Russ had put his foot down and said, 'We have to come home,' Caron would have died. He thinks her tenacity and determination won her those extra years, but she needed to be somewhere that gave her the courage to be strong. Before he had thought, What does it matter if people see her at the Lister Hospital? but he had seen now for himself the release she got when she was away from the family connection, television and the snappers. In the end, Paul thinks, her judgement was right: she had been right to go and right to stay. He tells anyone who will listen that Byron Bay is a place everyone should experience once and see what it has to offer. Although it is possible to go there and just surf, soak up the sun and have a really good holiday.

Paul saw Caron at the best she had been all year. I was not so lucky. By the time I got back Caron was on her little frame for support.

Just when I thought it had all turned round, it completely blew apart again, shattering all my ideas and beliefs about healing and what exactly was going on in the most incredible way.

Having struggled with my back for much of the year and finally got to a point where it seemed to be getting strong again, on Charlie's birthday I moved back on a day-bed and felt something give way. I thought I had just pulled a muscle but about a week later it started to really hurt. I was persuaded to have an X-ray, to eliminate stuff rather than prove it, and discovered I'd fractured my sternum and that several ribs weren't looking too healthy. This all gave me a bit of a shock and obviously hit my system a bit. Soon afterwards I started to feel not quite as steady on my feet.

I don't quite know what is going on. Every day my walking seems to become worse. Sometimes I need to hang on to Russ's arm walking down the lawn. I can no longer manage the steps at the front door. When I close my eyes in the shower I can feel myself start to wobble. My mum thinks I've just lost my confidence; my physiotherapist suggests strengthening my thigh muscles. Russ looks worried. It isn't until my GP bangs my knees with his small rubber hammer to test the nerve responses and suggests an MRI scan that we really discover what's going on.

It turns out the cancer has grown on a couple of spots on my spine and is now pressing on the spinal cord, making my balance and walking very unsteady. I'll need some radiotherapy treatment to free the nerves and I need it soon, before any more damage is done. Having had little medical intervention in the last two years I discover how closed I am to the whole notion of Western medicine, though at this precise moment I am very grateful that at least something can be done.

Everyone seems very worried about the possibility of me falling over and damaging my spine or breaking something so I go from staggering around the house as best I can to practically being wrapped in cotton wool . . .

This was the only time she vocalized her fear to me. When the doctor had said, 'The wrong move could cause problems,' she was terrified. The growths were so close to the nervous system that there was a chance she could become paralysed. She said to me, 'If I'm relegated to a wheelchair I couldn't stand it.' Caron was adamant: she could not, would not, live her life in a wheelchair. She'd put up with so much else but, looking back, I don't think it was really the wheelchair that frightened her so. I think it was the proverbial straw that broke the camel's back. It was all getting too much.

So, when it was confirmed that Caron needed radiotherapy on her spine, she accepted the situation more readily than we had expected: she was petrified of doing some permanent damage to her spine if the pressure wasn't lifted off her spinal cord.

The exploration was carried out at the John Flynn Hospital further up the east coast towards Brisbane. As hospitals go, it was a pleasant one, and again Russ made sure Caron was in a light, airy, room with a view. It was decided that she would be treated as an inpatient and probably go home at the weekend. Treatment began on 10 September. Stephen and I had been due to fly back to the UK, but decided to stay for as long as the radiotherapy lasted. We all took it in turns to be with Caron. The hospital was only half an hour from Byron Bay and we alternated shifts between school runs and the hospital. It seems ironic, but now, when I look back on all those hospital stays, I find that they left me with some wonderful, everlasting memories. One-to-one time during which Caron and I had our deepest conversations about life, youth, love, marriage, children, happiness, strife, illness – but, most of all, love. I remember the doctor saying how vital it was that Caron stayed in one place under supervision. He said that if we got her through the first three days she should do well. We were frozen in time, puzzled, frightened, trying to work out what he was really saying. Apparently radiotherapy can go one of two ways during those first crucial seventy-two hours. Well, she survived them and we all began to think she was invincible.

On the fourth day I took her out into the garden for tea. She was so looking forward to going home. I will never forget her face that day: she was smiling broadly. A much happier girl out in the sunshine and fresh air, and determined to remain an outpatient from then on. Russ made a cocoon of eiderdowns on the front seat of the car and that was how we travelled from Monday to Friday during the following two weeks until her treatment was finished. The cortisone tablets she was given to bolster her system made Caron a little fatter in the face. I'm surprised she didn't get fat everywhere because they also gave her a ferocious appetite. I had to make her a huge breakfast of buckwheat pancakes, scrambled eggs, smoked salmon, and afterwards she might have some of her favourite sheep's cheese with onion and fig marmalade. A curious combination, but food had become an obsession with her. We would while away the mornings by the pool, eating, chatting, making tea, more chats, another pancake or two, more tea, more chats. They were precious times, never to be forgotten.

I remember when Charlie was in the choir at school and Caron had very little strength. She was not well, but Charlie really wanted her to attend a concert he was singing in. Bless her, she made such an effort to get up the steps to go into that room. It upset me because people stared at her. The tumours on her spine were causing problems with her digestive system too: her tummy was distended, and she often swelled up. I will never forget walking into our favourite jewellery shop, Caron on her cane, and the owner asked Caron when the baby was due . . . You could have cut the atmosphere with a machete. I wanted to slap the woman, and we left without buying anything.

A few days later I made some excuse to leave the house and went back to the shop. I told the woman what I thought of her insensitivity since she was perfectly aware that Caron wasn't well. It was one of the worst trips. Sometimes when we went, we had the impression that things had been exaggerated, and then, like Paul, because Caron was so well, we were lulled into a false sense of security. This time it was as if she'd aged twenty years. I couldn't believe that Paul's wonderful holiday photos had been taken only two months earlier. Now I had to readjust everything to take in the sight of my daughter depending on a cane and sometimes a frame for extra support. In the end I rang Michael. I really wanted him to come over.

Michael asked, 'Why? What's changed? Be straight with me. Is she really bad?'

It was a fair question. We'd been at these desperate points before to varying degrees over the previous six years. Michael was going to Australia at Christmas anyway and it was September now: could it really not wait? I called back the next day. I was desperate, confused and scared. Michael, bless him, didn't need to be asked a third time: he walked out of the office, went home, packed and got a taxi straight to the airport. Only Stephen and I knew he was coming: we didn't tell Caron. I was so excited that I went to the airport far too early, needed to go to the loo but didn't want to miss him. When he finally came out of Immigration I had fallen asleep on the plastic table in the café. Michael remembers me looking up with a packet of sugar stuck to my cheek, seeing him and my face flooding with relief.

It was about three in the morning when we got to Taylors. Michael slept in the summerhouse. By six fifteen he was awake again, too excited to stay in bed so he snuck round the house commando-style, got to the playroom and found Charlie, who was overjoyed to see his uncle and ran into his arms. What with me at the airport and Charlie now, Michael knew he'd done the right thing in coming. 'Don't tell Mummy,' he whispered. They played until about seven, when he couldn't wait any longer. He made Caron green tea in her favourite Japanese tea-set, then walked to her bedroom door. He stopped outside, suddenly not so certain. Caron was intensely private: he didn't know whether to walk in or not. But he did. He walked in, shook his sister, said, 'Morning, darling.' Caron opened her eyes, a look of utter disbelief on her face, and said, 'What the fuck are you doing here?' Then she burst into tears. They both did.

Later she asked Michael in private if he'd come over because he thought she was going to kick the bucket. She was having another course of radiotherapy at the time, so Michael said quickly, 'Don't be silly. We're a close family and if anyone else was in hospital I'd be there.' She bought it, or allowed herself to buy it, and that was fine. Secretly, though, Michael, like me, was terrified. Caron rallied, as she did with any visit from the family. Her spirits rose, and she said later that if her brother, who was supposed to be on the other side of the world, could walk into her room carrying a tray of tea, anything was possible. It was all she needed to give her the courage to hope again.

Michael stayed two weeks, met the monks and saw for himself what joy they gave her. He supported me, supporting Russ, supporting her. He took over driving Caron to see Denise and the new reflexologist she'd found. Together, we would send the boys off to school with a wave, then help Caron back on to her day-bed. Moving was painful, awkward and difficult – she would swear blue murder as she lowered herself down – but once she was settled, the old Caron would return. Honestly, she was an inspiration to us all. Russ was under extreme pressure. Because Caron was so private, he was the only one allowed to care for her on an intimate basis. We tried to prop up everything else. People are trained to be carers, and now I know why. It is an incredibly difficult job. You walk a fine line between assisting and smothering. Caron was independent and hated being smothered. But we were all so terrified that those tumours would strike her down still further. She must have sensed our fear. When you see someone so vibrant, so beautiful, cut down like that and lose power, you can't hide how you feel.

We celebrated Caron's birthday early, on 4 October, the last day of Michael's holiday. She gave him a leaving present of a blessed monk's blanket for him to wrap himself in to feel protected. She had a matching one. Michael now has them both and wraps himself in Caron's often. She rallied for the day, but he left for the airport unsure of what the future held. He knew he was going back at Christmas for three weeks and tried in vain not to think beyond that.

The radiotherapy worked well and the pressure was off her spine, but her mobility did not improve as much as we had hoped it would. She and I went back to the man who had discovered that the cancer had gone to her bones, Professor Tattershall. He had not forgotten my words to him a year earlier, and even now, with her movement so questionable, he found a way to put a positive spin on some frankly disturbing results. We were driving home from the airport when he called with them: 'Thank God,' he said. 'I was really worried you might have holes in your bones, and I was going to have to put pins right down your legs to strengthen them but the good news is

I don't.' Immediately she was relieved. She hadn't even considered pins in her legs, but once he'd said it, she felt she was better off than she'd thought. It was cleverly done. He said, 'There is a little spot of worry, but we'll give it an extra boost,' and added that she'd responded well before to that treatment so she would again. She was made up: as always she hung on to the good news. There were a few areas in her legs that looked suspicious, but they were not as bad as he had thought they might be.

Russ continued to facilitate the monks' visits. When they came to visit, they stayed at Taylors. Sometimes they would chant right there in Caron's summerhouse. She didn't become a Buddhist, but they gave her so much joy, light and energy through the deep simplicity of unconditional love. They have nothing and didn't want anything from Caron. She benefited so much from their visits: she realized that she could find everything she'd ever been searching for in herself, which gave her the spiritual happiness and inner peace that she so needed at that time. Russ did an amazing thing to organize the monks. If there was any comfort to come out of this at all, it is that, at the end of her battle, she was spiritually in the right place. Completely. So, in the end, my resentment of Australia dissipated. I have to thank Byron Bay, where once I had detested it. She wouldn't have found that peace in the UK. Here, she would have continued to search and blame until the end. As Johnny has said, that last Christmas when her mobility had all but left her, she was still a joy to be with, still a laugh. The monks had taught her she had had that strength inside her all along, and Russ had brought them to her. It's just one more decision I will always remember.

Russ may have handed her wings but Byron Bay gave her the power to soar. It had been an incredible adventure, although unknown to us, it was coming to a close. Mountain air was calling: a new phase was beginning.

20. Hot Box

Those '*couple of spots on my spine*' that Caron referred to in her writing were in fact T2, T6, T7, T10, T11, T12 and L2. At T2 not only was there evidence of 'metastatic' disease (cancer), but she had a crush fracture at that point in her thoracic spine as well. Same again at T6 and T7, which had resulted in wedge deformities. At T10 there was severe cord compression, as at T11 and T12, although to a lesser degree. The last time, she had ten treatments of radiotherapy which concentrated on the T7–T9 area. As her medical records note, this 'preserved some motor functions in her legs, allowing her to stand and walk short distances'. The letter from the oncologist goes on to say: 'hopefully this will continue to improve as the treatment takes effect and with the help of her supportive family'. At this point the single blood test that she agreed to have showed an increase in her tumour markers, leading the oncologist to conclude that the hormone therapy she was on (Arimidex, Zoladex and Pamidronate) was no longer effective. There was more to worry about than just '*a couple of spots*', and it was getting worse.

From that point to the end, Caron had to dig deeper than ever before to find the strength to fight the pain. But she appeared to have that strength. Was it the monks who had given it to her? Or had they given her the key to find it in herself? I don't know. As scary as the loss of strength in her legs was, she also eased up on herself. For the six years Caron had been dealing with breast cancer, her concern had been whether it would move to her neck or lymphatic system. The fact that the cancer was now travelling through her bones at what seemed an alarming rate was something else. On that day back in July when Caron had eased herself up on one elbow from her day-bed and her sternum cracked, she knew she had entered another stage.

Russ and Caron started looking around for another crutch. Russ spent hours on the Internet searching the multitude of cancer-related websites and found something that looked promising: hypothermia, though hot rather than cold. The basic concept is that you heat your body up to 40°C and the heat kills all the weak cancer cells. They had been getting good results at various clinics around the world. Russ and Caron found a place in Switzerland which seemed to be the most progressive and boasted some good results. Frankly, there was not a lot to lose.

As one crutch was kicked away, Russ would make sure that another was swiftly found to replace it. The Paracelsius Clinic was that next crutch. They phoned me immediately to see if I could book her in. My friend Merrill Thomas, who speaks good French and German, made the necessary call and all was set.

With all the treatments Caron had tried, right from the beginning when she managed to get herself an appointment with Brandon Bays, or later with the body electronics or the sound healing in the rainforest, it was the fact that she was doing *something* to help herself that gave her the confidence to believe that everything was going to be all right. Latterly, getting to the appointment or meeting a new practitioner was almost always a letdown because things never worked out as they were supposed to. Russ thinks that, towards the end, he was searching the Internet for the 'next thing' because that would give them something to pin their hopes on during those dark hours when things started to look hopeless.

The first trip to Switzerland was planned late in the autumn of 2003. When I arrived at the clinic, it was with a mixture of excitement and trepidation. None of us had any experience of this place or knew anyone who'd been treated there. I needn't have worried. Typical of the Swiss, it was a pristine building over three floors, with doctors, nurses, practitioners and treatment rooms everywhere. They offered outpatient treatment by doctors and dentists trained in orthodox medicine, but combined with a very individual, holistic approach. At long last, we had found a place that straddled both worlds. They treated the person behind the illness.

I made my way into the clinic and discovered that Caron had already been through the registration process and was in the café having a typically healthy lunch. As I walked in and spotted them in the corner, I couldn't believe that they were at last back on European soil. There they were, my gorgeous little family unit – Caron, Russ, Charlie and Gabriel. There was so much exuberance at seeing each other again, and huge anticipation of what this clinic and its practitioners might do for Caron to strengthen her body.

Russ stayed for the first few days. I went back to Kent with Charlie and Gabriel until Russ returned and took them skiing. Then back I went to the clinic in Switzerland and the routine of days full of hour-by-hour treatment. Despite her often gruelling timetable, our evenings were very special times spent in Caron's hotel room. The family had found a cosy hotel nearby in St Gallen, their temporary home from home, tucked away in the Swiss Alps. We all took it in shifts so that Caron would never be alone. So tight was the schedule that at one point my sons passed each other on the train. The departing Michael couldn't warn Paul that what he was going to find on arrival in St Gallen was a very different sister from the one he'd left behind in Byron Bay six months earlier. Unaware of the physical change in Caron, Paul walked into her room and was completely thrown by what he saw. The person propped up in bed could not be his sister. The last he'd seen of Caron was her swimming and walking on the beach, laughing and singing in the sea, playing with the children. Now there appeared to be a walking frame next to her bed. He watched in total bewilderment as she took five to ten minutes to get herself from her bed to the loo. He had never witnessed her illness in such an unforgiving way. Finally it hit home. His sister was seriously, seriously ill – could it be that what some people had been trying to tell him was true?

There were sessions all day, every day, ranging from nerve and vitamin infusions to colonics, massage, cleansing her lymphatic system and even removing amalgam fillings from her teeth. They had special equipment at the clinic to remove the amalgam without the mercury leaking into the body. Paul found the next few days very disturbing. For that first session of the ultra-high-temperature 'hot box' treatment, he helped her to the clinic and noticed that everyone was looking. Because their progress was so painfully slow, there was more time to stare. The icy steps at the front of the hotel were a nightmare. At the clinic, Caron was placed inside a type of hot foil box which was then heated to 132°F so that the whole process of allegedly killing the bad cells could begin. The first time, Caron tried to claw her way out with claustrophobia.

Eventually she calmed down and started to cope better with the heat. But she wanted the music turned off, and swore blue murder until it was. Paul couldn't bear to see her in so much pain. Not only did he now know how ill his sister was, he was beginning to realize what being a carer entailed. What it was like for Russ. This was what we had all been doing at various stages, to various degrees, and Paul was knocked sideways. He would start chatting to people in the corridor, people who looked like fitness models, who told him they had colon cancer, bone cancer or brain cancer. Everyone was there for cancer. He found himself saying 'I'm here with my sister', so that people would stop looking at him and trying to work out what was wrong. One day he felt so uncomfortable and claustrophobic that he went on a long walk in the mountains. He met an old woman carrying two buckets on a yoke and she invited him into her wooden hut for tea. They didn't speak a word of each other's language, yet he remained there quite a long time. It was a very strange experience, but what was happening down the mountain was even stranger.

When any of us went over there, we would have room service with Caron. These were, for each of us, very intimate one-to-one chats. Like being in a time capsule, where nothing outside that room mattered. This really was living in the second. Paul remembers that he would watch her eat her regimented diet and found it almost impossible to be positive. He tried to make light of things but reality had crashed in and he couldn't pretend otherwise. Occasionally there would be flashes of Caron, and they would go out for lunch or shopping, but mostly it was someone else, someone not as spirited as his sister. Sometimes he would help her to the bathroom, then she'd shout at him to leave. Paul would sit on the bed listening just in case she fell: when it got too quiet, he would knock on the door or go in, only to feel the full force of her personality as she shouted at him again to get out. It was upsetting and frustrating not knowing what to do for the best. Paul admits that at times it felt unbearable to witness and it was a kind of relief to board the train. Three days finished him off and all he could think of on the journey home was that Russ had been doing that for months and months. It is hard to imagine what he did for Caron, he'd get her anything she wanted, without question, and there must have been times when it was mentally and physically exhausting. As for Paul, when he left Switzerland he was reeling. He knew the game had changed.

Russ returned to take over the baton. He did the next two sessions. It takes an awful lot out of you to see someone you love in that amount of discomfort, but to Caron it was yet another positive action to take. Just when you thought it was all getting too much, just when you thought she would be swamped by the enormity of the battle that was raging inside her, she would wake up smiling and want to go out. Johnny Comerford managed to go over there for a couple of days. He witnessed a quantum shift in her pain and saw how much it was troubling her, but she grabbed her old friend by the arm as she always had and dragged him off to the shops. She struggled down the street. Johnny wanted her to stop and go back, but she wouldn't hear of it. She insisted on getting something for his and Cathy's children. It was a beautiful gingerbread house.

Russ believes that Switzerland gave Caron a lot of support and the confidence that she could still beat this. However, she hurt herself. As the scans revealed, she had a massive amount of bone cancer. She was being prodded and poked, turned over and moved from bed to bed, so things were being aggravated. The pain scared her.

Paul was due to go back to take over again. On his way to Heathrow, he phoned Russ to see if they needed anything. Russ was obviously as scared and panicked as Caron was. He told Paul that they were already at the airport. They were heading home. It was simple really. Things had got worse and Caron wanted to go home. Paul turned back. He never saw his sister again.

The flight back to Australia was horrendous. Caron was in a lot of pain. Russ had to cope with the two little boys, Caron in agony and an interminable flight. They arrived in Australia with one more hurdle ahead of them. They were carrying bags of medication. Australia is very strict about immigration, Russ and Caron weren't nationals and they had thirteen full-size cardboard boxes of medication, a flimsy illegible letter from the clinic in the Swiss Alps, two exhausted children pushing overburdened trolleys, and Caron in agony balanced precariously on the front of a trolley pushed by Russ. The queue was endless. Finally the Lindsay family got to the front, Russ told the guard what was going on and, bless him, he just waved them through. I think Russ could have hugged the man. With the length of the queue, he'd envisaged being stuck there for hours arguing over the hypodermic needles and vials of meds.

It took two cars to get them all home, but as soon as they pulled up to Taylors Caron's spirits lifted once more. She was back in her own house, in her own bed, and could feel the sun on her skin and let the sweet smell of the frangipani trees drift over her. The panic slowly ebbed away. Even though the pain had worsened, even though they had fled again, Russ and Caron were glad they had gone. They believed it had helped to strengthen her system and agreed to return for more treatment six months later. Caron had really appreciated the cleanliness and freshness of Switzerland. It had given her a taste of being close to home.

From then on it was a medley of drugs and mood swings every day. I doubt Russ ever knew what he was going to wake up to. Sometimes Caron would wake up singing, loving, caring and understanding, in a fantastic mood. He would be blessed with every element of the woman he'd fallen in love with. On another day she'd be a nightmare. Those days he would try to help or, if he couldn't, he would batten down the hatches and just weather the storm. What else could he do? He understood her fear and pain. He empathized with her rages. No mother can bear the thought of not seeing their children again. That was the fear she was fighting now.

When they got home, they went yet again to the John Flynn Hospital, an hour's drive from their home, where Caron had had her radiotherapy in August. It was December. Her regular doctor there, David Christie, was on holiday and a different specialist took on Caron's further tests. After reading the MRI scan, she quietly confirmed to Russ that Caron had so many areas up and down her spine affected by the cancer that she thought it would be a waste of time and possibly unfair to put Caron through more radiotherapy.

However, there was no way Russ was going to tell Caron that, and kick away the vital crutch. For the first time in seven years, Caron was pressing for further orthodox treatment. She had reacted so well to earlier treatment that there was no reason to suspect it wouldn't work again. Once more, Caron felt in charge. She was doing all she could. The pain was frightening and anything was better than nothing.

Thankfully Charlie and Gabriel didn't see an awful lot of the negative side. They were so loved and cared for, the least Caron would do during those last few months was sit with them and do homework, draw, paint, play games. If she couldn't be up and about, she'd sit by the pool and watch them. And apart from that initial period of being an inpatient, most of her treatment took place as an outpatient. The odd occasion she did have to stay over, she hated. They'd do another scan, get the area they were concerned about irradiated, then Russ and Caron would go home and the pain would ease. For a while. They'd go back when the pain moved, to have the next area treated. Caron was rewarded for her tenacity – the radiation was working. As fast as the tumours were growing, the doctors were dealing with them.

Christmas was one of the good times. Russ says that he would watch in awe as Caron rallied when any of her family or friends arrived. She would literally go up two notches on the positivity scale. There was of course a bitter downside to that. The hardest time for Caron was when everyone left. There would be a tremendous drop as reality hit home. But then again, she always talked about the quiet time to meditate and heal.

Overall, Caron had come to the conclusion that there was no point in thinking that what she was doing, what the doctors were doing, wasn't going to work. She was doing everything she could from an oncology point of view and a complementary point of view, so why bring in the 'Am I going to live or die?' question. We all know she never wanted to enter that arena, she never drew up a will. None of us ever made any plans with

her about the children, certainly no specifics. That may seem
very strange for a woman who to the outside world was so
clearly fighting off death, but it reflects the essence of whom
Caron had become. She would live. Day by day, hour by hour,
minute by minute. As the monks said, where there is life there
is hope. She was alive. That was all she needed to know. So
thinking about leaving a legacy was not on the agenda. I think
she knew that Russ would do the right thing. Once she said,
'If anything happens to me, you wouldn't send the boys to
boarding-school, would you?' and Russ laughed and said, 'Of
course not.' Overall, she had enough trust in Russ's love for
their sons that he would never do anything other than dedicate
himself to looking after them. As he had done since the day
they were born. Nothing would change that. Caron didn't have
to worry about it. She didn't have to say 'This is how you cook
pasta', because he knew how to do all of those things. It wasn't
just Russ, it was all of us. She never said to Cathy Comerford,
'Will you do this or that for the boys?', even though they were
mothers with very close children. Caron lived for the present.
She wanted to get on with living. And if that meant packing
the boys' lunch, or sending them off to school with a wave, or
just lying down with them on her day-bed reading, then that
was what she would concentrate on. That was enough. Maybe
in hindsight you wish you'd said something, but it would have
gone against everything that Caron stood for. It would have
jarred. It would have been wholly inappropriate. She trusted all
of us to look after those precious children. And we all do.

Christmas arrived. It was special. Stephen, Michael and I were
due to travel on 21 December, but because Caron was in so
much pain and undergoing her radiotherapy I decided to go
earlier and arrived on 17 December.

Caron was having a therapy session in the summerhouse when
I arrived and about half an hour later, as I was changing in my
bedroom after the flight, there was a knock on the door and she

virtually fell into my arms, sobbing about her ongoing pain and fear. We clung to each other for what seemed like ages – perhaps it was better that we couldn't see each other's faces at the time. I was so petrified. However, after the initial outpouring, once again that incredible resilience of Caron's took over and we settled into a few unforgettable, magical days of enjoying our precious mother–daughter relationship, simply gaining strength from being in one another's company.

Obviously there was much Christmas planning. The toys for the boys were already bought and stored well out of reach. Caron wasn't in a position at this point to indulge in her favourite pastime of shopping and she was most anxious to get something special for Russ for Christmas morning. We settled on a top-of-the-range gas barbecue, which Russ had not so secretly coveted, and she even managed a short trip into Byron Bay to buy clothes and stocking fillers for him. Once that was done, she heaved a sigh of relief, and when Stephen and Michael arrived on the 21st we were well into the preparations. One of my lasting memories of what I now know was to be her final Christmas was down in the summerhouse, when the boys were well tucked up and asleep in bed, with Caron orchestrating a conveyor belt of present-wrapping and tying of ribbons, ready for Santa's arrival.

We had also rented a house on Belongil Beach for the Christmas period. We thought it might be too much for Caron at that stage to have all of us traipsing around Taylors all the time. It turned out to be a good decision, but not for reasons we could have foreseen. On returning from Switzerland Caron had begun to struggle with the rising heat. She missed the clean, cool air of the mountains. As the temperature soared to almost forty degrees, their lush garden felt hot and sticky. Our small rented house, however, looked directly on to the beach and was cooled by the ever-present sea breeze that rolled off the water. Caron loved it. It was a change of scene, a new focus. Every day we would roll out a bed on to the decking, plump it high with cushions and Caron would settle into it in a big floppy hat and stare out at her beloved ocean.

Christmas Day arrived. What joy to watch Charlie and Gabriel open their presents from Santa. We had the traditional early morning cups of tea as we all joined in with the flurry of ripped wrapping paper everywhere and the excitement of the boys getting what had been listed in their letter to Santa. The reindeer had eaten the carrots and Santa had even left a hurried note in the ashes of the fireplace. Then of course it was the turn of the adults' gifts which we had carried out in our suitcases, including, for Caron, a padded Christmas stocking which she had had every year since she was born. As is our family's wont, breakfast was the traditional Ulster Fry, this time by the pool. It seemed a little incongruous in the 40°C heat, but was a prerequisite none the less. Of course it was accompanied by a huge platter of fruit for Caron. Denny the gardener also joined the family, and it was the usual happy, animated Christmas morning but one which I know now to be so much more poignant than the rest and one which I have relived many times. After opening yet more presents, we all headed back to Belongil Beach to prepare Christmas lunch. We resisted the temptation to do turkey on the barbecue, settling instead for all of Caron's favourite food – fresh exotic salads and poached salmon. In the afternoon she rested, but was back in force for the nearest thing we could find to Christmas dinner: duckling with all the trimmings. It was amazing to see how, yet again, Caron's courage had seen off those bleak thoughts and fears of the 17th, how the treatment she was advised not to have had worked, and how, once again, she had risen from the brink. It was a happy, joyous Noel, one with many fixed images in my head, but none more so than Caron in that wonderful hat, breathing in the cool sea air, facing the horizon and whatever it held.

During the Christmas holidays, Johnny and Cathy Comerford came back up to Byron Bay for their second visit. They found something very touching about Caron during this visit that had been missing from their first. They arrived late after another long drive from Sydney and this time Caron was standing at the top of the path waiting for them. There was of course the tea ritual again and then Caron showed them to the summerhouse, where they were to stay. The fridge was stacked with healthy food, there were flowers in every room, the breakfast things were laid out and of course presents for all the children. But they also remember how frail she was and how difficult car journeys had become. We all had to drive incredibly slowly – the bumps would make her wince – and, just as in Switzerland, Johnny would think, Forget this, let's go back. But no. Caron would grab his arm and he knew he was in for more outings. Caron was amazing – amazing for all of us. As Russ said, we probably got the best of her, even when we thought we were seeing her at her worst. She would insist with tremendous bravery on continuing to do the things that she and her friends had always done together. They would go out to dinner and once she'd sat down and got settled with her favourite blue-checked cushion which travelled everywhere with her, the humour returned, she was the same girl. It was only when she stood up that her friends remembered she was ill. The last night of Johnny and Cathy's visit, Caron stayed up talking to them until midnight even though she must have been in great discomfort. She was just desperate for it all to be as it was, for nothing to have changed. That night when they said good night, they meant goodbye. Since they were leaving at such an ungodly hour in the morning, they didn't want to disturb her. There was another reason for taking the ceremony out of their departure. At that stage Johnny and Cathy were aware that it could be their last goodbye. But Caron wouldn't hear of it. At five thirty the following morning she staggered down the path, determined to say farewell to her great friends. With tremendous grace and willpower she walked out to the summerhouse.

Johnny and Cathy had arrived eighteen months before to find an agitated, irritable, distracted woman. A woman who talked of death in the middle of the night. This Caron, though clearly debilitated, obviously in pain and unquestionably in worse health, seemed happier and more at peace than she had been before. They were astounded and humbled by her bravery. Though physically quite shrunken, spiritually Caron soared. Cathy thought the words of the Rinpoche had set her free and regretted that someone of his weight hadn't said what he'd said earlier on. *You haven't been singled out.* There was nothing she had done or not done to deserve this. Maybe then she wouldn't have exhausted herself going so far down all those different paths in her quest to cure herself. But the same paths led her to the Rinpoche, so maybe she did need to go down them.

With the new year almost in place, Caron and I went down to Sydney to see the oncologist. It was a difficult journey and we were both silently afraid of what we would discover. We saw the doctor and then, as an added bonus, met Johnny and Cathy for lunch in the city, where they were staying for the famous Sydney celebrations. Caron was quite buoyant. The oncologist had told her she was pushing medical boundaries, and there was no reason to think that she wouldn't keep on going like this indefinitely. Her friends were thrilled. This was positive news. But at the end of lunch Johnny hugged Caron and over her shoulder he looked at me. The mask I had worn since leaving the oncologist, the mask I had fixed throughout lunch while she talked excitedly about defying the medical profession, the mask I had been wearing for seven years, slipped from my face. Johnny saw it fall. He saw me cry, he saw the terror in my eyes and held her frail body as tightly as he dared.

What Professor Tattershall had said off the record was that Caron had a slim chance of beating this. It was true she was defying medical predictions. It was true that they couldn't understand how she still managed to be up and about. It was true that he had said 'We'll see you next year then', it was even true that he'd challenged her with 'Let's see what you can do now'. But indefinitely? No. Whether I was prepared to accept it or not, there was nothing indefinite about it. But then something would happen to make you think, once again, that anything *was* possible. It was Gabriel's birthday, 28 January 2004, and as always Caron had made sure there was a party and a fabulous cake. She and Gabriel had decided on a theme which that year was a pirate ship. We also by tradition had to have my mother's special marshmallow and chocolate creation. I watched Caron from afar as Gabriel's friends piled into the garden at Taylors weighed down with colourful gifts. She was a proud and determined woman and at one point Caron somehow found the strength from deep inside her to leave the sticks that she now more or less relied on against the wall of the house. I stood in stunned silence as she walked all over the garden unassisted, talking to all the other mothers and greeting her son's friends. We were looking for miracles. That was one.

Russ and Caron battled through the rest of the new year with more visits to various clinics and hospitals, for blood transfusions, X-rays, vitamin injections . . . The pattern continued as it had done in the latter part of the previous year. Treatment was the precursor of an easing of the pain, but it would always come back. Caron was affected by the drugs she was taking. Her tummy remained bloated. Her face was fuller but her face was always exquisitely beautiful. She worried that she couldn't feel her legs sometimes. Fluid was building up on her lung. Her breath gurgled through the liquid. Some nights Russ would listen to the strange rhythm of his wife's breaths and hold his own if the pause between them got too long. Some nights he propped himself up on his elbow and stared at her through the darkness, not knowing what to think. Sometimes he reached over to her and gave her a little push and her viscous breath would return. One day it wouldn't. That was how he thought it would end. He thought he would wake up one morning next to Caron and she'd be gone. In March he agreed with the boys that they had to knock before coming into their parents' room in the morning so as not to disturb Mummy if she was sleeping. When he heard that knock, he would look across at Caron and watch as she opened a sleepy eye and smiled at him. That was how it continued until one day Caron decided, subconsciously or otherwise, that it was time to go home. Real home. Our home. England. It seemed that Byron Bay had woven its magic for so long, but had little more to give her.

11 March 2004

Going back to Switzerland on Tuesday morning. Had hope of going back healed (now know I won't). Still stuck – not walking properly – though I could and am strengthening up and having a very good day today. Acupuncture treatment with Neil – superb – he's a genius. Anxiety went and I felt much stronger. So much so, I decided I would like to work again: TV/Radio/Writing/Painting.

In truth what is my wish list – to write a book but then on what?

Should it be about life in Byron, healing, what?

Possibly interview people for radio about spirituality, searching, etc. – suitable for Radio Four?

Who knows? Anyway, the point is I'm so glad to be going – fed up just healing.

Time for structure and getting on with life.

This was the plan. Switzerland for further treatment. Sevenoaks for recuperation. Cornwall for the summer. Then back to Byron Bay in September. When she told me, I was overjoyed. It was everything I had prayed for. Caron was coming home. We could commence a full, comprehensive treatment plan under the guidance of her oncology team here, with all the support she needed. My baby was coming back.

21. In the End, These Things Matter Most

Caron didn't want the boys to be taken out of school early, so she flew with our great family friend Judith Doyle to Switzerland, where I was waiting. Judith, a successful businesswoman originally from England but now living in Sydney, had visited Byron Bay on holiday and fallen in love with it. Trading her high-heels and five-star lifestyle for sandals and beach huts, she set up temporary home there. Judith was incredibly generous with her time, support and love all through Caron's time in Australia. She helped out with the boys when Russ and Caron had to go to Sydney for treatment or examinations, or back to the John Flynn Hospital. She was a surrogate mother and granny in my absence and I love her for it. Russ and I agree that she is an angel in disguise.

Russ and the boys waved Caron and Judith off, along with half a dozen bags for her proposed six-month visit to England. He would follow a few weeks later as soon as school term ended. It is impossible to imagine how ecstatic I was that Caron was coming home. Finally my prayers had been answered.

It was Wednesday 17 March, St Patrick's Day. A good day, I thought, for Caron to come home. I went to Zurich airport to meet them. I was there a few hours early and literally paced up and down with endless cuppas and magazines until their flight touched down at one thirty p.m. I had also asked for extra help for the two of them to get to the baggage area. Caron was having none of it, however, and promptly placed her hand luggage in the wheelchair. To my delight, she was walking without the frame, but on two canes. As usual, she was energized by the thought of more progressive treatment. Energized at the thought that home was only a tiny flight away. Energized by the mountains, the change in scenery and the fact that she was returning to the bosom of her family. So once again, Caron rallied. Lulling us all into a false sense of security. Allowing the denial to continue despite what was obviously going on in front of us.

We had five days together before Caron's treatment at the Paracelsus Clinic began and once again we settled into life in the St Gallen hotel. Caron had the same light-filled corner room that she'd stayed in before and that first evening Judith, Caron and myself went upstairs to the top-floor restaurant for a cele-bratory dinner. The absolutely adorable *maître d'*, Fernando, welcomed us back as if we were family. He was thrilled to see Caron looking so well and remarked at the sensational way in which she was walking around. Remember, five months earlier she had left in agony, barely able to move, and now she was only having to use one of her canes to get about. It wasn't quite Soho House, but it was a good girly night and the three of us chatted non-stop until Caron's eyelids started to droop. Before Judith left for England, we all went across the border to Con-stance in Germany, where Caron bought herself a green heart-shaped ring that I have worn since her death and an extraordinary pair of red shoes. To my delight, that evening she arrived for dinner in fishnet tights and those fabulous red shoes. For five days we went out for lunch, shopped, chatted constantly and stocked up on warm clothes. Death was not imminent. It was not. On Sunday 21 March it was Mother's Day. We spent it together for the first time in three years. And for the first time since Caron was a baby, alone. Caron gave me a delightful picture of tulips she had painted and put it in a country frame. I was rendered speechless. Despite all the pain, frustration and fear of the previous months, she had sat herself down to paint something for me, knowing that we would be together on that day. Then she had packed it in tissue, tucked it carefully amongst her clothes in the suitcase and brought it with her from Australia. What a thoughtful and incredible piece of planning. Like my memories, it is another precious possession that is invaluable to me. We had a wonderful day and travelled up to a café high on Santis Mountain that Caron loved.

On Monday we registered with the clinic. On Tuesday, the prescribed treatments began in earnest. She called them her 'feelgood' treatments, which consisted of nerve infusions, reflexology, massage and vitamin injections. There were to be no more 'hot box' treatments during this visit. During a break we bought a pretty mountain walking-stick that was decorated with daffodils. One walking-stick. That was how good she was. Her passion for life, her enthusiasm for living, had returned. Everyone in the clinic reacted to her with the same genuine amazement as the *maître d'*. Caron had rallied again. On Wednesday she had an electronic back treatment. Forty-eight hours later, it all suddenly went into dramatic reverse. Caron was bent over the sink in her bathroom, clinging on for dear life. 'There is nothing from here to here,' she said, pointing to her hips and then her toes before grabbing the side of the sink again. 'Nothing. No strength. It's all gone.' As her strength left her, the severe pain returned. The daffodil stick was put aside.

The doctor at the Paracelsus Clinic said she had to go to the cancer hospital to check everything before they could carry out any more treatment and that he would send an ambulance for us. We pictured a small-town service. What happened next was like something out of a bad movie. Four burly men came striding down the hall to Caron's room. Stephen wouldn't let them in. There was an argument. I appeared at the door. At first they thought I was the 'sick woman' and wanted to take me. I told them my daughter was ill and she was in the bathroom and they would have to wait. I know they were simply doing their job, but their presence was a complete anathema to me and the cocoon we had built over the previous softly spoken five days.

The confusion was no doubt exacerbated by the language barrier. They wanted to lift Caron on to a hard stretcher. I was terrified they were going to damage her further. But they could not understand the fragility and complexity of the situation and I didn't have enough of their language to explain it. Finally, with much gesticulating, they agreed to a wheelchair.

The problems were not over. There was thick snow outside the hotel and they wanted Caron to walk to the ambulance. Walk over ice. How could I make these people understand? I couldn't. It would have been farcical if it hadn't been so utterly desperate. Finally they carried her in the wheelchair over the snow into the large waiting ambulance and Caron was taken to the place she hated most. Hospital.

We found ourselves once again in a small cubicle. There were new faces, new forms, new machines that Caron did not want to go in to. And once again I found myself waiting outside a doctor's office ready to doorstep the man until I made someone understand what was going on and got some answers. After the MRI scan was completed, I was brought into the neurologist's office. He was a tall, kindly man, and I will never forget the way he looked down straight into my eyes which at the time were filled with anticipation and terror, and he said, 'Do you realize how ill your daughter is?' Once again I heard the words tumble out of my mouth, 'Yes, of course I do,' but inside I still thought, You don't know Caron as we do. He told me in no uncertain terms that Caron needed more radiotherapy and should have it as an inpatient. She was endangering herself. I was watching the sand fall through my fingers, unable to stop the rapid change in events. Caron wouldn't have it. She checked herself out. She was not, simply not, going to stay in hospital. Our days changed again. From then on she made the difficult journey to the clinic for 'feelgood' treatments in the morning but returned to the cancer hospital for orthodox oncology treatment in the afternoon. Then she would rest. Then she would go out for dinner. She was amazing, absolutely amazing.

Sometimes I was with her in that bright corner bedroom in that little hotel in St Gallen. Sometimes Michael. Sometimes both. Whoever was there would sleep in the adjoining room so that Caron could ring in the night if she needed something. The doors were unlocked. Before going to bed there would be a routine of making sure she had water and the concoction of pills that she was taking were in the right place. Michael would set his alarm, knowing that Caron had to eat by a certain time because the drugs she was taking made her very hungry. She could get very irritable if she didn't eat. I didn't have to set my alarm. I was always awake at dawn. Off and on throughout the night. And always long after midnight.

Because the doctor had told me that Caron should not be walking around at all, particularly near snow and ice, it scared me whenever my daughter got that look in her eye that said 'I want to get out of here'. Out into the fresh mountain air. She was so stubborn, she wouldn't take no for an answer. I would be beside myself, saying to anyone who'd listen that Caron couldn't possibly go out walking. By now her strength seemed to be unravelling fast. Things were going very wrong. But Michael had other ideas. One day he was out and Caron rang him on the mobile to tell him to get her out of there. The town of St Gallen was completely covered in snow and ice, she had to cling to her youngest brother for support as they made their way over the precariously slippery surface and off they went. DVDs and books were the order of the day – top of the shopping list. Michael's words of warning were not well received. Caron would say 'Shut up, I'm fine' (or less printable words to that effect) and keep going. It terrified me that she would slip and hurt herself, but Michael wasn't going to sit in the hotel room with her and forbid her to go out. He knew she was a really sick girl at that point, and he thought, Damn it, if you want to go shopping, let's go. In his heart, he says, he knew she was going to die. He thinks she did too, but they never talked about it. Only once, when it became increasingly difficult to bath and wash herself, when getting her to the loo on time was an ordeal, did she mention the word death. She looked at me and said, 'This is no life, this is a slow death.' But I wouldn't have it. Once again I heard myself say words that now I don't know whether I believed or not. You reacted well to the radiotherapy before. You'll do it again. I couldn't undo the seven-year head job I'd done on myself overnight. Where there is life, there is hope. Where there is life, there is hope. Where there is life, there is hope, goddamnit.

Michael brought his DVD player and he and Caron would lie in the bed and watch movies. *Frida* was one they watched over and over again, there seemed to be so many similarities and Caron identified with her. Frida Kahlo, the Mexican artist, was bedridden at times and couldn't do the things she wanted to do, or the things she felt she still had in her to do. Immobility robbed Frida Kahlo of her mode of self-expression yet she had so much more to express. Her creativity had been dammed. The music in the movie alone expressed the deep rage and emotion that swirled inside the artist while she lay, like Caron, imprisoned in her bed. Michael and Caron would look at each other and there would be that knowing look, the one they'd been sharing all their lives, a silent nod to an unspoken truth. Death was stalking Caron. Sometimes they didn't even have to be looking at one another. On a couple of occasions when Michael was changing Caron's pain-relief patches, there would be a moment when time was suspended. For a second or two they were both looking directly into the eye of the future in full recognition of what lay ahead.

I could see that Caron was deteriorating fast. She was in so much pain, it would make her cry. It made us all cry and yet she was so incredibly courageous throughout. Eventually I gave in to my panic and rang Russ. I said, 'You have to come earlier.'

So he took the boys out of school, changed the flights, packed next to nothing and flew to Switzerland.

From Russ's perspective, Caron's deterioration wasn't actually very fast. It had been taking place slowly and steadily over the previous six months. When Russ arrived, he didn't think it was any different from the other bad times they'd been experiencing throughout early 2004. Caron had arrived excited to see us and anticipating a new phase of her feelgood treatment, but during her treatments something had been aggravated again and as a result the doctors had to increase her medication. The steroids which she had to take to help her cope with extra radiation had made her bloat up. Whatever had shifted, she was in deeper pain which meant stronger painkillers, so more drugs were administered. We were witnessing a very concentrated version of the vicious circle that Caron was caught up in. But Russ wasn't that thrown. He in turn gauged his reaction by the boys, watching them carefully when they came in to see their mother after a three-week absence. There was absolutely no register of any change in Caron's appearance from the boys. They just rushed at her like they always did, jabbering away about what they'd been up to, lots of hellos, kisses and hugs, and as always she rallied at the very sight of them. It confirmed what Russ suspected. Caron wasn't particularly worse; it just seemed that way to us because we'd never seen this level of pain before.

Caron was such a beautiful girl, it was sometimes hard to take on board how her body frame had changed, though Russ says Caron was never more beautiful to him than in those last months. Her courage radiated from within – her inner strength like a shining beam of true light. I don't think dealing with her looks was what really concerned her. I think it was that her looks belied the truth of her medical condition. A condition she was still, on the surface at least, refusing to accept.

If the gift of the tulip painting on Mother's Day had not been humbling enough, Caron then conjured up a surprise birthday breakfast for me that felt almost as carefree as any other. It was 10 April. Three days before Caron died. Three days. I still cannot believe that is true. The effort she made was extraordinary. Was she in more pain than I realized? Was I so in the thick of the fog that I couldn't see what was right in front of me? I don't know. She and Russ took over a private room at the top of the hotel and decked it out with streamers and balloons, flowers and cards and wonderful things to eat. Charlie and Gabriel were excited as usual at the prospect of a party. Presents were strewn over the table. She had been buying all of it over the previous weeks, every time she went into the town for treatment, and hiding them in her room. It was amazing to me that she was still even thinking of such things when each treatment consumed her strength and left her shattered. After breakfast we took the car back over the border into Germany, to Constance. Caron was determined for all of us to have a lovely day out. She was still purchasing, of course. On a previous visit, she and Michael had found a cute little restaurant that most importantly didn't have too many steps, and secondly had an easily accessible loo. By now the pressure of the tumours on her pelvic floor meant she had to get to the loo quickly. They had also found a nice art gallery there that Caron liked to visit. Maybe more than anything, it was an excuse to get out of the hotel. She loved the drive through the beautiful mountains, past vast opaque lakes and picturesque villages. So off we went, *en famille*, for a day trip to Constance. If that wasn't enough, when we came back she wouldn't hear of retiring to bed although she must have been exhausted. Instead she insisted that we all went back up to the private room and spent an hour together setting everything up for the next day's celebrations. Easter. The Easter Bunny always hid eggs for Charlie and Gabriel and this year would be no exception. We had booked dinner in a favourite Italian restaurant of hers just down the hill, but still a fair walk away.

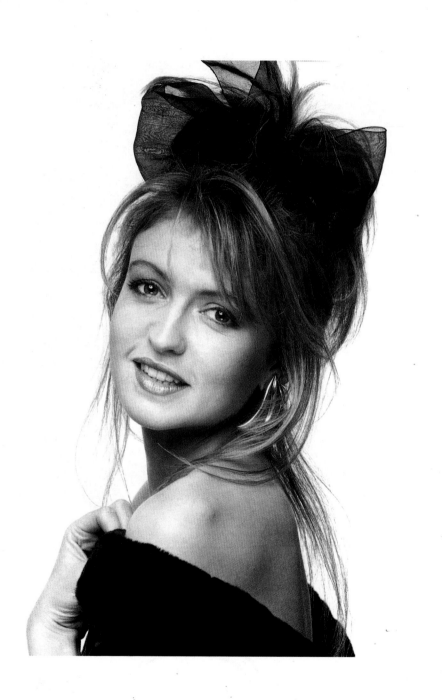

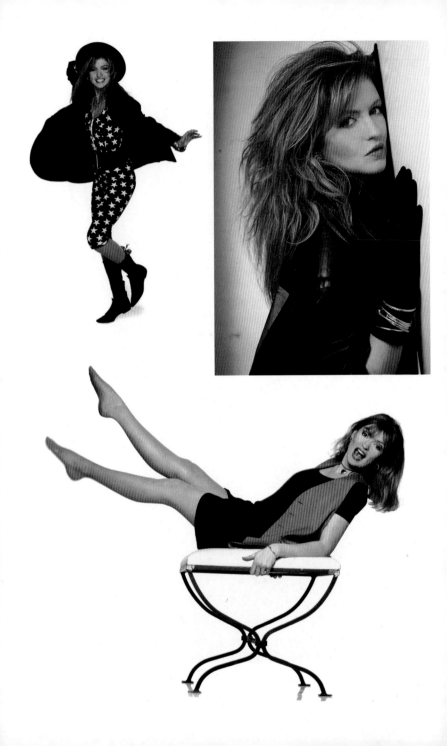

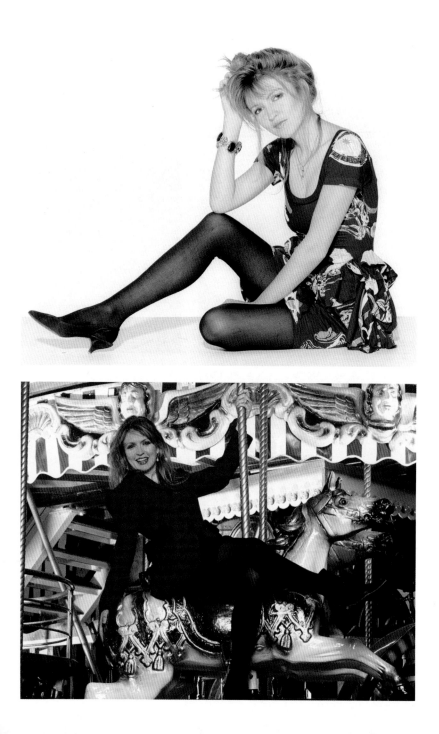

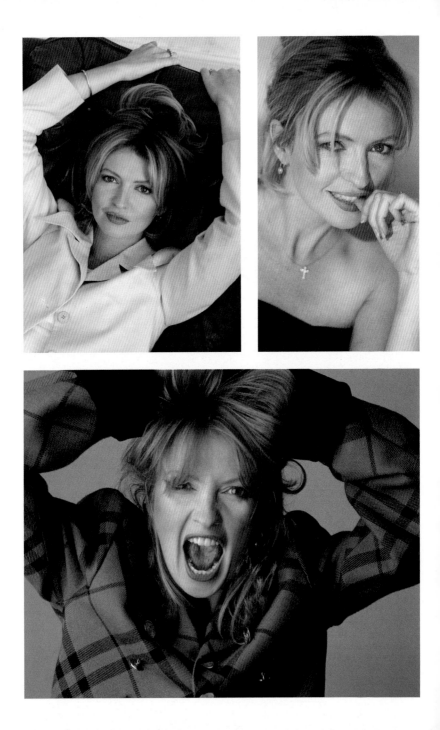

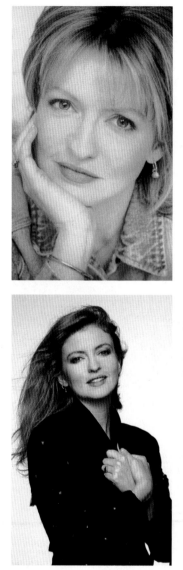
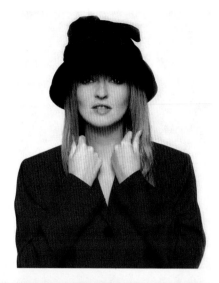
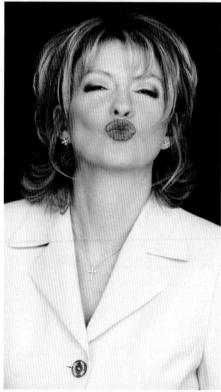

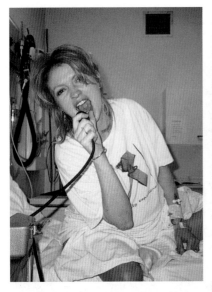
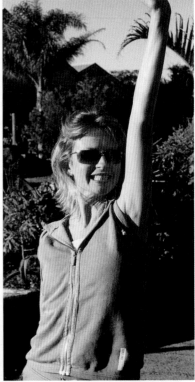
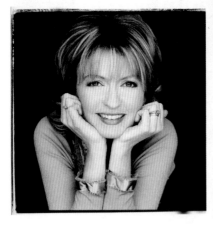
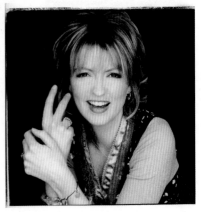

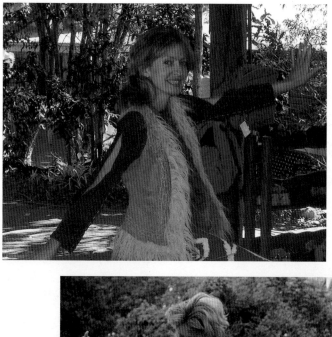

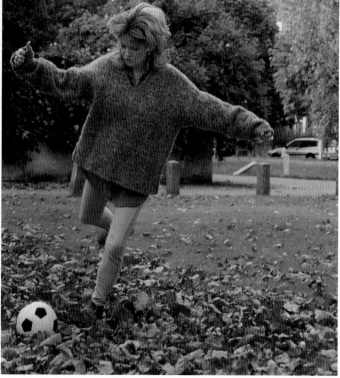

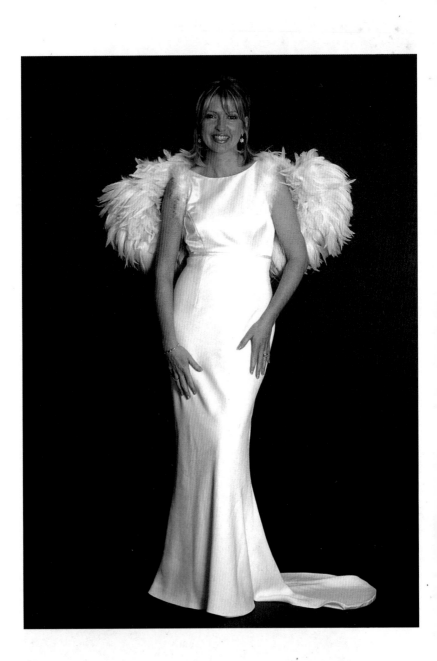

She would not be put off. Michael helped her get dressed. Putting on her new red shoes now caused her agony, but she struggled into them anyway, put on her coat and made it down the hill. That night she did have a sip of champagne, no one deserved it more. As at Christmas, settling her into her chair was the hard part. She complained about some people smoking a couple of tables away but it was probably to distract herself from the anger pain brings out. Once she sat down, she was fine. There she was again, the old Caron, chatting and laughing with the rest of us. But in reality the changes were coming thick and fast. I don't think Russ knew whether he was coming or going.

We awoke on Easter Sunday. We were all exhausted from my birthday celebrations the day before, but still my daughter was plotting and planning. Once again she wanted to go up Santis Mountain to let the boys have a snowball fight. We had to beg her to have a day at the hotel. Not one to take things lying down, Caron immediately threw herself into activity mode and convinced an easily swayed Fernando to part with a dozen eggs. An Easter-egg-painting competition began. There were paints everywhere, all of us trying to outdo each other with our designs. It would become the last family activity we would share with her. With hindsight it has become a morning of great significance. The egg-blowing, the mess, the laughs, my hopeless attempts to be artistic and Caron's wonderful creative streak still coursing through her. Three days later those silly eggs, like the tulip painting, were to become my most treasured possessions. For a year those eggs remained preciously placed on tissue paper in glasses on the mantelpiece in the dining room. Halfway through the painting competition, something in Caron changed. She appeared to become quite faint. We put it down to the central heating and eventually she agreed to return to her bedroom in the hotel.

At noon all the boys went into the town for lunch, leaving

my daughter and me alone for a couple of hours. We ordered up some room service and chatted about what we would do with Charlie and Gabriel in Cornwall that summer. For some days now, Caron had been complaining about fluid retention in her legs as well as the pain. She'd been finding it increasingly difficult to walk but now even the soles of her feet were painful. I suggested that while she was in bed I could massage her legs and try to ease the discomfort. I massaged Caron's legs on and off for two hours. It seemed to be helping. During that intensely personal time, we had the deepest and most extreme conversation that we had ever shared. Promises were made. Promises I will keep unto my death. I was rubbing her legs when suddenly she looked me right in the eye. 'Promise me one thing,' she said. 'Promise you'll never put me in a hospital or hospice.' I told her I would never allow that, I told her I would always keep her with me at home. She held my gaze. 'Promise me you'll always look after the boys.' I swore to her that I would. With those firm promises made, she lay back on the pillow and nodded her head. 'That's all right then,' she said quietly, closing her eyes. 'That's good.' It was as if I had witnessed a weight lift from her mind.

Did it raise alarm bells in my head? No. I just couldn't wait to get her home to Sevenoaks to get a new medical regime up and running, where she could be cared for in the bosom of her family. As for Caron, she was just very excited about going home.

The boys arrived back from St Gallen and Stephen took over with the massage. He was immediately worried about how Caron's legs felt. He thought they were cold and completely unresponsive to his touch. He knew that this had gone beyond anything they'd experienced before. He repeated his concerns to Russ. We had a family conference in the corridor. There we were, living in this hotel, and now we couldn't even get her the treatment she had come to receive. We were in a country we didn't really know, we didn't speak the language, we didn't know the experts. But in London maybe we could pull a few strings, we did know the doctors well and I had kept in regular contact with them when Caron was in Australia. We would have the ammunition to fight. And so it was decided, that after a two-and-a-half-year absence, it was time to get Caron home. Stephen and I were the first to leave. It was decided we should go back to Sevenoaks and get Caron's room ready and everything organized for her return. Michael took the boys home the next morning and he was well encouraged as Caron sat up in bed to kiss the boys goodbye as they headed off to the airport.

Paul was in France for a few days. He called for an update, as he did every day, throughout the day. He wanted to come to Switzerland and help Russ drive Caron home, but Russ said it made no sense since it would take the same amount of time for Paul to reach them. All those conversations were terrible for Paul. Caron would be bad. Then she'd rally. Then she'd dip again. We never knew what was going on from one moment to the next, so there was never a point when we said to him, 'Come now!' Instead, I told him to come home when his holiday ended and see Caron then.

That night, Caron was in a huge amount of pain. Russ listened to her agitated torment as she tossed and turned and mumbled in her sleep. She was almost delirious. Despite the harrowing previous few months, it seemed to Russ it was undoubtedly worse. Russ started packing up, and while Caron was having a final massage from Andrea at the hotel he started loading up the car. That was when she said to Russ that Caron had started to 'shut down'. Stephen had been right. Nothing was responding. Andrea believed all Caron's vital organs had begun to pack up. The nurse looked Russ in the eye and told him to get Caron home as soon as possible. It was eleven thirty a.m. on Easter Monday. By four p.m. they were in the car. Russ drove non-stop through Europe until they reached Sevenoaks.

I went into frantic overdrive as soon as I got home. We went shopping and bought everything we could think of that Caron might like when she arrived. Melon. Green tea. Spelt bread. Vegetables to juice. The ingredients for buckwheat pancakes. I rang the doctor. I changed the sheets and got the rooms ready for Caron, Russ and the boys. I rang all the specialists in the field that I knew to make appointments. I couldn't believe it. My daughter was on her way home. Russ pulled up at the house just after midnight on Tuesday morning. He and Stephen carried Caron on a chair through to the kitchen where she ate a little of the melon that I had bought and the organic vegetable soup that Stephen had specially made. Then they took her upstairs and finally, after such a long absence, Caron was back in her room, asleep on the bed I had made for her, home at last.

In the morning things did not improve. Russ called Paul. He told him to get back now. Luckily Paul hadn't gone up the mountain with the rest of his family, just in case Caron didn't rally this time. Suddenly there was a scramble to get to the airport. He packed, bought a ticket on the way down but couldn't get on a flight until six p.m. While Paul waited for his plane, Caron was dying at home. He rang us at Sevenoaks at five p.m., six p.m. our time. The boys had arrived home and Caron was already slipping away. What could I say? I just told him to get here as soon as he could. By the time he landed there was a message from Michael to call. His bags were late, he nearly left them, but when he spoke to his brother Michael just said, 'Get here when you can.' It didn't seem as urgent as it had been. It wasn't urgent. The worst had already happened. Poor Paul, his day got worse and worse. He took a cab home to pick up his car since it was on the way, but the battery was flat. He had to get a neighbour to jump-start the car, all the while thinking Caron was still alive and desperate to see her, hold her hand, tell her he loved her. Finally he got to the gates of our house. Before he even stopped the car, he felt something was different.

Something was wrong. Everything was very still. He didn't ring the bell, just opened the gates and walked in through the back door to the kitchen. There was no one there. The house was deathly quiet. He went through to the living room and there were the little boys watching television. Stephen was with them. All Stephen could do was look at Paul in terror, he couldn't speak. Paul knew but refused to believe what Stephen's silence meant, he wanted to shout 'Why aren't you talking to me, why aren't you saying anything?' But the boys were there. Staring at the television. Stephen was so shocked to see Paul, he didn't know what to say or do, but Paul sensed it. He'd sensed it the moment he pulled up at our gate. He watched himself walk through the familiar territory of our house in Sevenoaks with this unfamiliar sickening feeling, desperate for someone to break the limbo and tell him it wasn't happening. He went upstairs and there we were, Russ, Michael and I huddled on the landing, thrown into total confusion, shock and disbelief. I was in tears but could not find the words to tell Paul something that I couldn't fathom myself. Finally I heard these words: 'She's gone.' They came out of my mouth but I did not understand or believe them.

Where had she gone? Why had she gone? Who had taken her? I wanted her back. I wanted her back. I didn't want Russ to go downstairs and tell the boys that their mother had died. I wanted this nightmare to end. Enough. But it didn't. Russ went downstairs. The boys were shattered. Doctors came. Papers were signed. My daughter was dead. I went back into her room over and over again to check, but she was still there. She hadn't gone anywhere. Not then. Michael thinks his sister drifted away during the following week when we cocooned her in love, flowers, photos and memories. Others think that it was during her momentous funeral. Friends felt an uplifting sensation move through the congregation towards the end of the service. The heavy pall that had hung over the church pulled away and for a while it was easier to breathe. As for me, what do I think? I think that the answer lies with those angels that Caron believed in so profoundly.

I don't know how it started, but it built up over time, and long, long before she was diagnosed with cancer. On our many girly shopping days, before the mire of cancer hung over our heads, Caron would say to me when I was trying to park, 'Ask the parking angel . . .' I'd say 'Don't be silly, Caron,' but she would insist that there are angels for all sorts of things. Well, if I am going to pray I like to go direct, but Caron put me straight. God hasn't got time to deal with all those silly things, so ask the parking angel. Humouring her, I would say, 'OK, parking angel, where are you? Find me a space.' And sure enough, in the midst of my scepticism a meter would appear. We laughed about it then. But angels were to become a less frivolous subject once Caron had been diagnosed with cancer. Throughout her illness, Caron would pick up her angel cards and flick one over. The message on the card she'd chosen always seemed apposite. Whether real or imagined, her belief in angels helped Caron then and helps me now. When she saw a white feather, she always thought it was an angel leaving their calling card. Now of course, when I see a white feather I think it's Caron's calling card. I'm not talking about when you find five or six, where obviously a bird has been, I'm talking about a single perfect white feather that I have found in the most unlikely of places, and I've been finding a fair few.

The very first day I went off to work some months after Caron died, I didn't know whether I could do it, should do it, or whether I'd even be able to open my mouth, let alone smile and ask a coherent question. It was *This Morning*. I came home still demented with exhaustion and grief, made a cup of tea and dragged myself upstairs shattered by the very thought that I'd done it. The daily had been in, hoovered everywhere (I know because I checked with her) and the house was spotless. There on the landing, at the top of the stairs, was this perfectly placed single white feather, as if to say, 'Well done, Mum, you did it'. Back then it almost freaked me out, I was so raw with the pain of losing Caron. Am I imagining these things, as Caron did before me? Who knows? But I am not the only one.

Cathy Comerford was always the biggest cynic of all. When she and Caron were walking along the beach together, Caron would point out a white feather and say, 'An angel has been here.' Cathy, as ever, was swift to mock her. 'Caron, for God's sake, it's a gull, there is a gull in the air, a feather on the ground.' Nothing very spiritual about that. But earlier this year Cathy had agreed to do a twenty-six-mile walk for charity. It was dark and cold when she woke before dawn on the day of the walk. She hauled herself to the loo and had just decided that she couldn't do it when there on the floor of their completely tiled bathroom she saw this single perfect white feather. Cathy thought, 'You so and so . . . All right, all right, I'm going'. And she did.

Paul has had the boys over a lot recently, in fact he has been exceptional in the way he and Sandy have helped Charlie and Gabriel settle into their new life just a short distance away. While he was setting the table outside in his garden during the summer, I told him that Caron would be really proud of him and the way he was getting the four cousins together. From a cloudless blue sky a white feather fell and landed right on his hand. He was stunned. He said, 'Tell me what this is about.' I can't. I just believe, as Caron did, that it was the calling card of an angel. No guessing which angel.

On Gabriel's first birthday without Caron, we desperately wanted to do something different. So we decided to go to EuroDisney. Gabriel was so excited, we all went to Ashford from our house and as we were walking to the train, along the covered platform, there again, with nothing else around, was a white feather. I thought it was Caron saying 'This is a great idea,

I'm coming with you'. It's not just feathers either. On the night of our fundraising concert at the Albert Hall (A Night of A Thousand Voices) led by Michael Ball, James Galway and Cliff Richard, the tributes were exceptionally moving. It had been put together by our great family friend Hugh Wooldridge and turned out to be a celebration of Caron's life. We had a thousand voices from all over the country, all singing for Caron. Russ found it very hard, the dam burst and he was overcome with emotion. He had spoken to Maureen Lipman, whose husband Jack Rosenthal had recently died. Did she see white feathers? No. Jack communicated with her through the radio. Special songs floated over the airwaves at dire times to remind her of everything they had together and everything she had to be grateful for. Russ left that evening and sat in his car and cried. Overwhelmed by the enormity of what he had been – and was still going – through. He'd been looking after everyone for so long, Caron when she was ill and before, and the boys since they were born and since their mother had died. He and Caron had discussed every tiny aspect of Charlie and Gabriel's lives. Did he still have Caron's support that he was doing all right with the boys? Was he on the right path? Was he doing the right thing? Eventually he turned on the engine and the radio burst into life. The DJ said something that made it feel as if he were talking directly to Russ. Russ didn't drive away immediately, he sat and listened. Then the DJ played a song. It was Van Morrison singing 'Have I Told You Lately That I Love You?' Their wedding song. Their song. He sat, open-mouthed, and listened to the words like he'd never listened to them before.

We all went back to Cornwall for Charlie's eleventh birthday in July this year. A return to Caron's much-loved Alldays Field, the scene of many picnics and birthday parties while Caron was alive. It's what Charlie had really wanted to do for his birthday. Go back to where he had walked and played with Caron so many times and see his friends from Fowey. It had been grey and rainy for two days. At three o'clock, as many of Russ and Caron's incredibly supportive friends arrived for the party, the clouds moved aside. The sun shone through, the wind ceased to blow in from the sea. We were blessed with a perfect afternoon for the usual picnic, rounders and cricket. By seven that evening, the rain had returned. Are they signs? No one can ever know for sure, but I thanked Caron for our sunny afternoon none the less. The pain never completely subsides, but I get a very comfortable feeling every time I see a white feather. It certainly doesn't freak me out any more, because I believe my daughter is there. As Johnny Comerford says, cynic though he is, there is simply too much to disregard. So now when I see those white feathers in splendid isolation, and I see them all the time, I pick them up and put them in my pocket and say, 'Hello, Caron . . . Hello, Caron,' and, like seeing my grandchildren, it gives me the strength to go on.

Taylors, the house that Caron loved so much in Byron Bay, to which she sadly never returned, has been sold. But even there, her spirit remains. Amidst a twist of irony – or was it destiny – it was bought by a benefactor of those same monks who, in their own way, saved Caron's life. It will become a spiritual sanctuary, a place for the injured and lost to regroup and find peace. Caron's summerhouse, her own retreat, will be named after her. It will become a place where people can go to feel the force of unconditional love. Because in the end love is what Caron understood to be the ultimate cure. Love for her family and friends. Our deep and intense love for her. It is boundless and it transcends the human form. I will love her until I die. And beyond, even then I will love her, just as I still feel the force of her love for her sons today. She died with that knowledge and that, I believe, is why she smiled. She knew the power of her love would continue long after her physical being had gone. The last time Paul saw Caron, she handed him a card. On it she had written these words:

In the end these things matter most.
How well did you love?
How fully did you live?
How deeply did you learn to let go?

She loved well. She lived fully. And in the end, she let go.

22. How to Get By

A few weeks after Caron died, I received a letter from an elderly lady living in Wales. She wrote: 'I truly know how you feel – because I too lost a child – my son, but it is now 22 years since he passed on. I still think of him every single day and I'd like to tell you it gets better but it doesn't – you just have to learn to live around it and through it.' I remember reeling a bit when I read those words and thinking, What a harsh letter at this really vulnerable and raw time. But you know, I now realize she is right. You just have to learn to 'live around it'.

I want to make it absolutely clear that I am not under-estimating other losses. Grief is grief and it's all relative at the time. I have lost both my parents, a former husband, close friends and colleagues, but although it was deeply sad, not one of them comes close to losing a precious child whom you've carried inside you and given birth to.

When you lose a partner, it's not that you ever try to replace that person, but you can learn to love another, to share your life with them and be happy. Not that it seems possible at the time of death.

When it's a child, there is simply no way to capture ever again the bond and deep closeness experienced with your own flesh and blood.

The loss goes to the deepest core of your existence.

However, that same old lady who unwittingly knocked me for six also gave me advice which I refer to often. She said, 'The easy part is to sit in a room, weep, look at photos, read letters and so on' – but she pointed out that all that weeping isn't going to change anything and bring her back. That is the harsh fact.

She went on to say: 'Get yourself a new project, something to make you think of other things and people – keep yourself busy.' Being busy has never been a problem for me, I have always been 'a busy person'. Growing up in Northern Ireland, we were well indoctrinated with the Ulster work ethic. If we were ever sitting down doing nothing, we were chastised with 'What are you just sitting there for? Go off and do something.'

I now think that in the main that old lady was absolutely right. You have to have something to get out of bed for, to get dressed for, to put the old slap on for, to make you consider and think of other people and things.

Work for me has always been a therapy. I started work as that precocious and enthusiastic child singer at the age of eight. I have known nothing else, am still working and never expect anyone to work for me, so I have always been used to the routine and safeness of it. I suppose there's a solidarity about it which keeps you sane when everything else around you is flaky and breaking down.

Grief – particularly this endless emptiness of trying to cope with the loss of a child – is tough to get to grips with. People say, 'How are you coping?' The answer is, I don't really know, and it can all vary from virtually minute to minute. What I do know is that when you experience a huge loss like this, as I mentioned earlier in the book, it's a feeling of being completely flattened by a steam-roller and just when you're beginning to raise yourself off the ground, along comes that steam-roller again.

However, one day about three months after Caron died, I woke up and thought, I have to do something to keep Caron's spirit alive and something positive in her name. She had always hoped to write her own book and pass on to others some of what she had learned during her journey through cancer. So, I made up my mind that the book would be written and then, along with my sons Paul and Michael and son-in-law Russ, we launched the Caron Keating Foundation to raise money to aid cancer charities of all sorts. There is something extremely positive and mending about being able to hand over amounts of money to provide counselling services, because cancer is a very lonely business for patient and carer and family, and to provide complementary treatments and that feel-good factor which Caron so believed in. On top of that, we've also been able to contribute to buying vital pieces of diagnostic equipment and even a treatment room to be named after Caron in a log cabin for teenagers in the grounds of a holiday home in Northern Ireland, and we've made a contribution to the Royal Marsden Hospital for a lung-cancer project.

The reason I mention any of this is that everyone in their own way can do something positive to help their local hospice, hospital or drop-in centre. It is a very constructive way of trying to do something good in the midst of a negative situation. It's really irrelevant how small the gesture is, it is essential to the healing process.

Caron's death was such a shock to her friends, colleagues and people who loved her up and down the country. The mere fact that she had wanted her cancer to be kept secret meant that the shock of her death came from nowhere and, as a result, thousands of people very kindly wrote to us with their own thoughts and experiences. I can't begin to tell you how much those letters consoled us in the ensuing weeks and months. We, as a family, are so grateful for all of them, but the ones that proved to be a huge help to me personally came from people who had lost a child themselves, people who could say, 'I truly know how you feel.' It's not a club that one would ever want to belong to, but I find myself having deeply personal conversations with various parents I meet in my day-to-day life. For example, I was parking my car recently in London and a lady was putting her money in the next meter but came across to tell me about her own son who had died some seven years ago. We stood there for about half an hour, perfect strangers but bonded in a mutual loss, telling each other the most intimate of details of our lives, and most likely I will never see that woman again. It is amazing in the sharing of emotion and grief how we can all learn from each other.

May from Co. Down in Northern Ireland wrote to me to say, 'I lost my son of 38 years of age in 2003. He had an accident at work, he fell down from the first floor at a house where he and his brother were working. He left 4 little girls, his baby being only 7 weeks old.' She went on, 'People will tell you, you will have nice memories but it is these memories that make you cry. Funny little things will come to your mind in your daughter's childhood and one day, they will make you laugh as well as make you cry. Get yourself back to normal life as soon as you can. I am a great believer in daily routine, I really think it helps and of course talking about your child helps.'

Another mother from Hampshire said she felt compelled to write because Caron was very much in her head. Her advice was: 'The next chapter is still important, you must stop and listen to what needs to be done. Think about how Caron's life is to be carried forward and used to make some sense of her early passing, in some way. Place your faith, love, energy and skills to move Caron into another dimension for all of us to reach and touch the essence of her spirit. The world continues to search for a purpose but you have a key to unlock the treasure, the treasure that Caron brought with her into this world. It is not lost, she is not lost, you must believe this. The difference that can be made is huge – Caron's courage, kindness and days of pain will not be forgotten or lost for one second. You need to start work – this is a great opportunity to honour Caron, to move forward in a positive way, to make sense of something that on the surface has no sense at all.'

I have thought of that line over and over again: 'to make sense of something that on the surface has no sense at all'.

Cynthia from Suffolk lost her daughter a couple of years ago and a friend of hers who had also lost a child said to her, 'It gets easier but you never get over it and you learn to live with it. As time goes on you talk to many people this has happened to and you don't feel as if you're the only one. Remember you cannot alter the situation – you can do nothing about it.'

A letter from Yorkshire said, 'May I share with you a few things which have helped me through my dark days? The phrase which I have found very healing is where it says "I am I and you are you, whatever we were to each other, that we are still." A bit like the poem from Patricia in Primrose Hill who quoted:

They who are near me do not know that you are nearer to me than they are.

They who speak to me do not know that my heart is full with your unspoken words.

They who crowd in my path do not know that I am walking alone with you.

They who love me do not know that their love brings you to my heart.

Who walks that path of grief with you is so very important. A woman I know also lost her beautiful young daughter and she also subsequently threw herself into raising money for a cancer charity. One day her son stopped her as she was dashing out the door to yet another event, looked her straight in the eye and said, 'Mum – I am your child as well.'

What a defining moment. It's not that you ever forget for a second the rest of your family. In fact, they are your main strength and source of coping, but sometimes in the midst of being stripped to the core of your very being through the grief of losing your child, you can get side-tracked into not being able to take on board what those around you are also going through. As that old phrase has it, it's so vital to stop and count your blessings as well.

I genuinely don't know what would have happened to me if I hadn't had such strength, understanding, kindness and support from my sons Paul and Michael and naturally my husband Stephen. They have borne the brunt of my desperation and depth of sadness, but of course they too are coping with their own pain and loss.

I love them and admire them on a level over and above being my family.

You know that life will never be the same – it can't. A huge light has gone out and can never be reignited, but very, very, very slowly, bit by bit, you begin to stitch your life together again. For example, I have always been a very positive, upbeat, fairly jolly individual, but when Caron died I thought I would never be able to smile or laugh again. The lustre totally went from my life – I couldn't find the person I knew, I had lost Caron but I had also lost myself. The day-to-day coping can still change within minutes through a poignant reminder or memory or simply looking at a photograph, but slowly and subconsciously there comes a time when you're not totally consumed by your loss and grief – you begin to enjoy a taste of 'normal life', you don't cry so much, although scratch the surface and those tears are always there. Despite yourself, you start laughing again at the little things in life which have always amused you and, probably most significant of all, you begin to appreciate the riches you have had and shared with the one you've lost and the precious time you've spent together, in my case forty-one years of a treasured mother and daughter relationship. I now talk to Caron as I pass her photographs – I take her with me everywhere I go and consciously talk about how much she would have loved this or that situation. I recall very strongly meeting a deeply inconsolable young woman outside the Europa Hotel in Belfast. No one was with her and

I stopped to see if I could help her in any way. Through her sobbing she said, 'I know you, and you will understand how I feel, because recently I lost my baby girl – she just died in my arms. The difference is, you had your daughter for forty-one years, I only had my baby for seven weeks. I will never see her walk and talk and grow up.'

Of course, another person's loss doesn't take away your own, but I could see an element of truth in what she was saying. In fact, at the time I immediately thought of a piece of verse by Kahlil Gibran which Caron had pinned up above her desk in her own handwriting:

Your children are not your children.
They are the sons and daughters of Life's longing for itself.
They come through you but not from you,
And though they are with you yet they belong not to you.
You may give them your love but not your thoughts,
For they have their own thoughts.
You may house their bodies but not their souls,
For their souls dwell in the house of tomorrow,
Which you cannot visit, not even in your dreams.
You may strive to be like them, but seek not to make them like you.
For life goes not backward nor tarries with yesterday.
You are the bows from which your children as living arrows are sent
    forth.
The Archer sees the mark upon the path of the infinite,
And He bends you with His might that His arrows may go swift and
    far.
Let your bending in the Archer's hand be for gladness:
For even as He loves the arrow that flies, so He loves also the bow that is
    stable.

The illness and subsequent death of a loved one throws up so many, many emotions. In Caron's case, for seven years, as this book illustrates, we were all being positive for each other. We in a way couldn't allow ourselves to believe that the ultimate would happen. I know it isn't everyone's method of getting by and not the way everyone would want to play out life, but we all instinctively do what we have to do at the time. However, being totally honest, there have been occasions since Caron's passing when I was simply tired of trying to cope and tired of trying to be strong. I remember screaming at Stephen one day, 'It's my turn now, I just can't be that pillar of strength any more.'

We had seven years of respecting Caron's wish that people should not know about her cancer. Although we fully understood that, at the same time it meant there were very few people I could trust one hundred per cent with the information and any time thrust on them my deep fears, worries, sadness and terror of losing my wonderful daughter. Those who came to my rescue, apart from family, whom I could turn to at any hour or the day or night were two of my close girlfriends, Jackie Gill and Merrill Thomas. They were in contact daily and, not that I ever did call them at 4 a.m., the important thing was that I knew I could. The other good friend I could always depend on was Cliff Richard. I have known him for thirty-five years since meeting him in Northern Ireland and during these extremely difficult years he has been the most extraordinary sounding-board and source of advice on many levels – practical and spiritual. I have sharp memories of facing the first Christmas without Caron. I was chatting generally to him and said, 'I don't know how to even contemplate Christmas, which I love so much. I don't know how to get through, I just have no interest in putting up lights and decorations and sending happy Christmas cards.' I recall so clearly how he looked at me and said, 'Did Caron like Christmas?' 'Absolutely adored it,' I replied. 'Well then, do it for her, do it for your grandchildren, go bigger than ever. Have five trees, not one, decorate every room, hang those baubles everywhere.'

So it ended up, that's exactly what we did. We had a six-feet all-singing, all-dancing Santa, trees everywhere you looked and Blackpool would have been proud of our outside lights.

When Caron was in Australia, she didn't let too many visitors from home in. But Cliff was one who regularly came to stay when he was on tour or just visiting. Caron relished her chats with Cliff at the dinner table which lasted well into the wee small hours, long after the rest of us had given up and gone to bed. They were special times of revelation and sharing, and although neither totally revealed the detail of what they discussed, I do know those deep conversations meant a lot to them both. One of my favourite photographs of Caron is of her and Cliff dancing at a joint sixtieth-birthday party thrown by Stephen and myself. Caron had finished her chemo but her hair hadn't fully grown back and she hadn't really been out in the evening socially. However, as it was a costume party, she donned her big powdered wig and Renaissance gown and threw herself into the full fun of the evening. The significance of that photograph was huge.

Recently, I was at a dinner to celebrate the Caron Keating rose being launched at the Chelsea Flower Show (by the way, it's an exquisite peach/apricot rose which blooms profusely and Caron would adore it, roses being one of her top choices: she loved them). The sales of this rose go not to The Caron Keating Foundation but to Cancer Research UK. At the celebration dinner that evening, Professor Alex Markham had just come back from the States with the most exciting medical news straight from the world's biggest annual cancer conference in Florida. It had been delivered by Professor George Sledge, widely regarded as the world's leading spokesperson for the science of cancer. He had summoned the thousands of delegates to announce that a drug called Herceptin had achieved a dramatic reduction in breast-cancer deaths. The study involving 5,000 women world-wide began in 2001 and had achieved a

46 per cent reduction in the risk of recurrence in the early stage of an aggressive breast cancer and recent trials had shown similar results in women with an advanced stage of the condition. He concluded: 'These are the most stunning results in a clinical trial in my entire professional career. The findings are astonishing beyond belief. Biology has spoken, we should listen . . . A new age now begins.'

After the dinner, Professor Markham said to me, 'As I was delivering the brilliant and exciting news, I caught your eye a few times and I couldn't help but think about timing in life – the breakthrough came a few years too late to help Caron.' However, it goes back to the point which Caron herself never gave up on, the fact that you could never afford to give up hope, miracles do happen and new drugs are being developed all the time.

Caron was described by Russ as 'beautiful, intelligent, witty, fun-loving, caring, honest, loyal, loving and a most wonderful mother', and in trying through this book to bring you aspects of her childhood, her growing-up, her career, family life and subsequently her courageous quest for a cure to battle her breast cancer, it would be easy to make this sound like the end of the story. Although Caron is not with us physically, she is spiritually and her story is ongoing – a kind of new era. The work of The Caron Keating Foundation will be ongoing, and I know she would be thrilled and at the same time humbled by the number of organizations and individuals helped by the wonderful fund-raising which people are kindly undertaking all over the country in her name.

We have to live her dreams and aspirations. To look ahead, I only have to glance in the direction of my lively and gorgeous grandchildren, Charlie and Gabriel, and my son Paul and Sandy's boys, Jake and Beau. They are a constant source of joy, delight and discovery. I only have to see them to feel this huge surge of well-being. They are the biggest mender of a broken heart, they are the future.

I see so much of Caron's spirit and strength of character in her boys and I know she will live on through them. Everything Caron and Russ taught them, the combined love they gave them and impressions imprinted on them will only continue to flourish. As Caron herself said in recent years, she wasn't able to ride bikes, rollerskate, run and jump with them, but she was able to read to them, talk to them, tell them stories, paint, go to the movies, watch them swim, play cricket, be with and around them.

I often just sit and watch Charlie and Gabriel play with their cousins Jake and Beau and try to visualize them all growing up into their teens. What a *tour de force* they are, blond, bright-eyed, exuberant boys.

They really are the future – full of light and joy.

> Sometimes, when the sun goes down,
> It seems it will never rise again . . . but it will!
>
> Sometimes, when you feel alone,
> It seems your heart will break in two . . . but it won't.
>
> And sometimes, it seems it's hardly worth carrying on . . .
> But it is.
>
> For sometimes, when the sun goes down,
> It seems it will never rise again,
> But it does.
>
> Frank Brown, 'Sometimes'

My dearest and most beautiful Caron,

What a joy and privilege for over 41 years, to have you as my most precious and loving daughter.

I feel so proud to be your mum and I could not have wished for a more glorious daughter; spirited, caring, loving and full of fun.

You showered endless love and joy on our lives and brought light and rainbows to us daily. Although our relationship has always been exceptionally deep, during the last seven years there have been constant new depths and discovery, but through all your pain and suffering you have brought such warmth, love, laughter and friendship.

Watching you bravely battle with cancer has taught me so much about positivity, tenacity, dignity, spiritual growth and integrity. You are a total inspiration, not only to your family but to all those lives you have touched.

You and Russ have given us the precious and ultimate gift in two beautiful boys, Charlie and Gabriel, and you will live on through them. They will be a daily reminder of your spirit and individuality and all the values that you have taught them. Alongside Russ, Paul, Sandy, Michael and Stephen, I will forever love and look after your cherished boys, as you would wish.

I miss talking to you every day, you were the girl I loved talking to most in the world. The heartache of losing you will never be healed, but you have left us with millions of exquisite thoughts and memories.

In Australia you used to say that you could not wait to have a cup of tea out of your favourite cup, at the kitchen table in Sevenoaks, and with your incredible instinct and typical Irish timing, you made it back. Perhaps out of the endless memories, a few of the more recent ones will always shine out. Four weeks in Switzerland when, in the middle of concentrating on your healing and treatment, you also managed to organize my birthday celebrations, the Easter-egg-painting competition and a blissful Mother's Day, just you and me. It was the first time in three years that we had spent Mother's Day together and what a glorious day we had in the Swiss Alps, scoffing apple strudel and chatting non-stop.

How I treasure your gift, which you managed to paint in Australia despite your pain and frustration; beautiful tulips in a country frame which you carefully inscribed with love and kisses and lovingly placed in your suitcase for our special day together, which was yet another example of your generosity of spirit, which you radiated in abundance. You always did believe in angels and now you are one of God's brightest and most beautiful, so fly freely, my darling Caron, in your release from pain, and know that every second I will carry you in my heart.

With all my love for ever,

Mum.

The Book Bonus

In a way, we are so used to dealing with the future by referring to the past, it's the only knowledge we have and we drag it around with us, making it fit with totally different situations, allowing the past to keep reoccurring. The big learning for me has been to live IN THE NOW just in this present moment.

Caron's words

I had three main reasons for writing this account of Caron's life and her battle against this hideous disease which seems to affect virtually every family in the country.

First of all, to pay tribute to this gloriously beautiful free spirit of a young girl. I felt that her relentless but tenacious battle, and the way she dealt with it so courageously, was representative of thousands of people who have fought and are still fighting their own situation.

I also wanted to finish what Caron had started in her own diaries – two books. One about her Irish upbringing and the various family stories which have evolved over the years and the other concentrating on what she had learned about coping and dealing with cancer, and, of course, she was passionate about passing that information on.

However, probably the biggest driving force was to portray how hard she had fought to stay alive for her two wonderful sons, Charlie and Gabriel. As I am the only one around who knows

Caron's story intimately from birth to death, I feel it is my legacy to the two little boys, and when they are old enough and want to know more about their Mum, the story is here between covers.

What has been the huge, unexpected bonus is the way the book has taken on a life of its own and appears to be helping so many people in many, varying ways and on hugely different levels. It's as if Caron is carrying on her work and through this book is able to pass on what she learned and experienced through her own struggle.

Here is some of the reaction.

I am 39 years old – the mother of 5 children, ranging from 15 months up to 20 years. I have always worked and for the past 4 years I have been employed as an administrator in a breast-cancer clinic. I work part-time and my life is split between my job and family – close and extended – and I feel I have lost myself in routine and just 'getting things done'. In other words, losing sight of what is real.

Caron's story has made me re-evaluate what I have been taking for granted in my 'busy world'. I have spoken at length about the book with all who will listen and I wanted to share with you how it has changed me. Thank you for sharing Caron with all of us.

June
West Sussex

*

I want to let you know about the impact of your courageous book about your beautiful daughter, Caron. It's been part of my own search for comfort, solace and understanding in the few short weeks since my precious Mum passed away.

Since then, I have learned so much about Mum that I had not appreciated, but then I read your book and between the lines began to understand my Mum and how she loved me more than life itself, and I understand for the first time just how much she loved me for 'who' I am and that all was well between us.

I in turn treasure every precious moment with my three beautiful daughters and gorgeous son. I have resolved to work less and spend as much happy, treasured time as possible with my family.

Thank you for touching our lives.

Tessa
Kent

★

Miss me, but let me go

When I come to the end of the road
And the sun has set for me
I want no tears in a gloom-filled room
Why cry for a soul set free?

Miss me a little but not too much
And not with your head bowed low
Remember the love that once we shared
Miss me, but let me go

This is a journey we all must take
And each must take alone
It's all a part of God's perfect plan
A step on the road to home

When you are lonely and sick of heart
Go to the friends that we know
Bury your sorrows in doing good
Miss me, but let me go

(Author unknown)

★

I have no idea what it must feel like losing one's child, but I do know how it feels to lose a loved one as I lost my wife to breast cancer two months ago.

Reading your account of Caron's brave battle and the way you and the rest of your family are trying to come to terms with your loss has given me the strength to carry on. I now know I do

not need to feel bad about the mix of emotions I go through
every day. Anger, guilt, envy, even happiness sometimes, and
you've made me realize I'm not the only one.

We have something in common that we were both privileged
to love two very different, but equally brave women.

Ali

Northants

★

My own particular bugbear is FEAR. I seem to have been born with this inordinate amount of fear and, in the past, my mind became a master at concocting the most hair-raising scenes from what amounts to a tiny amount of storyline. I have known for two years about letting the emotions come and go, and yet, only last night, found myself thinking, Yes – but how do I deal with the fear? By allowing it, having no resistance, saying 'Look, you too are welcome.'

When I do this, it comes in like a cat and lies gently at my feet – when I resist, I think, Oh no, here it comes, look out. It forms like a tiger that wants to trap me, play games with me and fully devour me. So sometimes I choose to let it devour me and it sometimes feels like a fire burning up my body and then it goes. When we can finally allow WHAT is here to be here – know that those emotions will not destroy us – that we don't need to define ourselves by them – thinking, Oh, I shouldn't feel anger, sadness, frustration, whatever it is, we can finally allow ourselves to 'be'.

Caron's words

★

I have never been so touched by any book in all my life. My
young friend Nikki, who has just turned 30, has had a
mastectomy on one of her breasts and is currently having tests to
find out what the future holds.

You have equipped me with the understanding that I feel I
need to help her go through this. This book has helped me in
ways you will probably only ever begin to know.

Juliette Ratcliff

North Middlesex

Only the love is real – only that is healing – only that is ultimately *why* you are here, choose that in whatever situation you find yourself – that is ultimate freedom. How did Nelson Mandela cope whilst locked up – not knowing every day whether he would get out or not?

We must choose love, life, hope – not give up that trust which will carry us through to whatever. It is what I / we all have to do and face. Also, that power and strength, knowing and wisdom, is within us.

I have been confused as to what to do next. Wait, it will come whatever – you will know as you are 'here'. Stop harbouring the past. That is gone and will give you no more ideas and clues about the future – unless you allow it to shape it for you, which I presume is not what you really want.

Caron's words

★

I am a part-time nurse in the cancer field. When I held your book in my hands, I just knew instinctively it was special and full of emotion and love from the depth of your soul. It will help me in my field of work and help others in situations like yours all over the world.

Caron's soul is ENORMOUS and very much alive.

Mary Ronan
County Carlow, Ireland

★

I will walk properly again – I feel content and thankful my back is clearing and healing. All seems steady again.

I need to go slow – get a good healing programme. Now is the time to do that – no point delaying. Get on with it! No more distractions, excuses – do what you need to do now. Whatever that takes – give it to yourself now.

Everyone else is fine – you can't worry about them. They're all OK. You need it now – another chance. Seize it and the moment.

Do all you can – you will heal.

Caron's words

★

After reading Next to You, *I just felt I had to write. One of my brothers died aged 42 in 1991, so I sort of know the range of emotions that we as human beings go through. I know my mother, now 83, read your book in floods of emotion but I also know she gained great comfort from your words.*

I will treasure your book as it is haunting and it will stay with me for the rest of my life. I will never forget Caron and your book will never allow us to forget Caron.

Andrew Moore
Edinburgh

★

I dreamt I was kissed by an angel
Who knelt by my bed as I slept
Caressing my brow with a feather
And when I awoke, that I wept.
But a feeling of peace did surround me
A calmness that stilled all my fears
For when you are touched by an angel
Serenity comes through the tears.
The feather she left by my bedside
Reminds me her presence was here
So you'll know you've been
Kissed by an angel
When a feather is found lying near.
She'll open your heart to God's blessings
She'll open your heart to His love
Then you'll know you've been kissed by an angel
Direct from God's presence above

Sylvia Butcher
Strangford, Co. Down

★

Like Caron, I was diagnosed in my 30s. I am now 44 and my story has followed a very similar path to that of Caron's.

You would not believe how comforting it is to know that I am

*not alone in having some of the thoughts and emotions I go
through. I am really grateful to you for speaking of the fear
Caron felt. It is something that never leaves me.*

   *Reading about your pain, especially being unable to 'make
things better', has helped me to understand a little better how
my own mother must be feeling – something I had not always
had the energy to take on board.*

   *I now understand why she is so protective of me. I have two
beautiful daughters who have lived this nightmare with me – we
are extremely close and they are my miracle.*

   *I have gone through the full range of emotions having read the
book, but reading it has also inspired me enormously.*

Denise
Sussex

★

Choose a whole new future
Loving – family
Peaceful – time for them and you
Active – walking, swimming, yoga, music
Artistic – write
Choose – you have the potential
Goodwill for you is perfect peace, happiness, health. What do you *want*?

Know in yourself – I am the blessing – love this being – be the powerful
being you are.

Rest at this point – gather your strength.

Allow your body to heal and go forth and do your thing.
All is possible.

I will no longer limit myself with doubts.

Caron's words

★

*Your story of Caron's life and her battle against cancer has
touched me beyond any other story I have ever read. For this*

reason I feel it's important that I put these feelings in writing to you.

It wasn't just about Caron and her cancer but also about a wonderful family bonus you all have – the closeness and friendship and the amazing strength and support you all gave to each other through the good times as well as the bad.

I will never forget Caron's story and hope that if ever needed, I can draw strength from how she coped.

Diane Culpeper
Pembrokeshire

★

Next to You *is the most moving story I have ever read – brilliant, sad, emotional, heart-wrenching – but at the same time uplifting.*

I really wanted to read Caron's story because I was pregnant with my daughter when Caron died and it hit me like a ton of bricks the day it broke on the news.

I was having counselling sessions throughout my pregnancy as part of my training as a counsellor. I remember going to my session that week and spending an hour crying and talking about Caron and what had happened. However, I do think it is so important for people who are grieving to know that there is help out there for them if they need it and Caron's courageous and inspiring story of positivity will stay with me for ever and help me so much in my job.

Angela
Nottingham

★

My daughter Lisa bought me your book for Christmas – I only ever read biographies as I can't read anything that's not real. I tell you I have hundreds of books of this nature but I feel so wonderful reading this book because it reads like a Bible.

I think also when you have two children and a granddaughter, like me, I feel like I want to do more after this book – I feel everything that Caron went through inside me and thank God that my children, a 21-year-old and a 35-year-old girl, are both OK. I think it brings home the pain to us all and makes us truly appreciate what we've got.

David Peter Webster
Tenerife, Canary Islands

★

*When you get to the end of all the light you know
And it's time to step into the darkness of the unknown
Faith is knowing that one of two things shall happen
Either you will be given something solid to stand on
Or you will be taught how to fly*

Juliette

★

I have been so moved by Caron's story. I am a young woman of 42 and have battled ovarian cancer for the last five years. Thank God, I am doing well and I am now retraining to become a reflexologist. I trust my new job and my enthusiasm for life, just like Caron's, will help my fight.

My family can't understand why I would want to read a book about someone who had cancer like me, but I am finding the book hugely uplifting and provoking. I especially love the fact that you haven't glossed over the difficult bits. We don't all turn into angels when we get cancer and I am certainly no exception!!! I, too, am married to a wonderful man and know the emotions have sometimes pushed him near the limit, but we love each other deeply and have got through it. I am from a close Scottish family and they have supported me wonderfully.

Thank you for the inspiration as a result of the book.

Nina Roberts
London

★

I don't know what the future brings or means – I will 'expect' good. Try not to judge what is happening to me – remember it is always passing and live the best I can for me and others around me. Surrender to divine will –

whatever there is in as much generosity, humility, egoless attitude as I possibly can. I do not need to be perfect – on one level I am – but yeah, I'm here with all my shitty, like, ideas and faults – just like everyone else. I guess they love me for it anyway. Innocence, love, letting people in. Surrender to love. No more running and hiding, be brave – face all – know you are loved and supported. Expect the best – trust – it's a done deal. Ask and you shall receive. Just don't know how it's going to look, something will tell you. Write.

Caron's words

Considering Caron's deep passion and resolve to 'write', she would feel so thrilled and humbled to think that her story has hit a nerve with so many people, and, on top of that, was shortlisted for a British Book Award. Her vivid description of being diagnosed with cancer, the spiritual quest and subsequent journey she took in coping with and desperately trying to cure her cancer – alongside what she learned about the positivity of clinging on to hope and life and living for every second.

She arrived at a stage of enlightenment from the darkness of cancer – spiritual peace and calmness.

Ann from Tadley in Hampshire once wrote to me as follows:

The next chapter is important – you must stop, listen and think about how Caron's life is to be carried forward and used to make some sense of her early passing. Place your faith, love, energy and skills to move Caron into another dimension for all of us to reach and touch the essence of her spirit. The world continues to search for a purpose but you have to unlock the treasure, the treasure that Caron brought with her into this world.

Caron's courage, kindness and days of pain will not be forgotten or lost for one second – there is too much to lose. Make sense of something that on the surface has no sense at all.

Caron is not lost to you, her soul is bigger than death – death is never the end.

LIFE IS NOT WHAT WE THINK – it's not even what we make it. There's so much else and ultimately we can only love each other – help each other and extend that as much as we can. THAT'S IT. See that we are all one, no matter what is happening.

Have compassion – what else have we got? Faith, love, trust, just love.

Caron's words

Acknowledgements

There are so many people I would love to thank:

Russ, for his endless love and devotion to Caron.

Paul and Michael – two very special sons whom I love so deeply. They have always been and continue to be the most enormous support and joy in my life.

My husband Stevie, who has never wavered in his love and strength during very tough and sad times and continues to envelop me in that love.

Jake and Beau, great pals of their cousins Charlie and Gabriel – happy days of football, swimming and *The Simpsons*.

Sandy, for the way she supported Russ and the boys during the very difficult three months after Caron died, and still does.

Caron's friends – too many to list individually, but in particular:

Johnny and Cath Comerford, who were always there for Caron, in good and bad times – true friends.

Sonia Baillie and Janet Ellis. They shared such times with Caron – happy, sad, chaotic, muddling, but through everything, laughter.

The Soho Mafia: Yaz, Fiona, Deborah, Stephanie and Ainslie, for all the laughs and gossip.

The continuing strength of Richard and Judy, Roy and Maureen Heayberd and Karen and Simon Fowler, part of our family circle.

Eve and Dave Lindsay for always being there.

Many people in Barnes, Fowey in Cornwall and Byron Bay in Australia who took Caron, Russ and the boys to their hearts and homes. These include neighbours in Barnes like Nancy, George and Kate; Nick and Clare in Kew; and all the Barnes mummies at school and around the village. In Cornwall, Jono and Judith, Sarah Matthews, Bill and Clare, Graham and Wendy, Mallory and Mike, Nick and Navan, Barbara and Andrew. And finally in Byron Bay, Judith, Mark, Melinda, Frank, Susannah, Khalid, Kel, Satya, Denise, Brandon, Neil and Serge, Miten and Premal, who became their Australian family.

Those within the television industry who worked alongside Caron, ranging from her *Blue Peter* days to the *London Tonight* studios and *This Morning*.

Charles Lowdell, cancer specialist, who was always the most marvellous reference point, even when Caron was in Australia; and in Sydney, Professor Martin Tattershall. Jan de Vries, whom we live by as a family.

Special friends of mine, without whom I would not have coped: Jackie Gill, Merrill Thomas, Michelle and John Carlton-Smith, Libby Lees, Roberta McConville, Anne Thompson, Cliff Richard and Paddy Haycocks and Jo Carlton.

My manager, Laurie Mansfield, the 'wise buddha', always there with his constructive advice and guidance.

Thanks to Charlie and Teddie Pattinson, not only for their friendship but for their thoughts in a special letter which we received a matter of days after Caron died:

We were on a beach in Thailand when we heard the terrible news about Caron. April the 13th (the day Caron died) was Thai New Year – a time of reflection and in the Buddhist faith, rebirth – a time for the spirit.

We thought hard about you, about Caron, Russ and the boys that night. And can only imagine your grief. We lit a lantern for Caron and sent it up into the night sky. As it headed for the stars, fireworks played on the empty beaches down below. It was a beautiful sight and for us it represented everything we loved Caron for – her beauty, her peace, her spirit, all lit by the sparkle, crackle, energy and wit of the most exciting firework.

As with any book, there are a number of people to appreciate and acknowledge:

I am indebted to Gay Longworth for her dedication to Caron's story. Without her, this book might never have made its publishing deadline. Also for the extra research she carried out with Caron's friends and work colleagues, which added so much to the book. Thanks, Gay, for going the extra mile.

Ultimately, my total gratitude to Louise Moore, Publishing Director at Michael Joseph, for convincing me I could write the book in the first place, for nurturing me through every stage of the process, and for her total faith and devotion in this tribute to Caron.

Claire Bord, for the hours and hours spent sifting through countless family photographs, for sourcing others and especially for burning the midnight oil on changes to the manuscript in my horrendous handwriting.

Mary Clifford-Day and Vicky Tibbitts for typing up my ever-changing handwritten notes and never complaining.

Eugenie Furniss, literary agent and demon negotiator.

And everyone else at Penguin for their enthusiasm and commitment to Caron's story.

I'm indebted to Judy Tilbury, who so kindly sent me the poem 'Next to You'.

We have only been able to include a small cross-section of the huge number of letters that people have been kind enough to send to me about this book. I'd like to thank all those who took the trouble to write.

My love and thanks to you all.

Picture Credits

The author and publisher would like to thank all copyright holders for permission to reproduce their work, and the institutions and individuals who helped with the research and supply of materials.

'A very wet but happy day on a Cornish beach with our dear friends Richard and Judy and their son Jack' reproduced by permission of Richard Madeley and Judy Finnigan.

'All those years of practising with sticky-backed plastic and pipe-cleaners paid off' © BBC

'A *Blue Peter* escapade – one of hundreds' © BBC

'Christmas entertainment on *Blue Peter*: another snazzy song-and-dance routine. Yvette Fielding, Mark Curry and Caron' © BBC

'*Blue Peter* trip to Russia. No food but lots of shopping' © BBC

'Caron ahead of the fashion gang – before torn jeans were even trendy' © Neil Genower/Rex Features

'Gabriel looking slightly bored with his first photo-shoot' © Simon Fowler

'Beautiful boy. Charlie aged two' © Simon Fowler

'Consummate shoppers' © Mike Lawn/Rex Features

'Abseiling training with the Royal Marines. Caron was to abseil down the two-hundred-foot-high Bristol and West Building Society building, dressed as Snow White to turn on the Christmas lights. The marines were playing the seven dwarfs!' Reproduced by permission of Des Stewart

'Climbing Ben Nevis with Stephen Venables' reproduced by permission of Des Stewart

'Wing-walking at Cranfield Institute of Aeronautical Engineering during the open day and airshow' reproduced by permission of Des Stewart

'Re-enactment of the American War of Independence' reproduced by permission of Des Stewart

Photographic credits for the last inset section:

Pages one and two: © Simon Fowler

Page three: top photograph © Mike Wilson/Scope Features; bottom photograph © John Rogers/Stay Still

Page four: top photographs © Sven Arnstein/Stay Still; bottom photograph © Brian Moody/Scope Features

Page five: © Simon Fowler

Page six: bottom photographs © Simon Fowler

Page eight: © Neil Genower/Rex Features

Particular thanks to Charlie for the use of his special photograph album and also to Russ, Stephen, Paul and Michael for contributing to such a beautiful collection of photographs.

Every effort has been made to trace copyright holders and we apologize in advance for any unintentional omission. We would be pleased to insert the appropriate acowledgement in any subsequent edition.

The Caron Keating Foundation is a fund-raising partnership set up by Gloria Hunniford, Paul and Michael Keating. The foundation offers financial support to professional carers, complementary healing practitioners and support groups dealing with cancer patients, as well as individuals and families who are affected by the disease. It also financially assists a number of cancer charities with their ongoing quest for prevention, early detection and hopefully ultimate care.

For more information about The Caron Keating Foundation, please visit www.caronkeating.org, or write to
PO Box 122, Sevenoaks, Kent, TN13 1UB